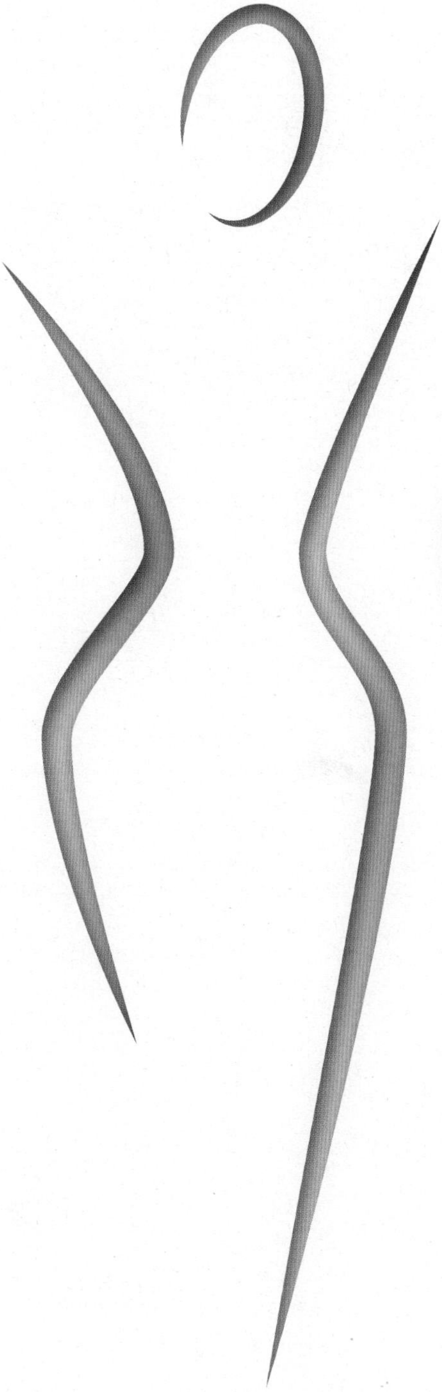

MINIMALLY INVASIVE AESTHETIC SURGERY

MINIMALLY INVASIVE AESTHETIC SURGERY

Donald W. Buck II, MD, FACS
Plastic Surgeon
Mercy Clinic Plastic Surgery
Mercy Hospital South
St. Louis, MO
United States

ELSEVIER

Elsevier
1600 John F. Kennedy Blvd.
Ste 1800
Philadelphia, PA 19103-2899

MINIMALLY INVASIVE AESTHETIC SURGERY
ISBN: 978-0-323-67987-9

Senior Content Development Manager: Somodatta Roy Choudhury
Content Strategist: Belinda Kuhn/Lauren Boyle
Content Development Manager: Ranjana Sharma
Publishing Services Manager: Shereen Jameel
Project Manager: Vishnu T. Jiji
Senior Designer: Patrick C. Ferguson

Printed in India

Last digit is the print number: 9 8 7 6 5 4 3 2 1

CONTRIBUTORS

Brayann O. Aleman, DMD, MSD
Craniomaxillofacial and Facial Cosmetic Surgery
Oral and Maxillofacial Surgery
Houston Methodist Hospital, Houston
Texas
United States

Babak Azizzadeh, MD
Associate Clinical Professor
Head & Neck Surgery
UCLA, Los Angeles;
Fellowship Director
Facial Plastic & Reconstructive Surgery
AAFPRS, Los Angeles;
Attending Facial Plastic Surgeon
Otolaryngology
Cedars-Sinai Medical Center, Los Angeles
California
United States

Jonathan Cabin, MD
Facial Plastic & Reconstructive Surgeon
Facial Plastic Surgery
SkinDC, PLLC, Arlington
Virginia
United States

Ruonan Chen, BA
New York Plastic Surgery Suite, New York
New York
United States

Steven R. Cohen, MD
Private Practice FACES+ Plastic Surgery Skin and Laser Center, La Jolla
California
United States

Armando Augusto Davila, MD
President & CEO
Plastic Surgeon
Pittsburgh Center for Plastic Surgery, Pittsburgh;
Clinical Assistant Professor
Department of Plastic Surgery
University of Pittsburgh School of Medicine, Pittsburgh;
Adjunct Assistant Professor
Department of Plastic Surgery
University of Nevada Las Vegas School of Medicine, Las Vegas
Nevada
United States

Adeeb Derakhshan, MD
Assistant Professor
Division of Facial Plastic and Reconstructive Surgery, Department of Otolaryngology - Head and Neck Surgery
Loma Linda University, Loma Linda
California
United States

Lara Devgan, MD, MPH, FACS
Department of Surgery
Lenox Hill Hospital, New York;
Manhattan Eye, Ear, & Throat Infirmary, New York
New York
United States

Caitlin Francoisse, MD
Resident Physician
Division of Plastic Surgery
Saint Louis University, School of Medicine, Saint Louis
Missouri
United States

Dennis J. Hurwitz, MD
Clinical Professor of Plastic Surgery
University of Pittsburgh Medical Center
Hurwitz Center for Plastic Surgery, Pittsburgh
Pennsylvania
United States

Omer Ibrahim, MD
Associate
Dermatology
Chicago Cosmetic Surgery and Dermatology, Chicago
Illinois
United States

Lisa E. Ishii, MD, MHS
Professor
Department of Otolaryngology-Head & Neck Surgery
Johns Hopkins University Medical Institute, Baltimore
Maryland
United States

Carolyn I. Jacob, MD
Medical Director
Chicago Cosmetic Surgery and Dermatology, Chicago
Illinois
United States

Linda N. Lee, MD, FACS
Facial Plastic and Reconstructive Surgeon
Department of Otolaryngology/Head & Neck Surgery
Harvard Medical School/Mass Eye and Ear, Boston;
Associate Chief of Plastic Surgery
Atrius Health, Wellesley
Massachusetts
United States

Tracy Leong, MD
Dermatology Rady Children's Hospital
Sharp Memorial Hospital, San Diego;
University California San Diego Medical Center, San Diego;
Private Practice, FACES+ Plastic Surgery, Skin and Laser Center, La Jolla
California
United States

Esteban Liscano
Corpus and Rostrum Surgery Center, Cali
Valle
Colombia

Gabriel J. Martinez-Diaz, MD
CEO
Dermatology
M D Aesthetics and Dermatology, Chicago
Illinois
United States

Farzad R. Nahai, MD, FACS
School of Medicine
Emory University, Atlanta;
The Center for Plastic Surgery at MetroDerm
Metroderm, Atlanta
Georgia
United States

Suzan Obagi, MD
Associate Professor of Dermatology
University of Pittsburgh;
Associate Professor of Plastic Surgery
University of Pittsburgh, Pittsburgh
Pennsylvania
United States

Briana Paiewonsky, MD
Charles E. Schmidt College of Medicine
Florida Atlantic University, Boca Raton
Florida
United States

E. Victor Ross, MD
Director of Laser and Cosmetic Dermatology Scripps Clinic, San Diego
California
United States

Ahmad N. Saad, MD
Private Practice FACES+ Plastic Surgery Skin and Laser Center, La Jolla
California
United States

Deniz Sarhaddi, MD
Plastic Surgeon
Plastic Surgery
St. Louis Cosmetic Surgery, Inc., Saint Louis
Missouri
United States

Sachin M. Shridharani, MD, FACS
Founder and Director
Aesthetic Plastic Surgery
LUXURGERY, New York
New York;
Associate Clinical Professor
Department of Plastic Surgery
Washington University in St. Louis, St. Louis
Missouri
United States

Grace M. Tisch, BA
LUXURGERY, New York
New York
United States

Lina Triana, MD
Medical Doctor
Scientific Director
Plastic Surgery
Clinica Corpus Y Rostrum, Cali
Valle Del Cauca
Colombia

PREFACE

The idea for this book developed in early 2019. My goal was seemingly simple at the time—to produce a quality text that highlighted the most commonly performed minimally invasive aesthetic procedures. I hoped that this book would serve as *the* reliable "how-to" guide for surgeons and providers wanting to add these options to their practices. I am truly grateful to the entire Elsevier team, especially Belinda Kuhn, who saw my vision and also felt this text would be a valuable addition to the Elsevier library. So, in late 2019, with the green light to proceed, we embarked upon an ambitious journey to bring together leading physicians from around the world to contribute to the book. Our enthusiasm grew as we received verbal commitments from key aesthetic opinion leaders and our table of contents began to take shape. Shortly after solidifying our stellar contributor list, and beginning to put text on blank pages, the world suddenly stopped. COVID-19 began to circulate the globe and the pandemic put normal life on pause; it was no surprise that chapter writing and book publishing dropped on most priority lists. Despite these incredible challenges, the Elsevier team and my amazing group of contributors never gave up. Although it took longer than anticipated, we persisted and have successfully put together a book that I believe has exceeded our expectations. It is my hope that you find this book to be a valuable and critical addition to your own libraries, and one that serves as the point of reference for your office-based aesthetic practice. I am confident that the anatomical and technical pearls within the text will equip you with the knowledge and confidence needed to provide the highest quality care to your patients.

ACKNOWLEDGEMENTS

To my contributors—thank you so much for your persistence, and your incredible effort despite the unexpected adversity. Your thoughtful and detailed contributions to this text will serve to educate providers around the globe, and positively impact the lives of countless patients.

To my Elsevier team—especially Belinda Kuhn and Ranjana Sharma—thank you so much for your belief in my vision and your support, persistence, and oversight. Despite the odds, you never gave up on us. This book is a testament to your determination. Let us hope that the subsequent editions are not affected by a global pandemic!

Last, and certainly not least, to my family—my beautiful wife, Jennifer, and my children, Ben and Brooke. Thank you for your unwavering support and encouragement. Without your love and support, none of this would be possible. The silver lining of this pandemic has been the extra time spent with you, and I am truly grateful to be your husband and father.

DWBII

TABLE OF CONTENT

VIDEO CONTENT

Video 2.1 Lecture video content on chemical peels.

Video 6.1 Demonstration of laser hair removal using a long pulse 1064-nm neodymium-doped yttrium aluminum garnet (Nd : YAG) laser.

Video 6.2 Demonstration of laser vein ablation using a long pulse 532-nm potassium titanyl phosphate (KTP) laser.

Video 7.1 Facial Assessment and Vector/Suture Markings

Video 7.2 Insertion of Sutures in the Face and Neck

Video 7.3 Tightening and Setting of Final Sutures

Video 8.1 40 Kilojoule BodyTite handpiece used to Tighten abdominal subcutaneous tissue

Video 8.2 Morphues8 of the abdomen

1

Basics of Skin Care

Lara Devgan and Ruonan Chen

THE IMPORTANCE OF THE SKIN

The skin is the body's largest organ, which maintains not only our homeostasis but also a physiologic environment for us to inhabit. Moreover, the skin has an important aesthetic function, as it reveals information about health, age, and environmental exposures. The skin has captivated people since the beginning of time: skin has been described in the canon of western literature as dewy, luminous, and beautiful. Similarly, when the skin is weathered, wrinkled, creased, or worn, patients may feel almost trapped in their own bodies.

Skin care can be a challenging topic in minimally invasive aesthetic plastic surgery, as it traverses the boundary between cosmetics and a medicalized approach to the dermis. Product marketing is not necessarily related to product efficacy, and consumer confusion is high. An academic approach to skin care requires focus on ingredients that have demonstrated clinical efficacy, and gradual incorporation of products, according to unique patient characteristics.

Topics related to skin and complexion have an increasing importance as people are celebrating the unique variance in their skin tones, colors, and textures. Understanding skin from a 21st-century perspective demands respectfully considering patients of all demographic backgrounds and skin colors. Approaches that may work well for one patient population may not work well for another, and the nuances of treating the skin of people of color cannot be underestimated.

THE FUNCTION OF THE SKIN

The skin serves many functions crucial to the body's normal operation, including barrier defense, ultraviolet (UV) protection, thermoregulation, and sensation.

Barrier Defense

The skin offers the body's first line of defense. As part of the innate immune system, it protects the body from external pathogens through mechanical and chemical mechanisms, including a waterproof barrier established by epithelial cells linked through tight junctions, secretion of lipids, and antimicrobial peptides. The healthy skin also houses a range of commensal bacteria that keep pathogenic bacteria from overpopulating.[1]

UV Protection

UV light from the environment is known to cause DNA damage, which relates to photoaging and carcinogenesis. The skin protects the body against UV damage through melanin, a peptide pigment that absorbs UV rays and neutralizes free radicals. Melanin is produced by melanocytes in the epidermis, "packaged" into melanosomes, and distributed to adjacent keratinocytes. The type of melanin and its organization in melanosomes contribute to the various skin colors in humans.[2,3]

Thermoregulation and Sensation

The human body can retain a stable body temperature in various environments because of the thermoregulation function of the skin, which is controlled by the autonomic (involuntary) nervous system. In hot temperatures, the body cools down by sweating, dissipating heat to the environment through evaporation of water on the skin. In cold climate, the hair on the skin stands up to form "goosebumps," a process called *piloerection* that prevents warm air from escaping.

The dermis of the skin contains a wide range of sensory receptors and free nerve endings, which allows us to feel pain, temperature, touch, pressure, stretch, and many other types of sensations.[1]

In addition to physiologic functions, the appearance of the skin, such as its color, elasticity, and texture, also reveals one's ethnicity, age, and general health status. This function of the skin has inspired the development of modern skin care, ranging from topical skin care products to in-office procedures to improve the skin quality.

THE LAYERS OF THE SKIN

The three main layers of the skin, from the outer to the innermost, are the epidermis, dermis, and the hypodermis, which is also known as the *subcutaneous fat.*

Epidermis

The epidermis consists of five sublayers and contributes the most to barrier protection.[4] The stratum basalis (basal cell layer) lies closest to the dermis layer and is the only actively dividing layer of the epidermis. It contains melanocytes and epidermal stem cells, which divide and differentiate into keratinocytes that make up most of the epidermis. As new keratinocytes continue to form in the basal cell layer, the existing move toward the surface of the skin into the stratum spinosum, stratum granulosm, and stratum lucidum. During this time, the keratinocytes continue to differentiate in a process called *cornification*, where they gain lipid granules and lose their nuclei. In the outermost layer of the epidermis, the stratum corneum, the keratinocytes have become dead cellular structures called *corneocytes* with barrier protection and water-loss regulating functions.[5]

Dermis

The dermis lies between the epidermis and the hypodermis, and it is the thickest layer of the skin. Unlike the epidermis, the dermis is innervated and contains blood vessels. It also contains hair follicles, sweat glands, and a range of innate immune cells, including mast cells and monocytes. The most abundant cell type dermis contains are fibroblasts, which secrete substances that make up the extracellular matrix, including collagen, elastin, and hyaluronic acid. Based on the arrangement of collagen and elastin fibers, the dermis is divided into the thinner, loosely packed papillary layer near the epidermis and the thicker, densely packed reticular layer near the hypodermis.[6]

Hypodermis

The hypodermis is located below the reticular dermis and the epidermis and mainly consists of adipocytes. It connects the dermis to the fascia.[7]

Fitzpatrick Skin Types

Fitzpatrick skin phototype categorizes people's skin types into six groups by their reactions to sunlight, specifically the ability to tan and to develop sunburns. A lower number for the Fitzpatrick skin type indicates lighter skin color and higher tendency of developing sunburn instead of tanning, while individuals with Fitzpatrick skin types IV–VI are more likely to develop hyperpigmentation. Clinically, the Fitzpatrick skin type is helpful in assessing the risks of patients in developing hyperpigmented scarring and determining parameters for laser treatment.[8]

INGREDIENT CLASSES

Several classes of ingredients have strong clinical efficacy as demonstrated in the medical literature.

Retinols and retinoic acid derivatives increase the rate of skin cell turnover. In so doing, they have been well established to reduce fine lines, decrease apparent pore size, decrease blemishes, and improve hyperpigmentation.

Vitamin C is a potent antioxidant that scavenges free-radical damage to the skin. It can be harnessed and topical skin care to improve fine lines, improve melasma, and improve hyperpigmentation. The use of vitamin C along with vitamin B, vitamin E, and ferulic acid has also shown to have improved efficacy.

Hyaluronic acid is the major component of the body's own collagen, and as such, it is responsible for an internal hydration and turgor to dermal quality. Conventional hyaluronic acid molecules are too large to penetrate dermal channels. A mixed-molecular-weight hyaluronic acid serum, therefore, becomes a powerful skin care ingredient because small fragments are able to penetrate into the dermis, while large fragments rest on the skin surface. The net result is an improvement in luster and hydration for the skin.[9]

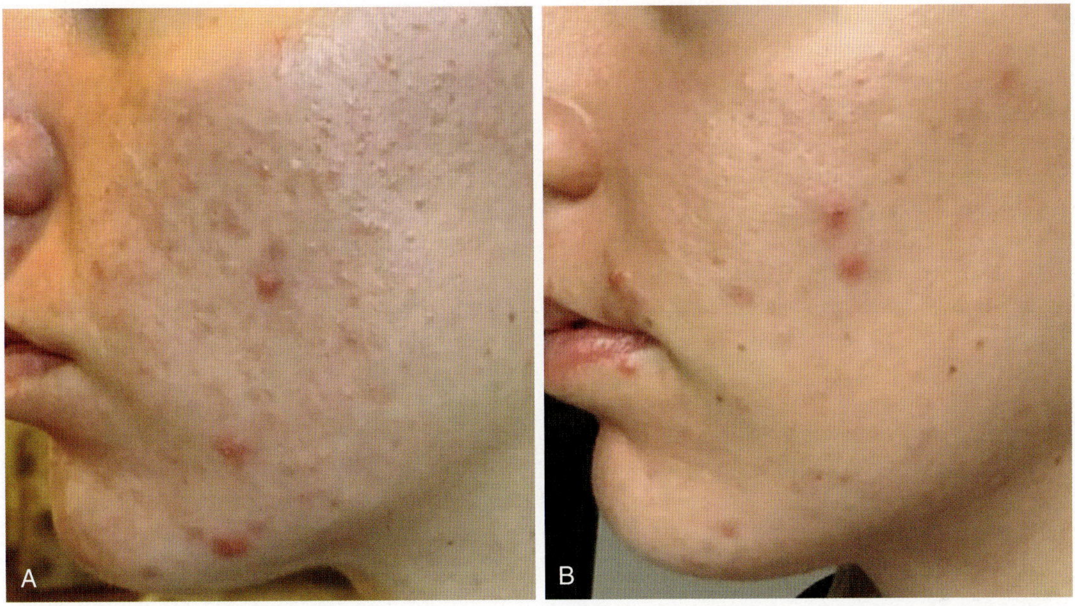

Consistent use of a skin care routine containing retinol, vitamin C, and hyaluronic acid improves the overall skin quality by addressing multiple common skin concerns. (A) Photograph of a patient's cheek showing inflamed acne lesions, clogged pores, and redness. (B) Photograph of the same patient's cheek 3 months after using a targeted skin care routine with over-the-counter retinol, vitamin C, and hyaluronic acid. Redness and shine have reduced after treatment. The skin texture appears smoother with fewer clogged pores. Scarring from the inflammation in (A) is barely noticeable in (B).

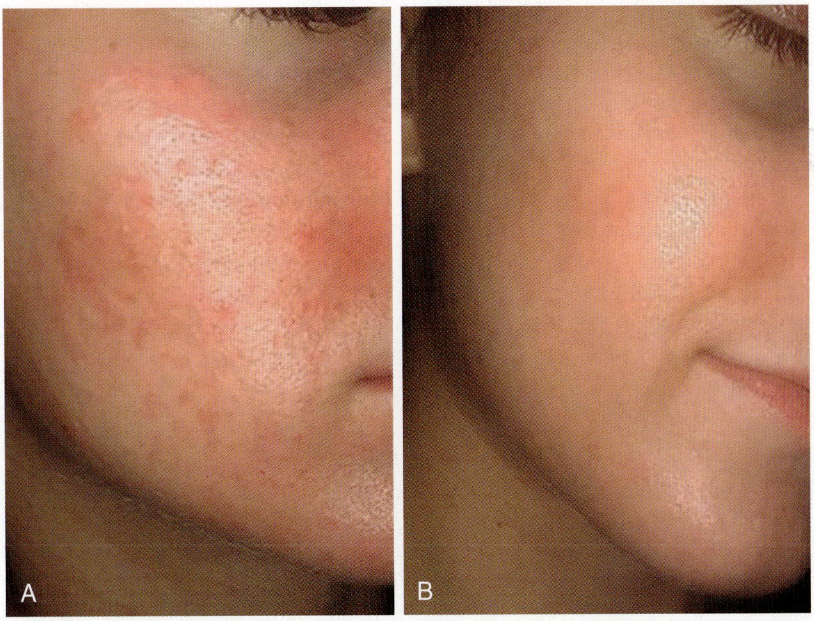

A skin care routine containing vitamin C, hyaluronic acid, and regular exfoliation effectively improves skin texture, reduces redness, and evens out the skin tone. (A) Photograph of patient's cheeks showing enlarged pores, redness, and mild inflammation. (B) Photograph of patient's cheek after incorporating serums containing vitamin C, hyaluronic acid, and weekly exfoliation with a facial scrub. After treatment, the skin tone becomes more even; skin texture is smoother, and pores become less visible.

Ingredients such as peptides and ceramides can help to soften the skin and improve light reflects on the dermis. While this is a subtle endpoint, this translates into a major cosmetic improvement in how the skin can be perceived. These ingredients are particularly powerful in the delicate and frequently moving tissues of the periorbital and perioral regions.

Cleansers and exfoliants also play an important role in the maintenance of skin quality. They can be used to mechanically and chemically exfoliate the top layer of the epidermis to allow more evenness of skin tone. Physical exfoliants such as microdermabrasion scrub, commonly based on granular sugar molecules such as sugar, salt, titanium dioxide, or solid wax beads, will create mechanical friction to achieve this goal. Chemical exfoliants like alpha- and beta-hydroxy acids, specifically salicylic acid and lactic acid, can gradually denude calloused skin and reveal a smoother complexion.

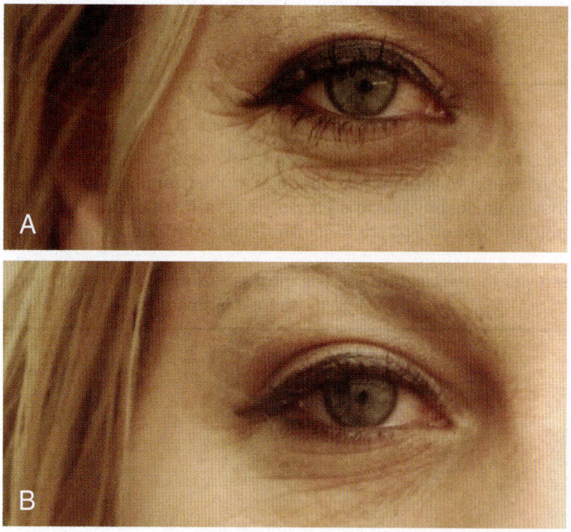

An eye cream rich in ceramids and peptides alleviates the appearance of periorbital rhytids. (A) Photograph of patient's periorbital region before treatment. (B) Photograph of patient's periorbital region after treatment with a peptide-rich eye cream. The appearance of crow's feet, under-eye wrinkles, and puffiness have all reduced.

Arguably, the most important and yet most frequently overlooked skin care ingredient is a zinc- and titanium-based sun protection agent. Sunscreens and sun blocks with mineral zinc oxide and titanium dioxide create a physical blockade against UVA and UVB radiation. This allows protection of the dermis from photoaging and the ensuing rhytids, hyperpigmented lesions, and loss of elasticity that come with it.

COMMON CONCERNS

Acne

Acne vulgaris, one of the most common skin concerns nowadays, is a type of skin lesion typically seen on the face, neck, chest, and back areas. Ranging from skin-colored closed comedones to inflammatory cysts or pustules, acne can affect both men and women from puberty through adulthood and can significantly impact one's self-image and quality of life. Many factors may contribute to the development of acne, including bacterial or fungal infection, overproduction of sebum, and hormonal imbalance. Other factors such as stress, diet, genetics, certain medications, and hormonal imbalance might also play a role in causing acne.[10]

Over-the-counter active ingredients are often sufficient to treat mild to moderate acne. Salicylic acid and

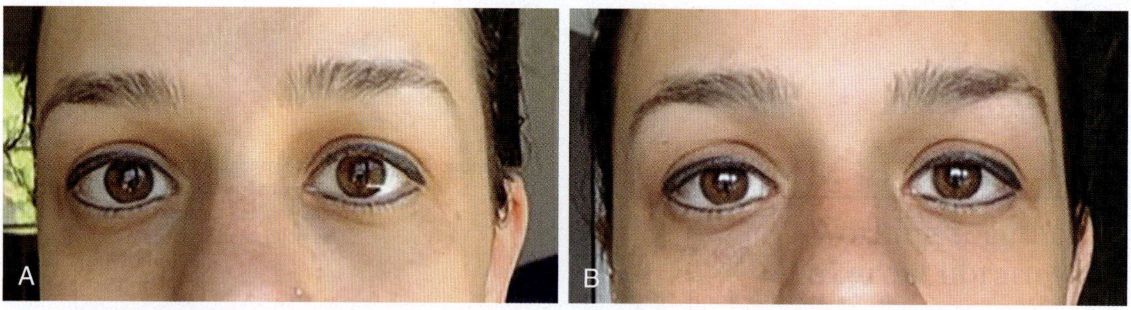

An eye cream rich in ceramids and peptides alleviates the appearance of dark circles. (A) Photograph of patient's periorbital region. (B) Photograph of patient's periorbital region after treatment with a peptide-rich eye cream. Under-eye hollowness and dark circles have both improved.

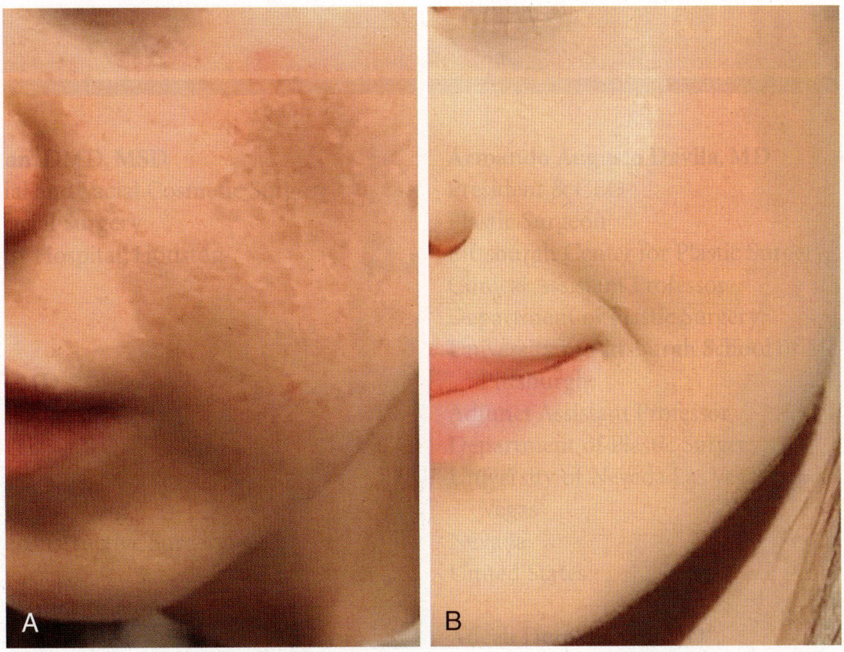

Consistent use of a physical exfoliant together with topical hyaluronic acid effectively reduces dullness, rough texture, and hyperpigmentation. (A) Make-up free photograph of patient showing rough texture, uneven skin tone, and hyperpigmentation on the cheek and nose. (B) Make-up free photograph of patient 8 weeks after incorporating a facial scrub with fine titanium dioxide particles and a hyaluronic acid serum to the skin care routine.

benzoyl peroxide have comedolytic and antibacterial properties and are the most commonly used ingredients to treat existing acne. Exfoliants such as alpha-hydroxy acids or mechanical scrubs can remove dirt and debris that may clog the pores and cause inflammation, preventing acne from forming. Over-the-counter topical retinoids such as retinol are also effective in treating acne and lightening postinflammatory hyperpigmentation (PIH) caused by acne. Other ingredients such as niacinamide and azelaic acid have also been shown to reduce acne and PIH.[11]

In the cases of moderate to severe acne, prescribed topical or oral medication, including retinoic acids, antibiotics, and hormonal agents, may be used alone or in conjunction with ingredients listed earlier.

Hyperpigmentation

Hyperpigmentation results in an uneven skin tone with excessive amount of pigment deposit on certain areas of the skin and has become an increasingly common skin concern. Hyperpigmentation can occur on any part of the skin from different causes, such as genetics (familial periorbital hyperpigmentation), inflammation (PIH), and hormonal changes (melasma during or after pregnancy).

Hyperpigmentation is best addressed from a multifactorial approach. Hydroquinone, topical retinoids, and vitamin C are safe and effective treatments for localized hyperpigmentation. Exfoliation facilitates shedding of skin cells and accelerates the resolution of hyperpigmentation. Common exfoliants include alpha-hydroxy acids, salicylic acids, and physical scrubs. These treatments, however, often come with the side effects of dryness, skin flaking, and irritation, which could contribute to PIH in some cases. Therefore, it is important to compliment these treatments with a skin care routine that focuses on barrier protection and repair. Sun protection is essential in any skin care routine, especially when treating hyperpigmentation. While effective at preventing photodamage when used appropriately, physical sunscreens containing zinc oxide and/or titanium dioxide are less likely to cause irritation or allergy compared to chemical UV filters with avobenzone, octinoxate, or oxybenzone.[12]

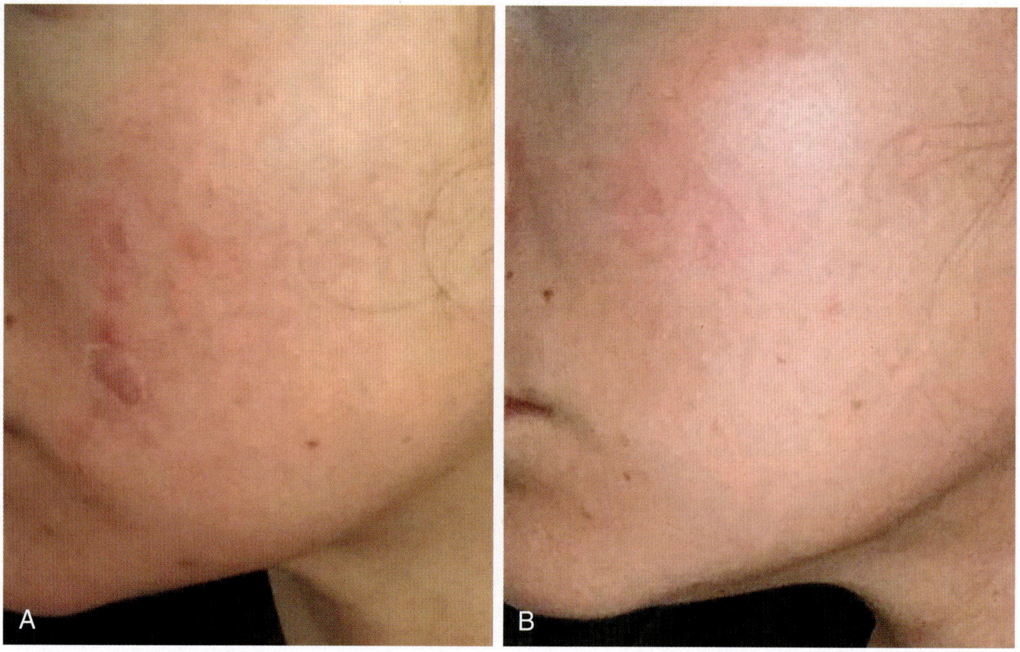

Over-the-counter combination treatment with glycolic acid, salicylic acid, benzoyl peroxide, and daily sun protection is effective against mild acne vulgaris. (A) Photograph of patient's cheek before treatment. (B) Photograph of patient's cheek after 2 months' treatment. Both active inflammation and postinflammatory hyperpigmentation have reduced. The general skin appearance is brighter and smoother after treatment.

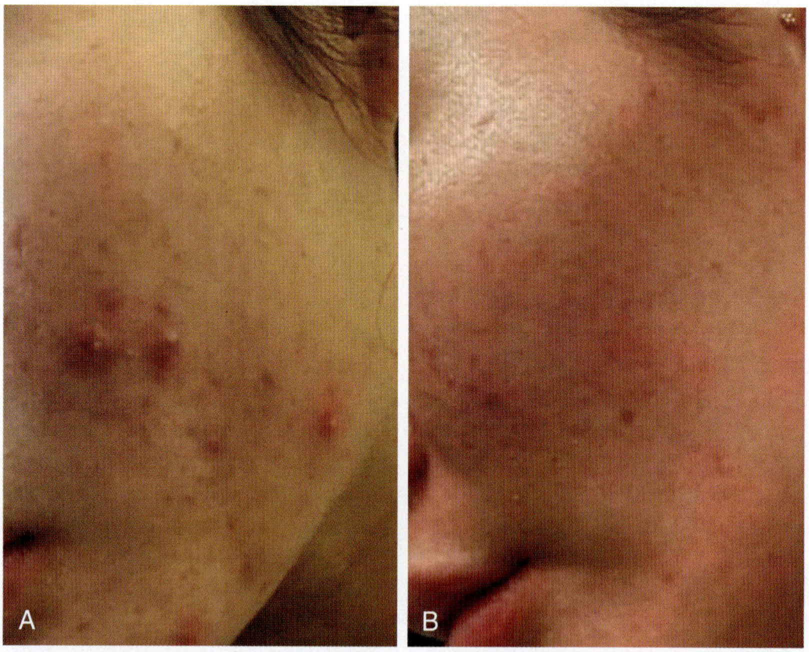

Over-the-counter combination treatment with glycolic acid, salicylic acid, benzoyl peroxide, and daily sun protection is effective against mild acne vulgaris. (A) Photograph of patient's cheek before treatment. (B) Photograph of patient's cheek after treatment for 8 weeks. Both active inflammation and postinflammatory hyperpigmentation have reduced. Scarring is minimal.

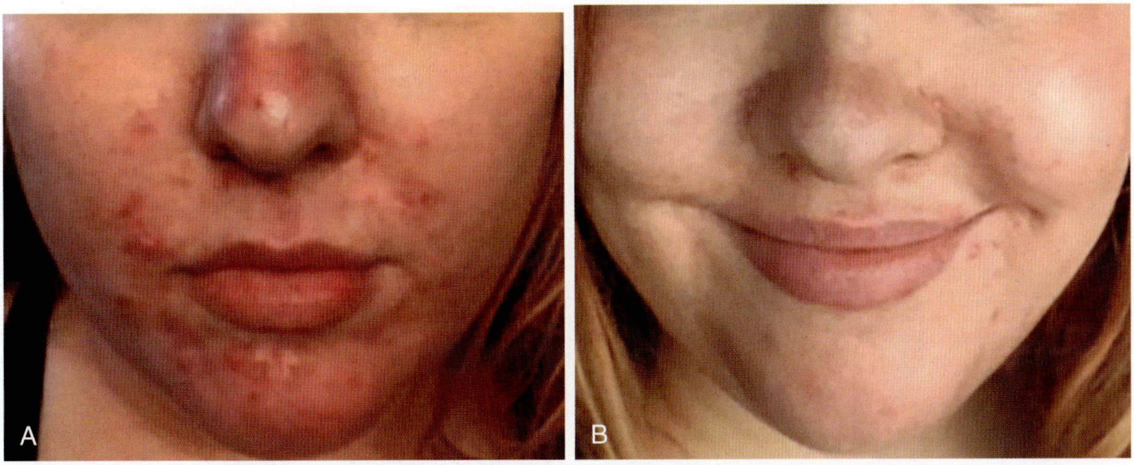

This patient is pictured in image (A) with moderate to severe inflammatory acne and rosacea in the lower third of the face, most prominent in the chin, nasolabial folds, nose, and inferior cheeks. She is pictured in image (B) after treatement with a combination topical approach of glycolic acid, salicylic acid, benzoyl peroxide, retinoids, vitamins C+B+E+ ferulic acid, mixed-molecular-weight hyaluronic serum, and zinc- and titanium-based SPF with a significant improvement in skin quality, texture, and evenness

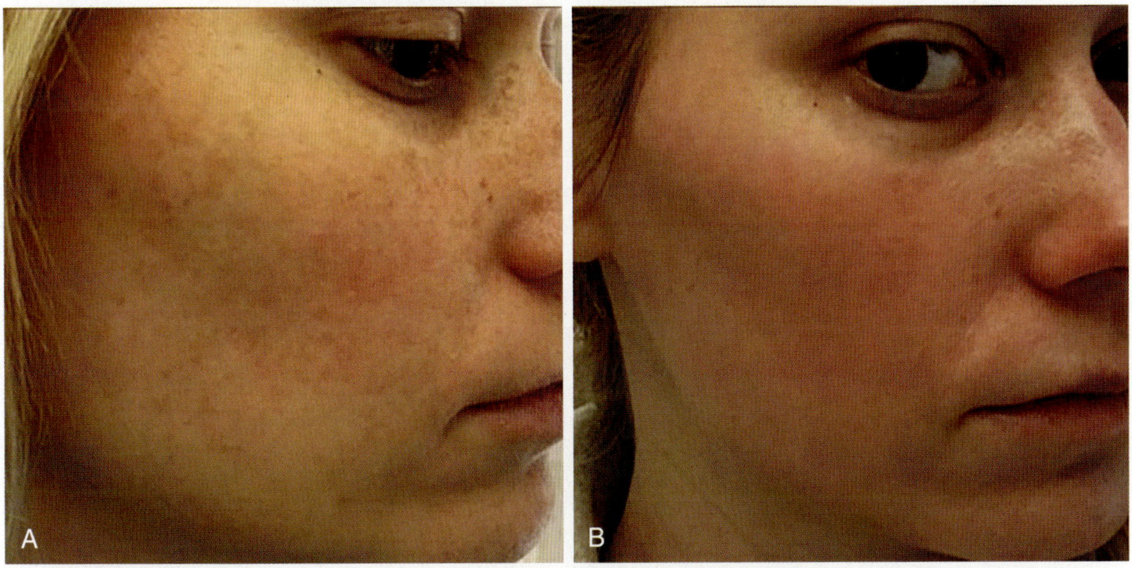

Photographs of patient with Fitzpatrick skin type II before and after a combination treatment with topical hyaluronic acid, vitamin C, topical retinoids, and daily sun protection. (A) Photograph of patient's cheek before treatment with hyperpigmentation (sunspots). (B) Photograph of patient's cheek after 3 months of treatment. Compared to Fig. 1.3A, the appearance of fine lines and wrinkles is reduced, showing a smoother complexion. Skin tone appears more even with less redness and dark spots.

An over-the-counter skin care routine incorporating skin resurfacing agents, depigmentation agents, and sun protection has shown efficacy across different types of hyperpigmentation in patients with different skin tones.

Aging and Rhytids

Aging is a natural process that occurs with time in all individuals. As the largest external organ, the skin is often the first place where people notice signs of aging. In the process of aging, the surface area of the epidermis-dermis junction

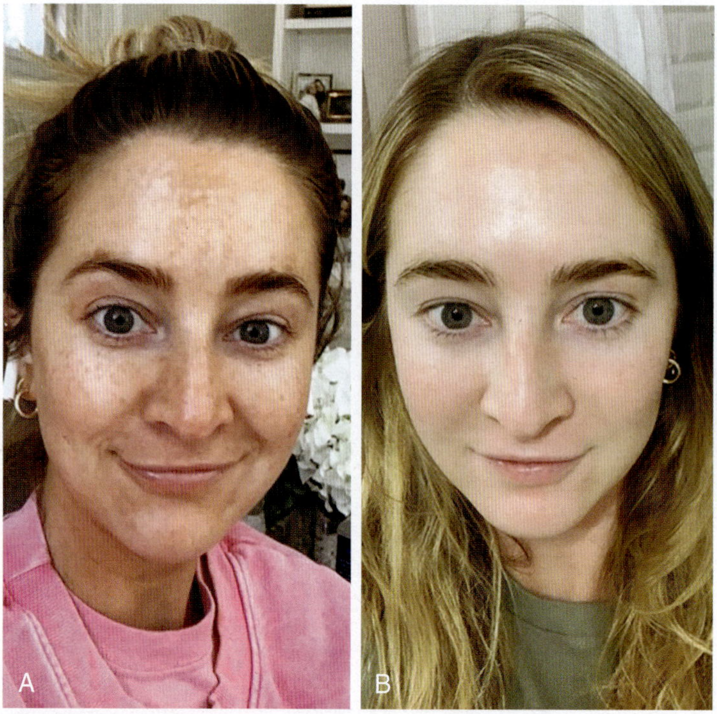

Photographs of patient with Fitzpatrick skin type III before and after a combination treatment with over-the-counter topical hyaluronic acid, vitamin C, topical retinoids, and daily sun protection. (A) Photograph of patient with photoinduced hyperpigmentation throughout the face and neck. (B) Photograph of patient a year after treatment. Hyperpigmentation has dramatically improved, resulting in a brighter and more even complexion.

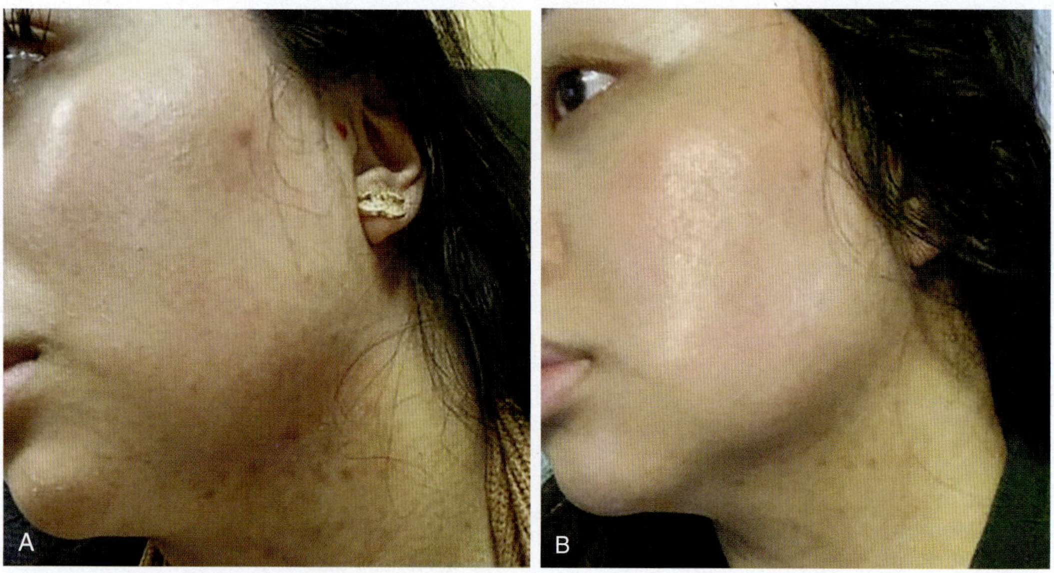

A combination treatment with over-the-counter topical hyaluronic acid, vitamin C, topical retinoids, and daily sun protection is effective at fading hyperpigmentation in patients with Fitzpatrick skin type IV. (A) Photograph of patient with rough texture on the cheek and hyperpigmentation on the neck. (B) Photograph of patient after treatment with hyaluronic acid, vitamin C, topical retinol, and daily sun protection. Skin texture appeared smoother, and hyperpigmentation on the neck had lightened.

decreases, resulting in reduced proliferation of basal cells and consequently a thinner epidermis. This change leads to weakened barrier protection and decreased ability of the skin to retain water. In the dermal level, the extracellular matrix made up of collagen and elastin fibers breaks down, leading to loss of elasticity and appearance of rhytids.

Besides the biological clock, many external factors can also contribute to premature aging, such as UV exposure, smoking, mechanical stress, hormonal changes, and diet. Therefore, an effective antiaging treatment should take a systematic approach addressing multiple causes of aging simultaneously. Common antiaging treatments include antioxidants, sun protection, and retinoids. Topical antioxidants such as vitamin C and vitamin E neutralize the reactive oxygen species in the environment and protect the skin from free-radical damage. Sun protection and sunscreens reduce UV exposure to the skin and prevent photoaging. Topical retinoids are fat soluble derivatives of vitamin A that can penetrate the epidermis and dermis and alter cellular genetic expressions. They promote proliferation of basal cells, resulting in strengthened skin barrier and reduced transepidermal water loss. By preventing collagen degradation, retinoids can effectively delay development of rhytids.[13-15]

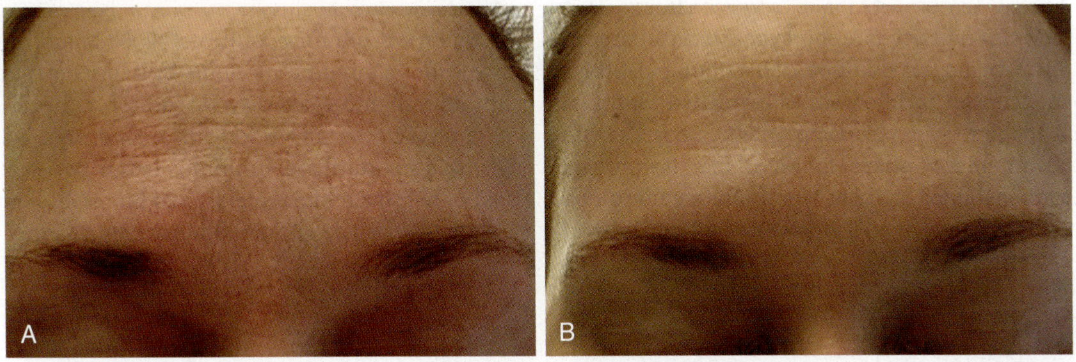

Over-the-counter retinol is effective in improving existing rhytids. (A) Photograph of patient's forehead showing fine lines, wrinkles, hyperpigmentation, and enlarged pores. (B) Photograph of patient's forehead after treatment with a topical retinol serum. Redness, fine lines, and appearance of existing wrinkles had all reduced.

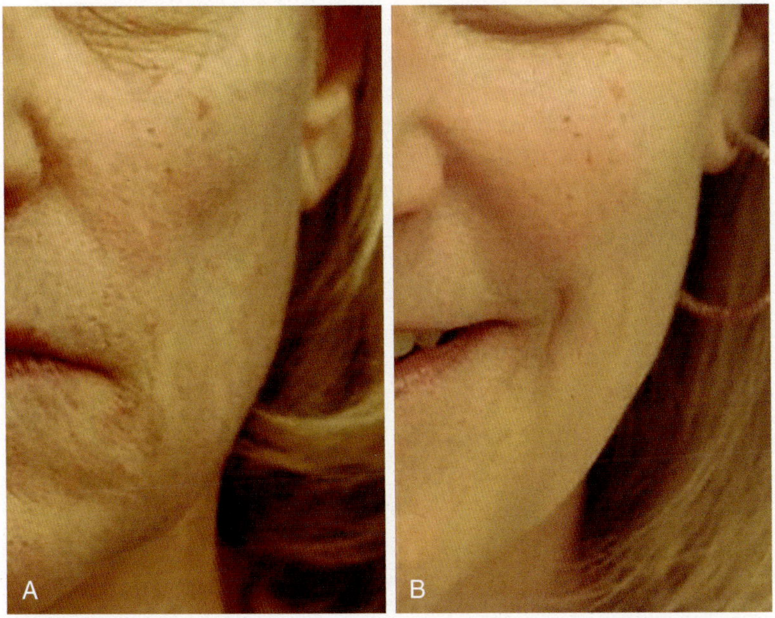

Over-the-counter retinol is effective in improving overall skin quality and reversing signs of aging. (A) Photograph of patient's cheek before skin care showing signs of aging, including dull complexion, hyperpigmentation, rhytids, and hyperpigmentation. (B) Photograph of patient's cheek after beginning an over-the-counter retinol together with hyaluronic acid, vitamin C, and physical exfoliation. This skin care treatment led to faded hyperpigmentation, improved luster and brightness, and an overall younger-looking complexion.

IMPLEMENTING SKIN CARE INTO YOUR PRACTICE

When speaking to my patients about skin care, I often use the analogy of going to the dentist: you get your teeth professionally cleaned twice a year, but you brush and floss your teeth every day. Topical skin care is like the daily dental maintenance we do at home: a tiny iterative daily step can make a profound impact on overall skin quality in the long run, and they can decrease the need for in-office treatments like lasers and peels. Several minutes of daily maintenance can accumulate into a lifetime of skin maintenance that often cannot be matched procedurally. While procedures such as erbium laser resurfacing, TCA chemical peels, and microinfusion microneedling can certainly accomplish more for the skin in a shorter period of time, it is not practical or advisable to do those things on a daily basis; skin care, on the other hand, can be.

A medical grade approach to skin care can help a patient maintain and preserve their plastic surgical and nonsurgical results. A simple and data-driven approach to skin care should be part of the lifelong care of any plastic surgery patient. Indeed, some aspects of patient management, such as lower eyelid crinkling after blepharoplasty, can be better addressed with a peptide-based eye cream than with injectable filler, neuromodulation, laser resurfacing, or surgical excision.

To that end, operational and logistical office flow should be set up to allow conversations about skin care with all patients.

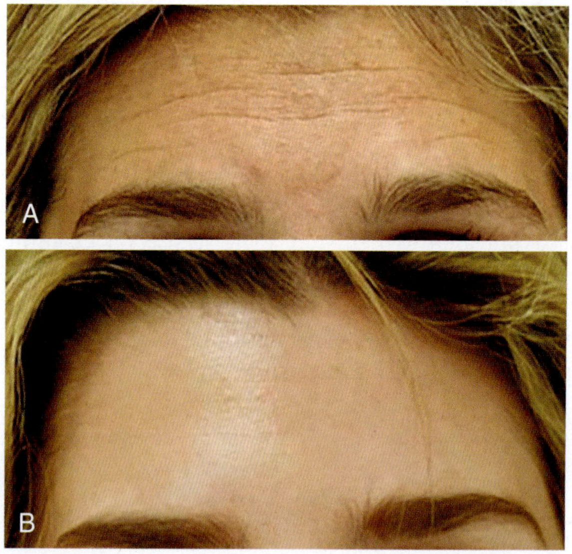

A combined skin care regimen containing topical retinol, hyaluronic acid, and vitamin C in conjunction with neuromodulator and microinfusion microneedling treatments is effective at improving overall skin quality. (A) Photograph of patient's forehead before neuromodulator and microinfusion microneedling treatments. Fine lines and wrinkles were apparent, and the skin appeared dull and dry. Patient was then given an at-home skin care regimen containing topical retinol, hyaluronic acid, and vitamin C. (B) Photograph of patient's forehead after treatment. The deep wrinkles on the forehead had reduced, and the skin appeared smoother, plumper, and brighter.

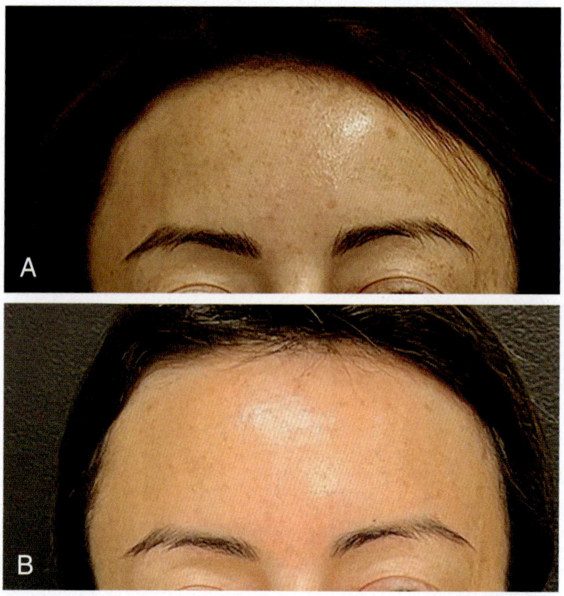

A comprehensive at-home skin care routine is important for maintaining the results from in-office laser treatments. (A) Photograph of patient's forehead before receiving erbium laser treatment for hyperpigmentation. After treatment, patient began an at-home skin care routine with hyaluronic acid, vitamin C, retinol, and sun protection. (B) Photograph of patient's forehead 5 months after erbium laser procedure. The skin tone appears even with greatly reduced hyperpigmentation. Result from the laser treatment was maintained.

REFERENCES

1. Kenneth M, Travers P, Walport M, Janeway C. *Janeway's Immunobiology*. New York: Garland Science; 2008.
2. Brenner M, Hearing VJ. The protective role of melanin against UV damage in human skin. *Photochem Photobiol.* 2008;84(3):539-549.

3. Stamatas GN, Zmudzka BZ, Kollias N, Beer JZ. Non-invasive measurements of skin pigmentation in situ. *Pigment Cell Res.* 2004;17(6):618-626.
4. Guyuron B, Chung KC. *Plastic Surgery: Indications and Practice.* Edinburgh: Saunders; 2009.
5. Agarwal S, Krishnamurthy K. Histology, skin. [Updated 2020 Jul 3]. In: *StatPearls.* Treasure Island, FL: StatPearls Publishing; 2021.
6. Brown TM, Krishnamurthy K. Histology, dermis. [Updated 2020 Jul 3]. In: *StatPearls.* Treasure Island, FL: StatPearls Publishing; 2021.
7. Gonzaga da Cunha M, Cury Rezende F, Gonzaga da Cunha AL, Machado CA, Fonseca FLA. Anatomical, histological and metabolic differences between hypodermis and subcutaneous adipose tissue. *Int Arch Med.* 2017;10-11.
8. Sharma AN, Patel BC. Laser fitzpatrick skin type recommendations. [Updated 2020 May 4]. In: *StatPearls.* Treasure Island, FL: StatPearls Publishing; 2021.
9. Jegasothy SM, Zabolotniaia V, Bielfeldt S. Efficacy of a new topical nano-hyaluronic acid in humans. *J Clin Aesthet Dermatol.* 2014;7(3):27-29.
10. Mahmood SN, Bowe WP. Diet and acne update: carbohydrates emerge as the main culprit. *J Drugs Dermatol.* 2014;13(4):428-435.
11. Oge' LK, Broussard A, Marshall MD. Acne vulgaris: diagnosis and treatment. *Am Fam Physician.* 2019;100(8):475-484.
12. Keyes E, Werth VP, Brod B. Potential allergenicity of commonly sold high SPF broad spectrum sunscreens in the United States; from the perspective of patients with autoimmune skin disease. *Int J Womens Dermatol.* 2019;5(4):227-232.
13. Zasada M, Budzisz E. Retinoids: active molecules influencing skin structure formation in cosmetic and dermatological treatments. *Postepy Dermatol Alergol.* 2019;36(4):392-397.
14. Mukherjee S, Date A, Patravale V, Korting HC, Roeder A, Weindl G. Retinoids in the treatment of skin aging: an overview of clinical efficacy and safety. *Clin Interv Aging.* 2006;1(4):327-348.
15. Zhang S, Duan E. Fighting against skin aging: the way from bench to bedside. *Cell Transplant.* 2018;27(5):729-738.

2

Chemical Peels*

Suzan Obagi

BRIEF INTRODUCTION

Skin resurfacing procedures have continued to increase in popularity as the worldwide trend in noninvasive to minimally invasive procedures increases. Chemical peels are a low-cost yet highly effective means by which skin resurfacing can be achieved. Peels are a great alternative to laser resurfacing for certain indications and a great adjunct to laser resurfacing in other instances. With the proper patient evaluation, skin preparation, and correct treatment plan, skin rejuvenation results can be remarkable.

Chemical peels are increasing in popularity as the trend toward noninvasive or minimally invasive procedures grows. The American Society of Plastic Surgery 2014 Survey data show that surgical cosmetic procedures since 2000 have decreased by 12%, and noninvasive outpatient cosmetic procedures have risen by 154%.[1] The most common cutaneous concern in darker skinned patients is the issue of dyschromia. The ability to safely resurface, with peels or lasers, patients of a wide ethnic diversity hinges on the knowledge of skin anatomy, the depth of the issue they present with, and the proper performance of the procedure.

It is important to recognize that the skin undergoes aging both intrinsically (chronologic passage of time) and extrinsically (environmental damage). Intrinsic aging shows that with the chronologic passage of time, the epidermis and dermis atrophy and the turnover of skin cells slows down. Collagen, elastin, and glycosaminoglycan production declines steadily through the years starting from about the age of 18 years. Furthermore, the combined effect of tanning and cigarette smoking is more deleterious than either one alone.

PREPROCEDURAL CONSIDERATIONS

Patient Selection

Indications for chemical skin resurfacing include textural changes such as acne scars, enlarged pores, and wrinkles, to pigmentary concerns such as freckles/lentigines, and photodamage (Table 2.1 and Fig. 2.1). In addition, peels have been used in the management of precancerous changes in the skin.

As with any cosmetic surgery procedure, evaluation, preoperative consultation, and proper patient selection are crucial. Patients who seek treatment for barely noticeable skin anomalies are likely to be unhappy with postoperative results, even when the physician considers the outcome a success.

Patient History

A thorough history and physical examination should focus on medications and illnesses that could impact wound healing (Table 2.2). These would include medications such as prednisone, immunosuppressants, or D-penicillamine, along with conditions such as diabetes or scleroderma. Smoking or "vaping" (electronic nicotine use) or prior radiation treatment to the face and neck can also impair wound healing, as resurfaced skin requires intact and functioning pilosebaceous units and a good blood supply to reepithelialize correctly. Furthermore, tanning the skin and/or cigarette smoking will diminish the duration of any improvement that is achieved. See Video 2.1 for lecture video content on Chemical Peels.

*Adapted from Suzan Obagi; Plastic Surgery, Volume 2: Aesthetic Surgery, Fourth Edition

TABLE 2.1 Clinical Indications for Skin Resurfacing

Anatomic Skin Level	Clinical Presentation	Treatment Options
Epidermis	Epidermal melasma actinic keratosis Seborrheic keratosis[a] Solar lentigines (sun spots) Ephelides (freckles)	Topical products Superficial peels Pigment lasers
Dermis	Dermal melasma Wrinkles-depth varies Scars-depth varies Telangiectasias[b] Sebaceous hyperplasias[a] Syringomas[a]	Medium-depth resurfacing to deep peels Vascular lasers
Epidermis and dermis	Mixed-type melasma	Medium-depth resurfacing

[a]Best treated with electrodessication (using an epilating noodle for dermal lesions).
[b]Best treated with chromophore-specific lasers.

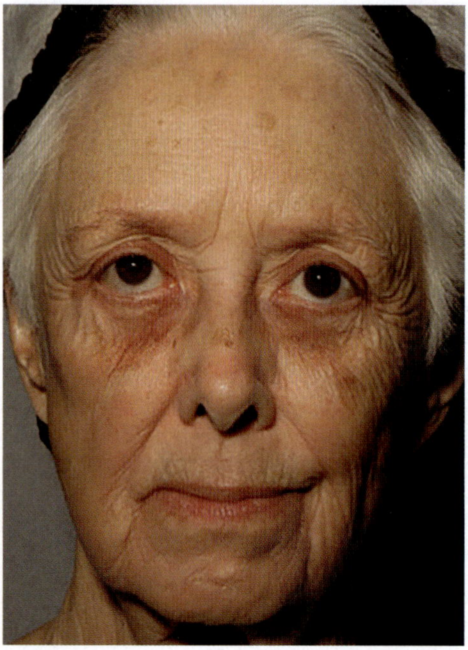

Fig. 2.1 Photoaged skin showing rhytides, dyschromia, and volume loss.

KEY POINTS

1. Knowledge of skin anatomy is crucial for proper resurfacing.
2. Chemical peels can be tailored to various patient concerns.
3. Knowledge of the various peeling agents allows for proper selection of the peeling modality for each patient's needs.
4. Proper performance of chemical peels allows patients of darker skin types to be safely treated.

The general health and nutritional status of the patient is also an important consideration for appropriate wound healing, especially in a time where the number of bariatric surgery patients is increasing. Often, post–bariatric surgery patients are deficient in vital nutrients or protein. The physician should inquire about previous poor wound healing, hypertrophic or keloid scars, or a tendency to develop postinflammatory hyperpigmentation (PIH). Seborrheic dermatitis, atopic dermatitis, and rosacea indicate the presence of inflammation in the skin, thus increasing the risk for postoperative complications secondary to alterations in the skin's normal barrier function. Melasma is a very common dyschromia for which patients seek treatment (Fig. 2.2). However, if the patient is taking estrogen or oral contraceptives, is using a hormone-containing intrauterine device, or is exposed to sun or heat during the recovery phase, they may be prone to a relapse of melasma or a temporary issue with PIH during the healing stages of the procedure.

Concurrent or recent (within the last 6 months) oral retinoid use has been generally considered an absolute contraindication to resurfacing because of reports of prolonged healing and hypertrophic scarring. A number of recent studies have brought into question the validity of this concern and challenge the conventional thinking that isotretinoin impairs wound healing with regard to skin resurfacing and laser treatments.[2-6] Until clear-cut guidelines emerge, the author stops isotretinoin 3 to 4 months before resurfacing and does not restart it until 2 to 3 months postoperatively. If the patient develops an acne or rosacea flare, antiinflammatory

TABLE 2.2 **Patient Social and Medical History**

	Pertinent History	Relative Contraindications	Absolute Contraindications
Medical	Medications Systemic illnesses Psychiatric illnesses • Depression • OCD • BDD MRSA history Radiation to the treated area HSV or VZV tendency	Active acne, rosacea, CTD, vitiligo Bariatric surgery with nutritional deficiency Diabetes Isotretinoin use recently	Active infection at the treatment site History of keloids at the treatment site—avoid reticular dermis level procedures Pregnancy
Social	Smoking history Chronic sun exposure	Smoking/vaping/nicotine use	Inability to follow instructions Unrealistic expectations

BDD, Body dysmorphic disorder; *CTD*, connective tissue disease; *HSV*, herpes simplex virus; *MRSA*, methicillin-resistant *Staphylococcus aureus*; *OCD*, obsessive-compulsive disorder; *VZV*, varicella zoster virus.

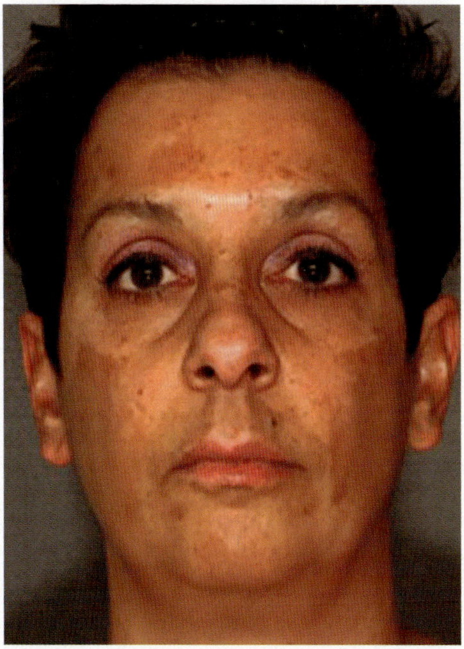

Fig. 2.2 Melasma—hormonal pigmentation aggravated by heat, trauma, and hormone supplementation.

antibiotics (doxycycline) can be used to quiet this down without impairing wound healing.

A similar question arises with regard to the safety of simultaneous skin resurfacing and cosmetic surgery. In the past, it was thought that combining these procedures increased the chance of impaired wound healing.[7] Newer studies have reported safe outcomes combining fractionated laser resurfacing with short-flap rhytidectomy,[8] full-face laser skin ablation combined with rhytidectomy,[9] fractionated CO_2 laser has been used to complement and enhance the results of endoscopic eyebrow lifting and surgical blepharoplasty,[10] and simultaneous facelift and laser resurfacing over skin flaps with decreased laser energy settings, and reduced number of passes, has achieved excellent aesthetic results.[11]

While most patients can safely undergo skin resurfacing, absolute contraindications include pregnancy, active infection at the treatment site, significant tendency to develop keloid scars, and the inability to adhere to postoperative instructions.

Evaluating Skin Type

Older skin classification systems such as Fitzpatrick skin type or Glogau skin type do not provide the physician all the information needed to select the best treatment modality. In particular, these scales were devised before the emergence of nonablative and fractionally ablative technologies and fall short in addressing patients with thicker skin or darker skin types. The author uses the Obagi Skin Classification (Table 2.3) to help with proper procedure planning.

Particular attention should be paid to the patient that has skin that freckles, develops melasma, or is prone to PIH. Regardless of ethnic background, the presence of these issues heralds the risk of postprocedure hyperpigmentation. These patients can be treated safely if the duration of both pre- and postresurfacing skin conditioning is extended to at least 8 to 12 weeks.

TABLE 2.3 Obagi Skin Classification

Skin Variable	Skin Conditioning—Pre- and Postresurfacing	Suitable Procedures and Potential Complications
Color	Conditioning varies with skin color More aggressive with darker White skin and with lighter Asian or lighter Black skin	Complications related to depth and skin color Darker skin: Hypopigmentation: • Superficial procedure: rare • Medium-depth procedures: possible • Deep procedures: more likely Hyperpigmentation: • Common regardless of depth
Oiliness	Increased skin surface oil interferes with effectiveness of skin conditioning It may contribute to postoperative acne flares Topical or systemic therapy to control or reduce surface oiliness preoperatively[a]	Excessive oil hinders chemical peel acid penetration Laser resurfacing is not affected by oiliness
Thickness	Thin skin needs papillary level procedures to thicken the papillary dermal collagen layer Thick skin needs reticular dermis level procedures to effect a textural change	Thin skin: light- to medium-depth peels Medium-thick skin: good for peels, dermabrasion, fractionated lasers Thick skin: deeper chemical peels, dermabrasion, fractionated lasers
Laxity	Lax skin requires long-term collagen stimulation to prevent further laxity	Differentiate between skin and muscle laxity: Skin laxity: medium-depth peel to the level of the papillary dermis Muscle laxity: facelift alone or in combination with a medium-depth peel (to correct any associated skin laxity)
Fragility	Goal is to maintain or possibly increase skin strength	Fragility correlates with postsurgical scarring Procedure depth should be limited to the papillary dermis in fragile skin

[a]If systemic isotretinoin is used, it is prudent to delay medium or deep skin resurfacing by at least 3 months (medium-depth resurfacing) to 6 months (deeper resurfacing).

SKIN CONDITIONING PRE- AND POSTRESURFACING

Proper skin conditioning should be started at least 6 weeks (8–12 weeks or longer for darker skinned individuals) before resurfacing.[12] Typically, the patient will use this regimen up until the night before the procedure. Tretinoin 0.05% to 0.1% or retinaldehyde 0.1% cream promote collagen synthesis, enhance hydroquinone penetration, restore normal epidermal thickness and maturation, and improve solar elastosis.[13,14] Studies have shown faster wound healing from skin resurfacing in patients pretreated with tretinoin.[15] Since many retinoids are photolabile, it is suggested that they be applied at night. Patients are instructed to apply 0.5 to 1 g of tretinoin or retinaldehyde to the entire face nightly, including the lower eyelids with feathering to the hairline, jawline, and preauricular areas. The corners of the eyes and mouth should be avoided. The upper eyelids should be treated one to two times per week. If there is significant retinoid dermatitis, the topical agents can be stopped 4 to 7 days before skin resurfacing.

Hydroquinone 4% cream reduces the risk of PIH. Since the half-life of hydroquinone is 12 hours, it requires a twice-daily application. Patients are instructed to apply 1 g twice daily to entire face, with a second light application to areas of darkest pigmentation (sun spots, melasma).

A topical polyhydroxy acid/lactobionic acid or alpha-hydroxy acid 6% to 8% can be applied in the mornings to help minimize acne flares and to enhance the penetration of hydroquinone or tretinoin. These are especially important for patients with thick or oily skin. However, these agents can oxidize tretinoin; thus it is not recommended to apply them in the evenings along with the retinoids. Photoprotection with sunscreens is important to protect the skin against deleterious effects of ultraviolet radiation. In addition, there is new interest in the effects of visible light on the aging process. Therefore, we may see an evolution in sun protection to be effective in the visible light spectrum.

Sunscreens have been divided into chemical absorbers (organic) and physical blockers (inorganic) on the basis of their mechanism of action. In the author's practice, physical sunscreens are the only recommended type of photoprotection. These contain zinc oxide and titanium dioxide, which are chemically inert and therefore less irritating and less allergenic.

Newer, micronized zinc or titanium formulations have improved the elegance of sunscreen products and may virtually replace moisturizers for patients.

The use of proper skin conditioning before a procedure helps reduce the risk of hyperpigmentation afterwards. Furthermore, the improved skin texture motivates patients to proceed with further procedures to enhance their skin (Fig. 2.3A, B). Lastly, the ability of a patient to adhere to a skin care regimen helps to predict which patients are most likely to be compliant with postoperative instructions.

All patients should receive prophylaxis against herpes simplex virus (HSV) or varicella zoster virus (VZV) to prevent reactivation and potential scarring regardless of their personal history of previous viral infection. Valacyclovir is the author's preferred medication; the usual dose is 500 mg twice daily, starting the day before surgery and continuing until the skin has fully healed (7 days for chemical peel resurfacing and 15 days for laser resurfacing). If a patient has a significant history of HSV or VZV, a dose of valacyclovir 1 g twice daily is used. This dose can be increased to three times a day if needed to control an outbreak. Antibiotics and anti-*Candida* agents are reserved for use only when an infection develops. However, topical mupirocin ointment is prescribed to patients to apply to the nares three times a

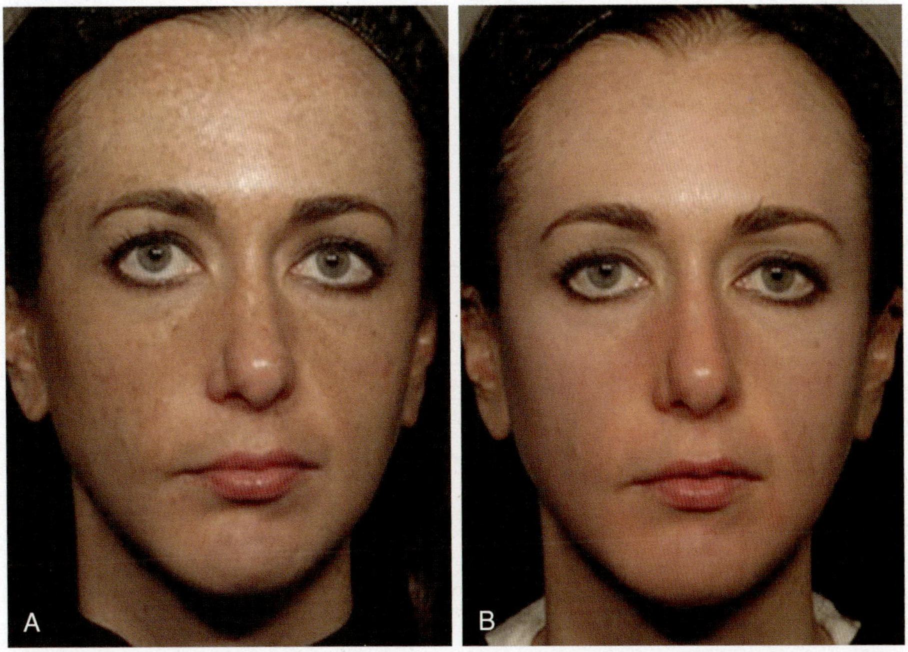

Fig. 2.3 Skin conditioning before (A) and after (B) 6 weeks of a topical skin care regimen consisting of tretinoin, hydroquinone, alpha-hydroxy acid, and sunblock.

day starting 1 week before their skin resurfacing and continuing until their skin is fully healed.

BACKGROUND INFORMATION/ ANATOMIC PEARLS

Terminology

This chapter will categorize peels according to their depth of penetration into the skin rather than strictly referring to the acid used (Table 2.4). Exfoliation will refer to wounds confined to the epidermis (basal layer and above). Peels reaching the papillary dermis but not entering the reticular dermis will be classified as light, while medium-depth peels will refer to peels that have entered the superficial aspect of the reticular dermis. Deep peels extend into the mid-reticular dermis. It is imperative to monitor the intraoperative signs to assess the depth of penetration. This will be discussed further.

MECHANISMS OF ACTION

There are a few key factors to be aware of with regard to skin–acid interaction and penetration. These are the type of acid used, the concentration of the acid, the force by which the acid is rubbed into the skin, the volume of acid applied to the skin, whether or not the skin is preconditioned properly to enhance penetration, and in some cases, the duration of contact of the acid on the skin[16] (Table 2.5). Selection of peeling agents should be based on the mechanism of action of the solution and not on acid concentration. Chemical peeling agents are classified as keratolytics or protein denaturants. Keratolytics are primarily used for superficial, exfoliative procedures, whereas the protein denaturants can be used for superficial or deeper peels. As will be discussed later, keratolytics can be used in combination with protein denaturants to enhance peel penetration.

TABLE 2.4 Chemical Peel Formulas

Acid Properties	Commonly Used Concentrations and Formulations
Keratolytics	Salicylic acid peels 15%–30% Glycolic acid 50%–70% Jessner's solution Phenol 25%–50%[a]
Protein denaturants	Trichloroacetic acid 15%–100% Phenol 60%–88% Baker-Gordon phenol peel: 50% phenol, 2.1% croton oil Hetter phenol peels: 50% phenol, 0.7% croton oil Hetter "all around": 35% phenol, 0.4% croton oil Hetter VL (neck and eyelid): 30% phenol, 0.1% croton oil Stone V-K: 62% phenol, 0.16% croton oil Stone 2: 60% phenol, 0.2% croton oil

[a]Phenol at concentrations below 50% has keratolytic properties

TABLE 2.5 Key Points for Acid Penetration

	Enhanced Penetration of Peel Solution Into the Skin
Acid properties	Protein denaturants penetrate deeper than keratolytics Higher concentrations penetrate more than lower concentrations Higher volumes of acid applied penetrate more than lower volumes Keratolytics applied before protein denaturants results in deeper acid penetration
Skin properties	Acid will reach deeper into the skin in thinner skin Properly retinized skin will absorb acid faster and more evenly Applying the solution with greater force results in deeper penetration Degreasing the skin enhances peel penetration Open wounds in the skin will absorb the acid quickest[a]

[a]Caution is required when combining pools with dermabrasion and laser resurfacing. The pool should be performed first, the acid then washed off, then the laser or dermabrasion is performed.

Keratolytics

Keratolytics act as exfoliating agents based on their ability to disrupt adhesions between keratinocytes. Glycolic acid, salicylic acid, and Jessner's solution are the most commonly used keratolytic peeling solutions. Jessner's solution is comprised of 14% each of resorcinol, salicylic acid, and lactic acid mixed in ethanol. These agents are primarily used for superficial conditions such as roughness, acne, and mild dyspigmentation.

Salicylic acid and Jessner's solution have an advantage over glycolic acid in that salicylic acid is lipophilic. Therefore, these two peel solutions penetrate acne lesions or oily skin better than a hydrophilic agent such as glycolic acid. Another advantage they have over glycolic acid is that salicylic acid and Jessner's solution do not have to have the skin contact time closely timed.

All three of these peels have the benefit of little to no "downtime," no anesthesia requirement, and they are easy to perform. Because of the superficial nature of these peels, results are seen only after a series of peels, spaced several weeks apart. However, because of the superficial nature of these peels, deeper issues such as wrinkles, acne scars, or dermal melasma will not improve with these, regardless of how many peels are performed.

Protein Denaturants

Trichloroacetic acid peels. Trichloroacetic acid (TCA) can be used to reach a variety of depths and is therefore considered the "workhorse" of chemical peels. As TCA penetrates through the skin, it causes protein coagulation and denaturation of the cells in the epidermis and dermis as well as the blood vessels. TCA is self-neutralizing, thus it is not one that can be neutralized. This means that once TCA is applied to the skin, it will keep penetrating until it has been used up during the coagulation of a certain amount of protein. This is a key concept, because subsequent applications of TCA will drive the peel deeper, regardless of concentration, until the acid has coagulated proteins deeper down in the skin. Based on this knowledge, it is incorrect to refer to TCA peels as light or deep according to acid concentration.

Another key point is that there are four ways in which TCA can be formulated.[17] Therefore, to avoid errors in formulation, it is of utmost importance to purchase the acid from a reliable source using the weight to volume (W: V) method. The author uses a 30% TCA solution, which is then modified as part of the Blue Peel to create a 15%, 20%, 22%, or 25% solution.

While many physicians have switched from chemical peels to the perceived "safety and reproducibility" of lasers, peels can be approached in a systematic manner, making them very powerful tools in skin rejuvenation. In an attempt to obtain more consistent results while giving the physician more control over the peel, variations of the TCA peel (Jessner–TCA peel, glycolic acid–TCA peel, Blue Peel) have been developed. Anatomically, they are designed to peel through the papillary dermis and into the most superficial aspect of the reticular dermis. Their main indications are for epidermal and upper dermal pathology: photodamage, actinic keratoses, large pores, lentigines, ephelides, fine rhytids, and very superficial, nonfibrotic scars. Deeper pathology such as deep wrinkles or deep scars are not amenable to correction with these peels.

These combination TCA peels can be categorized as being "accelerated" or "decelerated." In an attempt to speed the penetration and depth of TCA peels, two modified peels were created that incorporate the use of a keratolytic agent. The Jessner–TCA peel uses Jessner's solution (keratolytic), applied before the application of TCA.[18] Application of the Jessner's solution allows for faster and deeper penetration of the subsequently applied 35% TCA. A similar mechanism is used with the glycolic acid–TCA peel, which uses 70% glycolic acid (keratolytic) before application of 35% TCA.[19]

The Blue Peel is unique in that instead of increasing the speed and depth of the peel, the process is slowed down.[20] This allows the physician better control of depth during the peel. The Blue Peel incorporates a nonionic blue dye, glycerin, and a saponin with a specific volume of 30% TCA to yield a 15%, 20%, or higher percentage of TCA–Blue Peel solution. Use of TCA, a colorless solution, requires close attention to avoid reapplication over previously treated areas. Therefore, the blue dye is advantageous as it stains the stratum corneum and helps the physician to visualize even application of the peel. Since TCA is hydrophilic, the use of a saponin as an emulsifying agent creates a homogeneous TCA–oil–water emulsion that penetrates the skin in a slower and more even fashion.

PHENOL PEELS

Phenol peels are inherently categorized as deep peels because of the predominant effect of phenol on the skin. Similar to TCA, phenol works through protein denaturation and coagulation. However, phenol differs from TCA in that it penetrates quickly to the level of the reticular dermis.[21] Phenol is partially detoxified by the liver and excreted through the kidneys. The percutaneous absorption of phenol can lead to a rapid elevation of serum phenol levels, resulting in systemic toxicity and cardiac arrhythmias. Therefore, all patients should be cleared from a cardiac, hepatic, and renal standpoint preoperatively. In addition, intraoperative cardiac monitoring and at least 1 L of intravenous (IV) hydration are imperative.[22]

Because of the depth of penetration of phenol peels into the mid-reticular dermis, the risk of scarring, prolonged erythema, and depigmentation is extremely high. This limits the utility of this peel to a small subset of older, fair-skinned individuals with significant rhytides and laxity. Although any resurfacing method that reaches the reticular dermis may cause permanent hypopigmentation, the traditional Baker–Gordon peel resulted in unacceptably high rates. Weaker solutions of phenol (25%–50%) can be used to achieve lighter peels; however, the results are not better than TCA and there is still the risk for systemic toxicity.

Modifications of the Baker–Gordon phenol peel formula with reduced levels of croton oil have significantly reduced the amount of postoperative hypopigmentation, postoperative erythema, and scarring. Both Hetter and Stone independently described modifications of phenol peels (lower phenol acid concentration and/or lower croton oil concentrations) that allow better control over depth of penetration,[23,24] allowing patients of a variety of skin types to be treated. These newer formulations have contributed to a renewed interest in phenol peels, as they provide physicians with clinically and financially effective alternatives to laser resurfacing.

PROCEDURAL CONSIDERATIONS

Techniques

Glycolic Acid Peels, Salicylic Acid Peels, Jessner's Peels

> **HINTS AND TIPS**
> **Glycolic Acid Peels, Salicylic Acid Peels, Jessner's Peels**
> These lighter-peeling agents must be applied to clean skin. Have the patients cleanse their skin of all make-up and lotions. The skin is first degreased with 70% ethanol (ETOH). However, if the desire is to push the peel deeper, the skin is degreased with acetone instead.

Glycolic Acid Peels

Glycolic acid must be applied quickly (within 15–20 s) to the treatment area, and the contact time must be measured. Glycolic acid is started at a lower concentration, and with subsequent treatments either a stronger concentration is applied or the contact time with the skin is increased. Typically, 50% to 70% glycolic acid is applied with gauze or a large cotton-tip applicator swab. The acid is left in contact with the skin for 30 s, and with subsequent treatments the contact time is worked up to 1 to 2 min. The peel is then diluted with copious amounts of water or neutralized with sodium bicarbonate. Close timing is important since a study has shown that glycolic acid left on the skin for 15 min created a dermal wound identical to that seen with 35% to 50% TCA.[25]

Salicylic Acid Peels

Salicylic acid is applied to acetone- or alcohol-cleansed skin in concentrations of 20% to 35% using gauze or cotton-tip applicators. Multiple applications can be applied to problematic areas to enhance the depth of penetration. The peel is washed off with water after 6 min. Salicylic acid does not need to be neutralized as it precipitates into a powder on the surface of the skin after the solvent evaporates. Application to a large surface area or the use of occlusion should be avoided because of the risk of salicylism.

Jessner's Peels

Jessner's solution is also applied to alcohol- or acetone-cleansed skin. The solution is applied in multiple coats to problem areas. After 6 min, the peel is washed off with water.

TRICHLOROACETIC ACID PEELS

TCA is usually used to achieve medium-depth peels. The recovery time can range from 5 to 10 days and the procedure can be associated with significant discomfort while the peel is performed. However, the pain usually subsides before the patient goes home. Patients receiving intramuscular or IV sedation tolerate the procedure better and allow the peel to proceed at a faster speed. Additional pain control can be achieved with the use of strong fans or cooling units with refrigerated air and oral sedation. Topical anesthetics should not be used before skin peels because they enhance the penetration of the TCA and may result in an undesirable depth of peel.

Skin resurfacing, whether with peels or lasers, is all about reading the skin depth signs properly. Regardless of the type of TCA peel performed, the evolving clinical depth signs remain the same. The only difference between the various peels is the speed by which these signs appear.

Physicians with minimal peeling experience are encouraged to start with relatively slower peeling techniques before proceeding to faster peels. Combination peels using a keratolytic peel followed by a TCA peel will speed up the penetration of the TCA, therefore carrying the risk of penetrating deeper than expected. Just as with laser resurfacing and dermabrasion, physicians must keep in mind the anatomic variations of skin thickness before resurfacing.

Residual oil or thick scale may lead to a patchy peel; therefore, it is essential to cleanse and degrease the face well before proceeding. Clinical depth signs are very important to monitor during the peeling process.[26] Frost appears on the skin gradually as a result of coagulation of epidermal and dermal proteins by the action of TCA.[20] As TCA is first applied, a light, nonorganized frost begins to form (level 1 frost) (Figs. 2.4A and 2.5A).

Further application results in the frost being solid but with a diffuse pink background (vasodilation; level 2 frost) (Fig. 2.4B); this level of frost indicates a peel to the level of the papillary dermis. The pink background of the frost is referred to as the "pink sign"[20] (Fig. 2.5B). The "pink sign" will be apparent as long as the blood vessels of the papillary dermis are still intact with normal blood flow. This "pink sign" is the endpoint for the standard, papillary dermis-level peel.

Additional chemical peel solution application will result in further protein coagulation, a more solid white frost, and the loss of the "pink sign" indicating coagulation of the papillary dermis vascular plexus (level 3 frost) (Fig. 2.4C).

The "pink sign" is difficult to see in darker skin. When peeling dark skinned individuals, the "epidermal sliding" must be used to gauge depth.[20] The "epidermal sliding" sign shows up as exaggerated wrinkling of the skin that occurs before complete precipitation and coagulation of papillary dermis proteins (see Fig. 2.5B). At this point, papillary dermal edema and disruption of anchoring fibrils allow the epidermis to be more freely movable, resulting in wrinkling in an exaggerated fashion when the skin is pushed or pinched. This sign will disappear when the papillary dermis protein becomes coagulated and adherent to the epidermal coagulated proteins, thus indicating that the peel depth has reached the superficial reticular dermis (Fig. 2.5C). At this point, the pink background also becomes lost. In thick skin, "epidermal sliding" may not be very obvious, and the "pink sign" alone has to be used to indicate the peel depth.

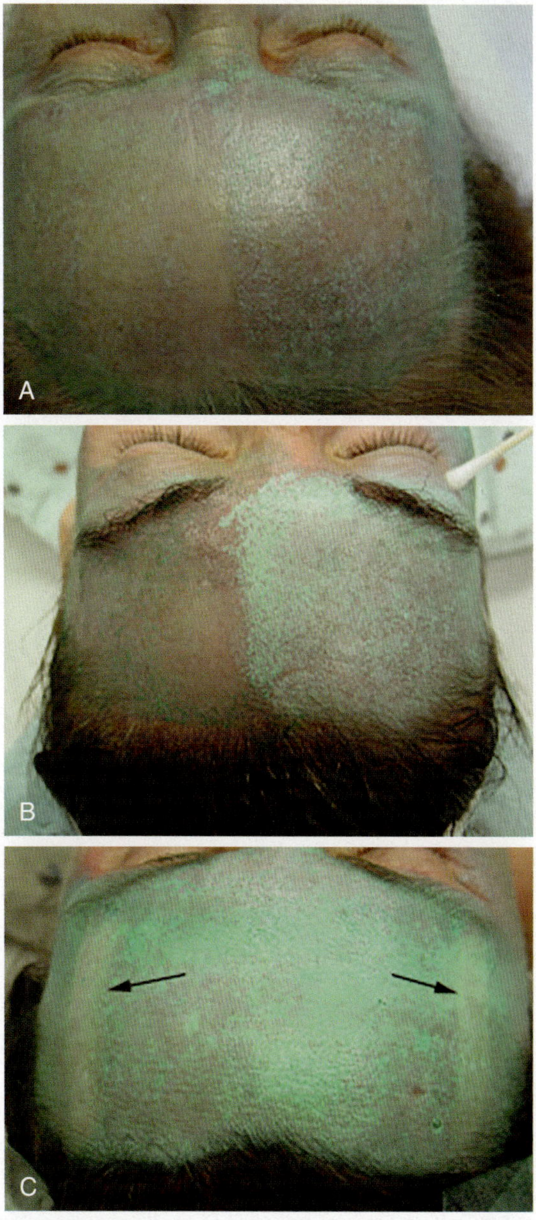

Fig. 2.4 (A) Level 1 frost: light, nonorganized frost on right-hand side of forehead. (B) Level 2 frost: even frost with a pink background, "pink sign," on right-hand side of forehead. (C) Level 3 frost: solid frost with no pink background on lateral parts of forehead *(arrows)*.

Further TCA application will penetrate the upper reticular dermis and clinically show a solid frost with a loss of the pink background (level 3 frost) (see Fig. 2.4C) and the presence of dermal edema upon pinching the skin. Reaching this level implies that the whole papillary

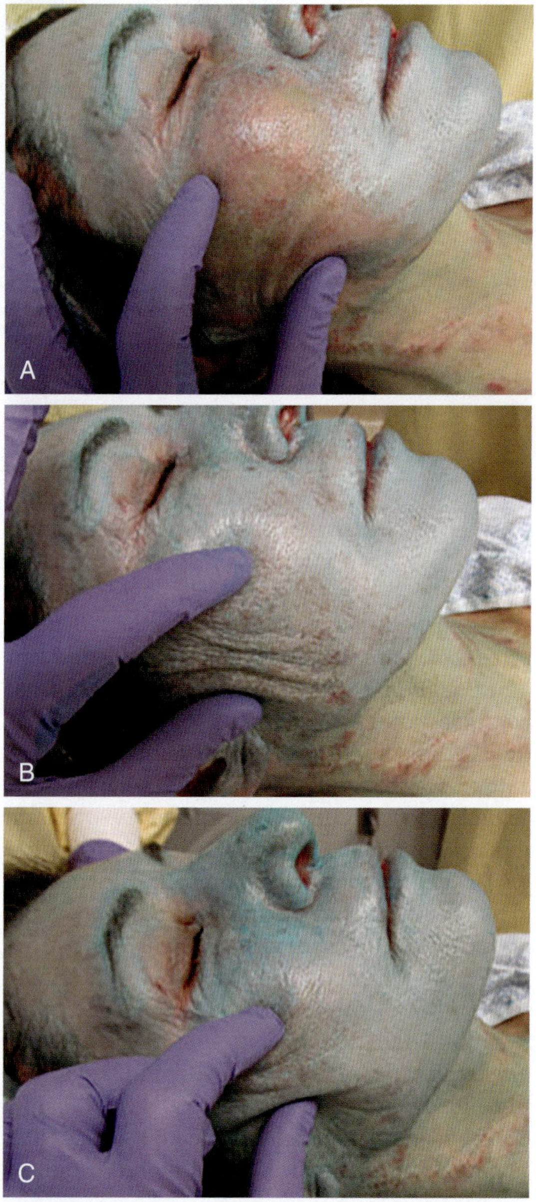

Fig. 2.5 Peel progression signs: (A) Minimal frost, no edema, no epidermal sliding sign. (B) Level 2 frost, minimal edema, almost solid frost, with pink background and epidermal sliding. (C) Level 3 frost, deeper, frost more solid, edema present, epidermal sliding gone.

dermis is involved with the peel and the upper reticular dermis has been reached but not yet involved. This is the endpoint for most peels. Beyond this level, the solid frost begins to take on a gray color, and this correlates with an increased incidence of scarring and hypopigmentation.

JESSNER–TRICHLOROACETIC ACID PEELS

After the skin is cleansed, acetone is used to degrease the face further. With either 2 × 2 gauze or cotton-tipped applicators, the Jessner's solution is applied evenly until a very light frost develops. A small amount of 35% TCA is then applied to the skin with either cotton-tipped applicators or gauze in even strokes. Two minutes are allowed to pass before further application so that the depth of TCA penetration can be assessed. Areas of inadequate frosting can be carefully re-treated. Sharp demarcation lines should be avoided by feathering out the solution to the hairline, ears, and jawline.

GLYCOLIC ACID–TRICHLOROACETIC ACID PEELS

The skin is first cleansed with soap and water only. Seventy percent unbuffered aqueous glycolic acid is rapidly applied to the skin and left on for 2 min. It is then washed off with water. Next, a small amount of 35% TCA is applied in even strokes to the face with gauze or cotton swabs. After allowing 2 to 3 min for the acid to neutralize, areas of poor frosting can be carefully re-treated.

TRICHLOROACETIC ACID–BLUE PEELS

The skin is gently cleansed with alcohol. The Blue Peel mixture is then prepared by mixing the Blue Peel base with 2 mL, 4 mL, or 6 mL of 30% TCA to create a mixture of 15%, 20%, or 22%, respectively. This mixture is applied evenly to one quadrant of the face if the patient is awake or can be done on the entire face if the patient is sedated. After a 2 to 3 min waiting period, a subsequent coat is applied. The amount needed for thinner skin will be less than that needed for thicker skin. An even blue color, even frost, and a pink background indicate that the papillary dermis has been reached. Additional coats will result in loss of the pink background, thus indicating penetration beyond the papillary dermis and into the superficial reticular dermis. This is the maximum recommended depth of a facial TCA–Blue Peel.

PHENOL PEELS

Hetter VL Peels

The modified, lighter phenol peels, like the Hetter VL solution, can be used to treat a single cosmetic unit without the need for cardiac monitoring or IV hydration.

However, if a larger area is to be treated, or a stronger solution of phenol is used, the patient must have appropriate cardiac clearance, good hepatic and renal function, and receive appropriate IV hydration and cardiac monitoring.

The skin is degreased with alcohol. The phenol mixture must be swirled before each application as the oil and water components of the solution have a tendency to separate. The solution is applied to the skin with a cotton-tipped applicator. Care must be taken not to let the solution drip or run down the face. Once the solution is applied, the skin will frost quickly. The endpoint is an even white frost (Fig. 2.6). The frost dissipates quickly, so one must pay close attention to make sure that one does not apply more solution and peel the skin too deeply.

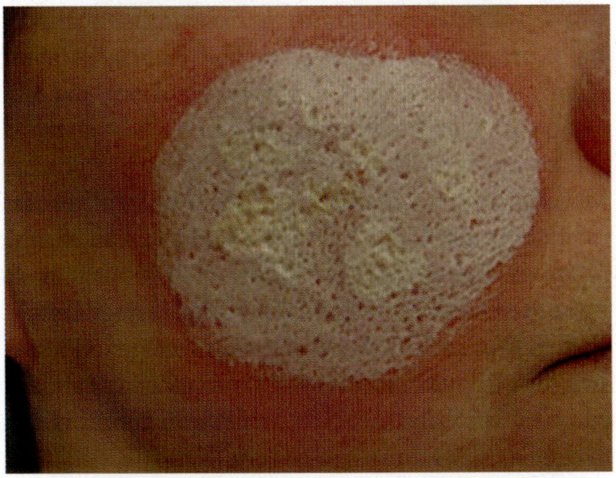

Fig. 2.6 Phenol peel frost—more solid frost on deeper scars, less solid frost at periphery.

COMBINATION PROCEDURES

Chemical peels can be successfully combined with laser resurfacing and surgery, with certain precautions. When performing chemical peels with laser procedures, the following guidance should be adhered to: (1) nonablative or minimally ablative lasers (vascular or pigment lasers) or electrodessication is performed first; (2) the medium-depth peel is performed next; (3) if a phenol peel is to be used in certain cosmetic units, this is then performed; (4) the skin is cleansed to remove all residual acids; and (5) the laser resurfacing of certain areas can then be performed (Fig. 2.7). If peels are done in combination with a facelift, care is taken to avoid peeling beyond the superficial papillary dermis over the undermined skin flap.

POSTPROCEDURAL CONSIDERATIONS

Postoperative Care

Light Peels

Patients will experience minimal erythema and a variable amount of desquamation. They are instructed to avoid sun exposure during the healing phase. Patients should gently wash their face twice a day and apply a

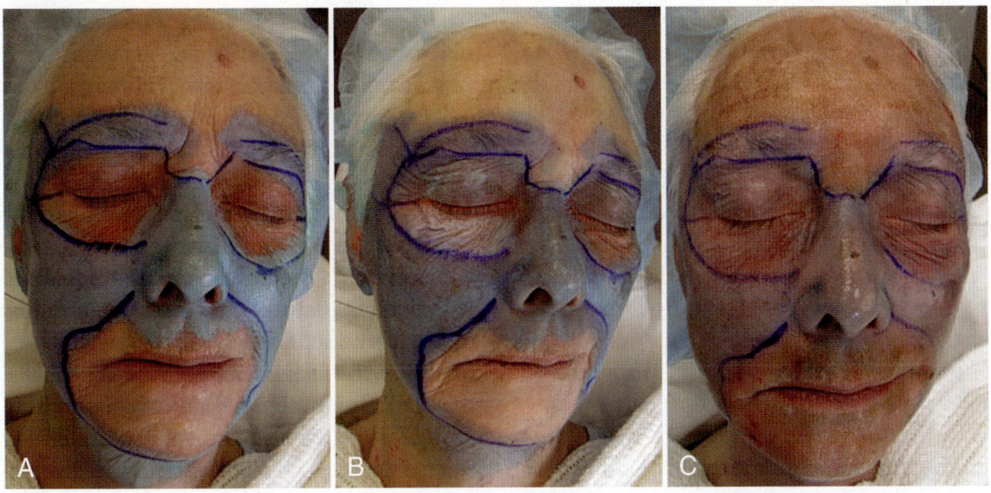

Fig. 2.7 Combination resurfacing: (A) Trichloroacetic acid (TCA)–Blue Peel performed first, (B) periorbital Hetter VL phenol peel is performed next, the skin is then cleansed, and (C) fractionated laser resurfacing to the perioral and forehead region is performed last.

light moisturizer and a sunscreen. They should hold off on applying their retinoids or alpha-hydroxy lotions until the skin has fully healed.

Medium-Depth to Deeper Peels

Every patient will have a different postoperative course, but, for the most part, patients should be fully healed within 7 to 8 days of the procedure (Fig. 2.8). Rarely, 10 days may be needed in areas of deep resurfacing. Patients will experience a moderate amount of facial edema between 24 and 48 hours. If a phenol solution or a resurfacing laser is used, those areas will also have a fair amount of proteinaceous exudate. While every physician will fine-tune the postoperative care to their patient, the author's 15 years of experience have resulted in a many modifications and, ultimately, in simplification of the postoperative care.

Patients are instructed to begin topical mupirocin ointment three times a day to the nostrils, starting 1 week before the procedure and until the skin has fully healed. Patients will wash their face twice a day with a gentle cleanser using only their hands (no washcloths). In addition to the soap cleansing, twice a day (at midday and late afternoon) patients perform an astringent soak for 10 min using gauze soaked in Domeboro's Solution (Moberg Pharma, Cedar Knolls, NJ). After each wash or soak, patients apply an inert emollient to the skin such as Vaniply Ointment (Pharmaceutical Specialties, Rochester, MN) or Aquaphor Ointment (Beiersdorf, Hamburg, Germany).

Patients continue this regimen until the skin is 100% reepithelialized. Once reepitheliazed, patients can slowly reintroduce their routine skin care. It is important during this time that patients avoid exercise and sun exposure. Furthermore, they are instructed not to pick, rub, or scratch their skin during the healing process (Table 2.6).

COMPLICATIONS AND OUTCOMES

With the correct patient selection, skin preparation, and procedure performance, results can be very gratifying. Patients will see more skin firmness, clarity, and a reduction in precancerous changes (Figs. 2.9–2.11).

Infections need to be recognized and treated early to avoid the risk of scarring. Infections are most commonly bacterial (*Staphylococcus aureus*, community-acquired methicillin-resistant *Staphylococcus aureus* [MRSA]) followed by virus (HSV, VZV) and less so by

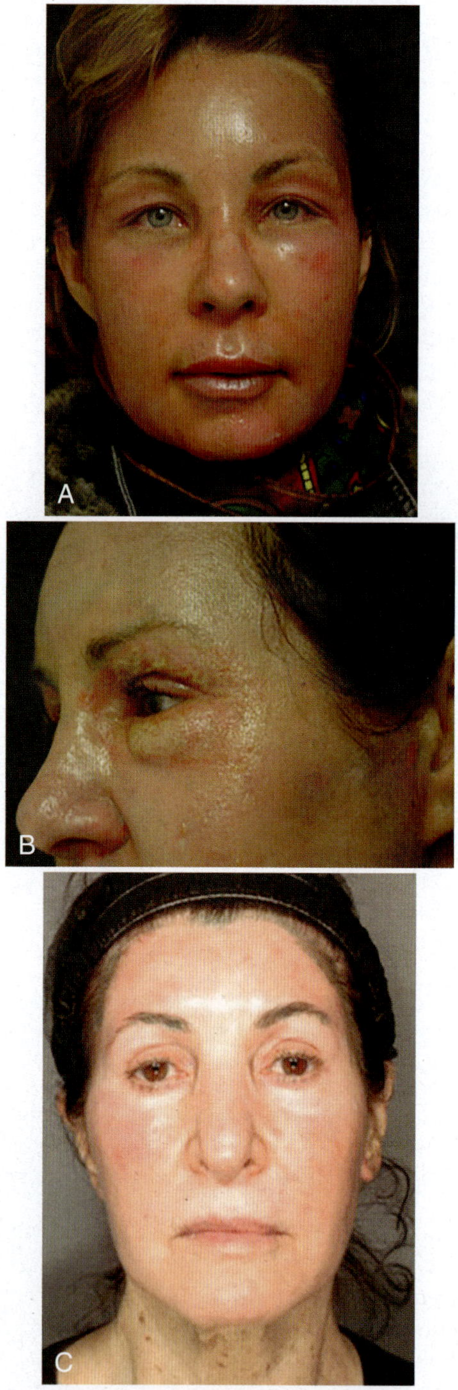

Fig. 2.8 Wound healing stages: (A) First 48 hours: medium-depth peel, swelling peaks. (B) Laser resurfacing and phenol peel areas show proteinaceous exudate (periorbital). (C) Postoperative day 7 full-face medium-depth peel, neck still healing from electrodessication of lesions.

TABLE 2.6 Hints and Tips: Peels

Ways to Enhance Peel Depth	Ways to Enhance Comfort
Degrease the skin with acetone	Cooling air units or strong fans
Apply firmer pressure when applying the peel solution	Oral analgesics: ibuprofen, meperidine, hydrocodone
Apply more peel solution volume	Music or relaxing atmosphere
Apply a higher acid concentration	Intravenous sedation
Perform a light peel or microdermabrasion before applying the deeper peel solution[a]	Nerve blocks[b]

[a]Caution is recommended with more aggressive techniques.
[b]May not give complete analgesia.

yeast (*Candida*).[27] A potassium hydroxide (KOH) slide prep can be performed in the office to confirm a yeast infection if one is suspected. If a patient is on a systemic antibiotic and develops an infection, consider *Pseudomonas aeruginosa* and other gram-negative organisms as the most common etiology.

HINTS AND TIPS

Whether the skin is treated with lasers, peels, or dermabrasion, the complications are identical (Fig. 2.12). Complications such as hypertrophic scarring, prolonged erythema (over 3 months), and pigmentary changes are related to wound depth and not specifically to the modality used. In contrast, complications such as infections and contact dermatitis occur from the impaired skin barrier function seen with resurfacing.

Cultures and sensitivities should be performed as indicated to identify the bacterial organism. Appropriate systemic therapy should be directed at the most likely etiology while results are pending.

Although the use of herpes prophylaxis has greatly decreased the incidence of viral infection, some patients can experience an outbreak even while on suppressive treatment. If a viral infection is suspected, a direct fluorescent antibody test (DFA) can quickly confirm a herpes or zoster infection. However, patients should be treated with antiviral therapy dosed as if treating a varicella zoster infection (i.e., valacyclovir 1 g three times a day for 10 days) until results are finalized.

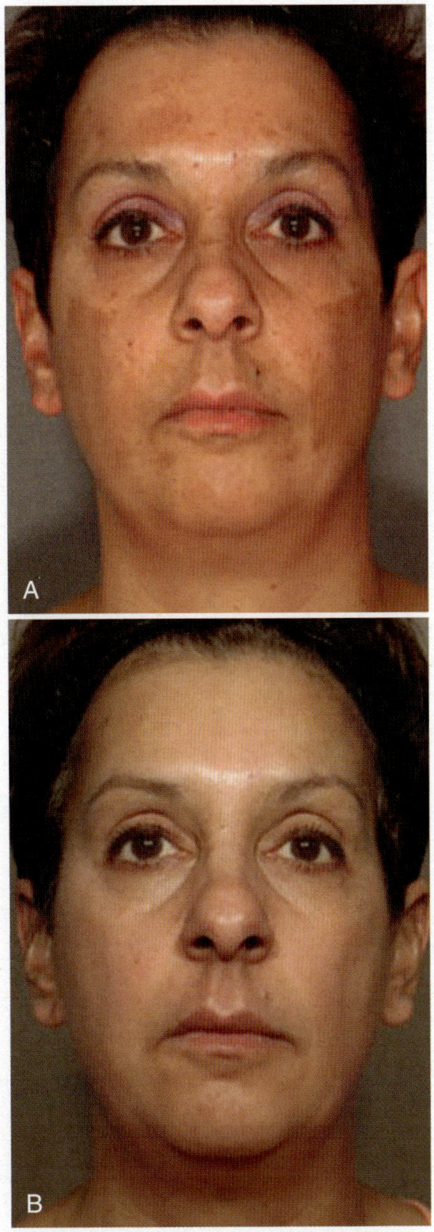

Fig. 2.9 Skin resurfacing before and after: (A) Patient with melasma baseline and (B) after skin conditioning and a medium-depth Blue Peel.

Allergic contact dermatitis to the postoperative skin care agents is often a challenging diagnosis. Patients will

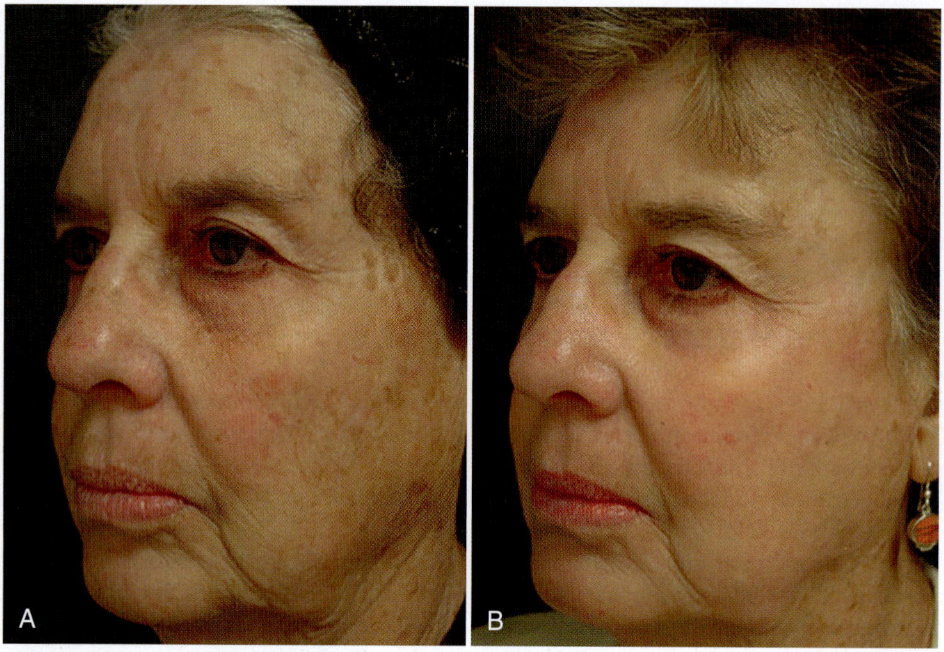

Fig. 2.10 Skin resurfacing before and after: (A) Patient before and (B) after 3 months full-face medium-depth Blue Peel and electrodessication of adnexal lesions.

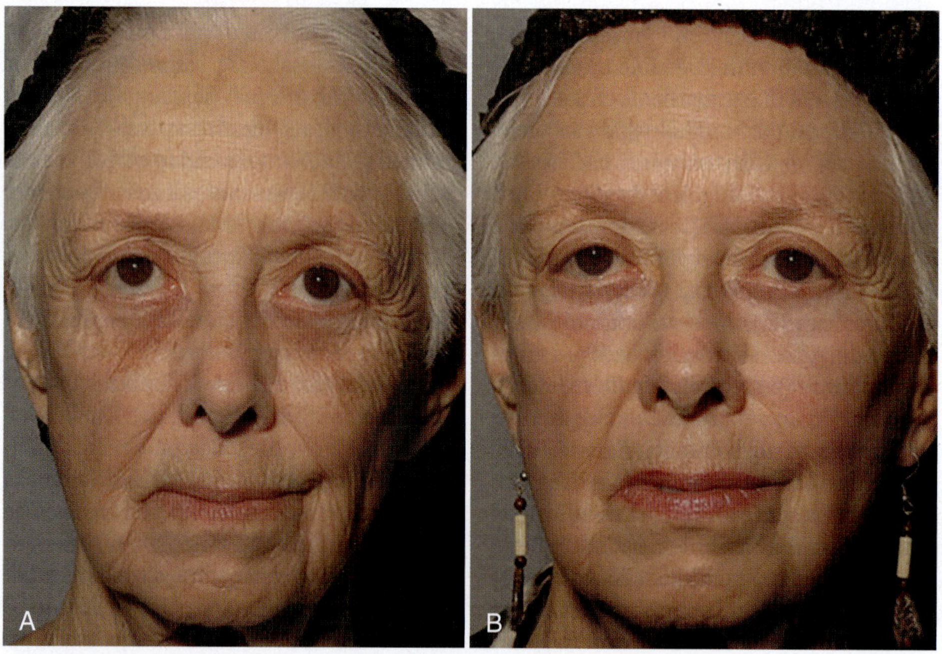

Fig. 2.11 Skin resurfacing before and after: (A) Patient shown in Fig. 2.1, before and (B) 4 months after medium-depth Blue Peel, fractionated laser forehead, and perioral and periorbital Hetter VL peel.

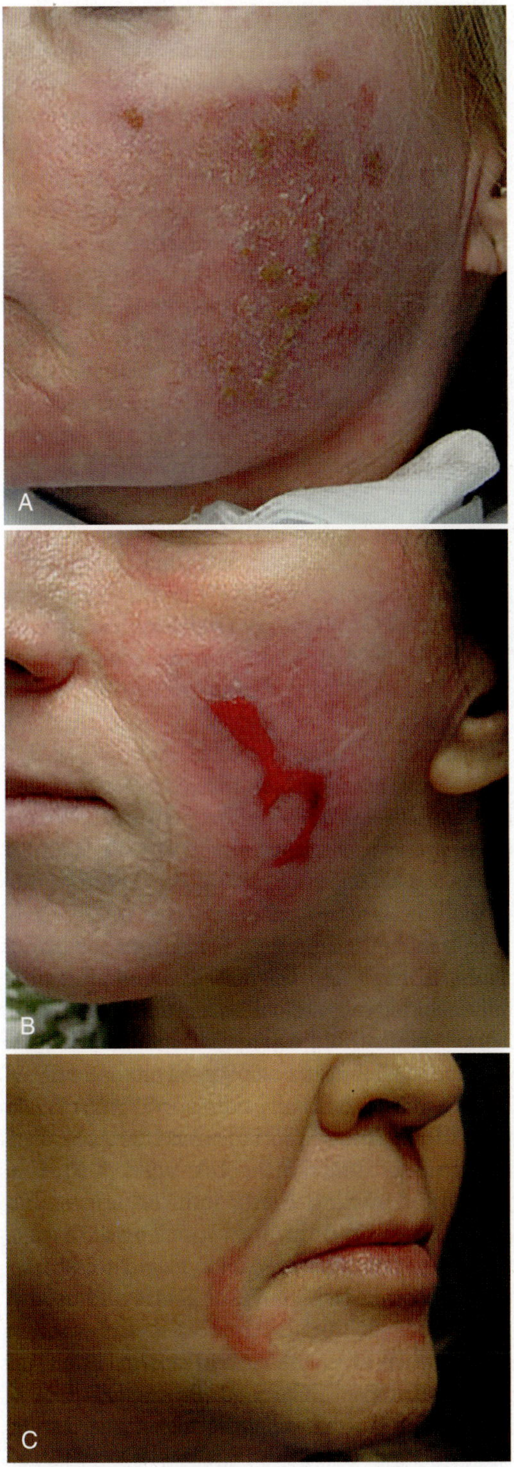

Fig. 2.12 Complications: (A) impetigo, (B) delayed wound healing, (C) hypertrophic scar formation.

usually complain of itching or burning of their skin along with increased redness. Patients may have been healing well only to show a setback in wound healing. The most likely culprits are propylene glycol or lanolins. One must rule out an early, disseminated viral infection or *Candida*. If an allergic contact dermatitis is still the most likely diagnosis, the patient should stop all offending agents, cleanse the skin with water, and apply only white petrolatum to the skin. A topical mid-potency steroid ointment can be used, as long as it does not contain propylene glycol. These patients need to be followed up every couple of days to monitor the wound healing process.

Hypopigmentation can be very disconcerting to the patient. Any procedure that reaches the reticular dermis can result in permanent hypopigmentation. While the color discrepancy may not be as apparent in lighter skinned individuals, darker skinned patients are more likely to notice any color discrepancy. Therefore patients with darker skin should be warned of this possibility. This must be differentiated from the pseudo-hypopigmentation that is seen in patients with heavily photodamaged skin. Pseudo-hypopigmentation is when the resurfaced skin looks lighter than the adjacent, un-resurfaced skin, but this is because the sun damage has been removed, and not because the skin is actually lighter.

PIH can occur in all but the fairest of patients. PIH can overshadow the results of resurfacing; thus, it is better to anticipate this and treat it before it manifests. PIH can be minimized or avoided by having patients resume their skin reconditioning regimens once the wound has healed fully. This is most often by postoperative day 8 or 10. However, if PIH occurs and is resistant to the topical agents alone, salicylic acid peels biweekly can help speed up resolution.

Patients with acne or rosacea can experience a flare-up during the postoperative period. Systemic antiinflammatory antibiotics can help resolve this before scarring occurs. Systemic antiinflammatory antibiotics (tetracycline, doxycycline) should be used in combination with appropriate topical therapies to quickly quiet down these conditions.

Erythema lasting more than 2 weeks postoperatively is less common with peels than with laser resurfacing. It is seen commonly for several months following aggressive laser resurfacing, dermabrasion, and modified phenol peels. Close observation of areas of persistent erythema is important as it can portend an impending scar. Usually, this occurs at areas where the wound has penetrated the reticular dermis (deeper resurfacing) or

TABLE 2.7 Complications of Chemical Peels

Complication	Comments
Infection	Bacterial[a] Gram positive (*Staphylococcus aureus*) Gram negative (if skin was occluded) Viral[b] Herpes simplex virus Varicella zoster virus *Candida*[c]
Contact dermatitis	Eliminate all possible offending topicals Switch to water to cleanse and bland emollients Consider a mid-potency topical steroid ointment[d]
Scarring	Areas of delayed healing Areas of "angry" redness Consider intralesional steroids Consider a mid-potency topical steroid ointment Consider pulsed dye laser series
Dyschromia	Postinflammatory hyperpigmentation Resolves with topical agents and light peels Postinflammatory hypopigmentation Can be permanent. May be improved with fractionated laser or microneedling.

[a]Culture and sensitivities necessary to rule out MRSA (methicillin-resistant *S. aureus*).
[b]Direct fluorescent antibody test gives a quick diagnosis.
[c]KOH prop of a skin scraping can help identify the presence of this yeast.
[d]Very cautious use of topical steroids during the reepithelialization stage.

at sites of infection and trauma. These areas can be treated 2 days out of each week for several weeks with a mid- to ultrapotent topical steroid (triamcinolone acetonide or clobetasol). Too much steroid use can have adverse effects; therefore, close patient monitoring is needed. The use of pulsed dye laser (nonpurpuric settings) early on can resolve the erythema and halt the progression of scarring, often without the need for a topical steroid. The laser treatments can be spaced 2 to 4 weeks apart until the erythema resolves.

The most dreaded complication of skin resurfacing is scarring and textural change. Scars can take a variety of morphologies such as atrophic, hypertrophic, or keloid-like. As was previously mentioned, areas of delayed healing or infection can then progress to scar formation. The importance of early detection and intervention cannot be emphasized enough. If the skin has already begun to thicken or become fibrotic, it should be treated with an ultrapotent topical steroid twice a day for 3 to 4 weeks. Care should be taken not to apply the steroid to normal skin as it may result in atrophy, telangiectasias, and skin fragility. Early intervention with a pulsed dye laser should be the next step. This laser can greatly improve skin texture, erythema, and can sometimes halt the progression of scarring.

Intralesional steroid injections and manual massage should begin if the topical steroids fail to improve the scar. The thicker areas of the scar are injected at 2- to 4-week intervals with triamcinolone acetonide 1 to 10 mg/mL. The concentration used is based on scar thickness. A combination of triamcinolone acetonide and 5-fluorouracil can be used as well, with the advantage of allowing for less steroid to be injected. The 5-fluorouracil is an antimetabolic agent that helps to slow down scar fibrosis (Table 2.7).

REFERENCES

1. American Society of Plastic Surgeons. *2014 Plastic Surgery Statistics Report*. Available at: https://d2wirczt3b6wjm.cloudfront.net/ News/Statistics/2014/plastic-surgery-statistics-full-report- 2014.pdf.

2. Khatri KA. Diode laser hair removal in patients undergoing isotretinoin therapy. *Dermatol Surg.* 2004;30:1205-1207.
3. Chandrashekar BS, Varsha DV, Vasanth V, et al. Safety of performing invasive acne scar treatment and laser hair removal in patients on oral isotretinoin: a retrospective study of 110 patients. *Int J Dermatol.* 2014;53:1281-1285.
4. Picosse FR, Yarak S, Cabral NC, et al. Early chemabrasion for acne scars after treatment with oral isotretinoin. *Dermatol Surg.* 2012;38:1521-1526.
5. Kim HW, Chang SE, Kim JE, et al. The safe delivery of fractional ablative carbon dioxide laser treatment for acne scars in Asian patients receiving oral isotretinoin. *Dermatol Surg.* 2014;40:1361-1366.
6. Obagi S, Obagi Z, Bridenstine JB. Isotretinoin use during chemical skin resurfacing: a review of complications. *Am J Cosmet Surg.* 2002;19:9-13.

   A retrospective study of chemical peel patients looking at the incidence of hypertrophic scarring in patients that recently took isotretinoin, were on isotretinoin, or took isotretinoin during the perioperative period. The study found that past, current, and postoperative use of isotretinoin did not result in hypertrophic scarring if the depth of the peel was kept to the papillary dermis.
7. Dingman DL, Hartog J, Sieminonow M. Simultaneous deep-plane face-lift and trichloroacetic acid peel. *Plast Reconstr Surg.* 1994;93:86-95.
8. Taghizadeh F, Leibowitz A, Ellison T, et al. Short flap rhytidectomy and fractional CO_2 laser rejuvenation of the aging face. *J Cosmet Dermatol.* 2013;12:49-56.
9. Jackson IT, Yavuzer R, Beal B. Simultaneous face lift and carbon dioxide laser resurfacing: a proven technique. *Plast Reconstr Surg.* 2001;108:802-803.
10. Trelles MA, Brychta P, Stanek J, et al. Laser techniques associated with facial aesthetic and reparative surgery. *Facial Plast Surg.* 2005;21:83-98.
11. Koch BB, Perkins SW. Simultaneous rhytidectomy and full-face carbon dioxide resurfacing: a case series and meta-analysis. *Arch Facial Plast Surg.* 2002;4:227-233.
12. Spencer L, Obagi S. Cosmetic dermatologic skin care: the essence of our training. *J Cosmet Dermatol.* 2007;20:663-669.
13. Weinstein GD, Nigra TP, Pochi PE, et al. Topical tretinoin for treatment of photodamaged skin. A multicenter study. *Arch Dermatol.* 1991;127:659-665.
14. Didierjean L, Tran C, Sorg O, et al. Biological activities of topical retinaldehyde. *Dermatology.* 1999;199(suppl 1):19-24.
15. Hevia O, Nemeth AJ, Taylor JR. Tretinoin accelerates healing after trichloroacetic acid chemical peel. *Arch Dermatol.* 1991;127:678-682.
16. Moy LS, Howe K, Moy RL. Glycolic acid modulation of collagen production in human skin fibroblast cultures in vitro. *Dermatol Surg.* 1996;22:439-441.
17. Bridenstine JB, Dolezal JF. Standardizing chemical peel solution formulations to avoid mishaps: great fluctuations in actual concentrations of trichloroacetic acid. *J Dermatol Surg Oncol.* 1994;20:813-816.
18. Monheit GD. The Jessner's–trichloroacetic acid peel. An enhanced medium-depth chemical peel. *Dermatol Clin.* 1995;13:277-283.

    Details the indications for Jessner's-trichloroacetic acid peel and how to perform the peel. Describes the rationale behind using Jessner's solution before TCA application.
19. Coleman WP, Futrell JM. The glycolic acid and trichloroacetic acid peel. *J Dermatol Surg Oncol.* 1994;20:76-80.
20. Obagi Z, Obagi S, Alaiti S, Stevens M. TCA-based blue peel: a standardized procedure with depth control. *Dermatol Surg.* 1999;25:773-780.

    Details the mechanism of action of TCA peels while describing the rationale behind the TCA-based Blue Peel. In addition, explains in detail how to perform the TCA-based Blue Peel.
21. Brody HJ. Deep peeling. In: Brody HJ, ed. *Chemical Peeling and Resurfacing.* 2nd ed. St. Louis, MO: Mosby; 1997:137-160.
22. Truppman ES, Ellenby JD. Major electrocardiographic changes during chemical face peeling. *Plast Reconstr Surg.* 1979;63:44-48.
23. Hetter GP. An examination of the phenol–croton oil peel: part I. Dissecting the formula. *Plast Reconstr Surg.* 2000;105:227-239, discussion 249-251.

    Describes the factors affecting the depth of penetration of phenol acid peels. The author breaks down the various components of the phenol peel solutions and identifies the role each of them plays. He further details the important role of croton oil in driving the phenol peels deeper.
24. Stone PA. The use of modified phenol for chemical face peeling. *Clin Plast Surg.* 1998;25:21-44.
25. Moy LS, Peace S, Moy RL. Comparison of the effect of various chemical peeling agents in a mini-pig model. *Dermatol Surg.* 1996;22:429-432.
26. Johnson JB, Ichinose H, Obagi ZE, et al. Obagi's modified trichloroacetic acid (TCA)–controlled variable-depth peel: a study of clinical signs correlating with histological finding. *Ann Plast Surg.* 1996;36:225-237.
27. Zhang AY, Obagi S. Diagnosis and management of skin resurfacing-related complications. *Oral Maxillofac Surg Clin North Am.* 2009;21:1-12.

    An overview of the common and rare complications associated with skin resurfacing. Evaluation, diagnosis, and management are discussed in detail. Photographs are shown to illustrate these complications.

3

Chemodenervation

Farzad R. Nahai, Deniz Sarhaddi, and Caitlin Francoisse

INTRODUCTION

Botulinum toxin type A injections represent the single most frequently performed minimally invasive aesthetic procedure in the United States, totaling an estimated 7.7 million procedures in 2019 alone, according to the American Society of Plastic Surgery. Neuromodulators represent a cornerstone of minimally invasive surgery with 150% more procedures performed annually than the next three leading procedures (soft tissue fillers, chemical peels, and laser hair removal) combined. Their popularity only continues to surge with an over 850% increase in volume in the past two decades.[1] Moreover, noninvasive procedures serve as an important gateway to attract patients to more invasive options; one study estimated 15% of patients who sought noninvasive treatment underwent an invasive surgery an average of 19 months later.[2] Given their critical role, mastery of neuromodulator technique has become an essential skill for any plastic surgeon.

BACKGROUND

Botulinum toxin derives from the bacterium *Clostridium botulinum*, which produces seven serotypes (A, B, C1, C2, D, E, F, and G).[3,4] Although both botulinum toxin A and B are commercially available for use, botulinum A (BTA) represents the workhorse of injectable neuromodulators and the only one currently approved for cosmetic use.[5] Initially reported in the 1970s as a novel method to weaken extraocular muscles for treatment of strabismus, BTA gained traction throughout the 1980s for facial spasmodic disorders including blepharospasm and hemifacial spasm.[6-12] In 1989 the U.S. Food and Drug Administration (FDA) officially approved the use of onabotulinum toxin A, commercially known as *Botox*, for the treatment of facial spasmodic disorders.[13]

Botox's relative obscurity as a niche ophthalmologic drug was short-lived, however. In the late 1980s, Dr. Carruthers, an ophthalmologist by training, noted the incidental improvement of dynamic glabellar rhytids in patients receiving Botox for management of blepharospasm. Recognizing a potential application in aesthetic surgery, she partnered with her husband, a dermatologist, and the pair published the first landmark study showing its use for improvement in dynamic glabellar frown lines in 1992.[14] A decade later, the FDA officially approved cosmetic use of Botox in the treatment of glabellar rhytids; this was followed by approval for the treatment of crow's feet in 2013 and forehead lines in 2017.[5,15]

BTA ameliorates dynamic wrinkles by inducing flaccid paralysis. The protein disrupts the synaptosomal-associated protein 25, located on the presynaptic cell membrane. This inhibits synaptic vesicles containing acetylcholine from fusing with the presynaptic membrane, blocking release of the neurotransmitter into the synaptic cleft.[5,16,17] Although motor endplate activity ceases within hours of injection, maximal clinical effects take up to 2 weeks to manifest because of spontaneous, nonvesicle associated release of acetylcholine. The toxin's results are irreversible; attenuation of effects is attributed to sprouting of new axons and the formation of new neuromuscular junctions.[5,16]

FORMULATIONS

Four formulations of BTA are approved for aesthetic use by the FDA: abobotulinum toxin A (Dysport), incobotulinum toxin A (Xeomin), onabotulinum toxin A (Botox), and most recently prabotulinum toxin A (Jeuveau).[18] Although each drug shares the common active ingredient responsible for muscle paralysis, the three differ in purification and processing, yielding slight variation in the products.[19]

Each drug has its own unique dosing regimen, with no universally accepted exchange ratio.[20-22] Although the conversion ratio of Xeomin-to-Botox is generally considered as 1:1, the ratio of Dysport-to-Botox remains under debate.[17,23] The reported Dysport-to-Botox ratios range from 1.3:1 to 11:1, although the majority of studies settle on a ratio somewhere between 2:1 or 3:1.[4,21,22,24-27]

The lack of consensus for conversion standards undermines clinical efforts to scientifically compare the different products.[18,28] Some studies, including a randomized control study by Lowe et al., report Botox affords a superior result to Dysport in terms of glabellar line severity with a conversion rate of 2.5 units Dysport:1 unit Botox. However, these studies are criticized for being underpowered or inadequately randomized in terms of patient age.[29,30] Other studies by the same author contend Dysport is, in fact, better; Lowe et al. reported that Dysport is significantly more effective than Botox for upper face lines, but this time with a 4:1 ratio.[31] A different study by Karasi et al. argues that Dysport used in a 3:1 ratio of Botox has a longer duration of action when measured by serial electromyography.[32] This lack of conversion consensus makes it difficult to compare products directly. As a result, there is no overwhelming evidence arguing the superiority of one product to another.[19]

Besides relative efficacy, the diffusion profiles of each drug are also contested. Diffusion differs from spread; spread refers to the more technique-dependent movement of the product from the original site of injection. Differences in spread could be attributed to the volume, speed, or angle of injection.[33] Diffusion refers to the movement of the toxin beyond the original site as a result of kinetic dispersion, dictated by the toxin subtype's unique properties as well as the property of the surrounding tissues. For example, diffusion can differ with the receptor density of a particular area, since areas with a high density of receptors will bind more of the toxin, limiting overall diffusion.[33] This was demonstrated by Hexsel et al. when examining hyperhidrosis. Three women received 5-unit injections at three points on their back at three depths (2, 3, and 4 mm), and the field effect of each injection (the area where the toxin prevented sweating) was measured. Interestingly, location mattered more than depth, with injections at the midline having a smaller field effect no matter the depth. This highlights how the same dose in a different anatomic area can elicit a different response because of receptor density.[34]

Diffusion is not a desirable quality with BTA. Relatively less diffusion allows for precise, intentional product placement and decreases the risk of the toxin spreading systemically and causing adverse side effects.[16] Differences in diffusion are sometimes attributed to the different molecular weights of each of the toxins, which are attributed to the different protein load of each toxin. When BTA is produced naturally by bacteria, it is complexed to a series of proteins that help to protect the toxin from destruction inside the gastrointestinal tract.[35] For equivalent clinical doses, the protein content of Dysport is 40% lower than Botox (5 ng protein per 100 units Botox vs. 4.35 ng per 200 units Dysport). Xeomin is reported to be completely free of complexing proteins with an estimated weight of 0.44 ng per 100 unit vial.[36]

Early studies initially postulated that larger protein complexes could limit the diffusion of BTA. One such study was a randomized control study of 12 patients by Cliff et al. where 4 units Botox were injected into the one side of a forehead, 12 units of Dysport on the contralateral side, and saline in the center. The resulting anhidrotic halo was measured to yield the field effect (and thus the extent of diffusion).[37] Dysport was found to have a larger field effect by a mean of 77%. Another, similar study by Trindade et al. used this same anhidrosis model to measure the extent of diffusion. Twenty patients received one medial and one lateral injection of Botox to one side of face and Dysport to the other, with laterality randomized. Patients were also randomized in respect to conversion ratios, receiving either 2.5:1, 3:1, or 4:1. Anhidrosis was subsequently measured over time for up to 6 months, indicating that the anhidrosis halo was larger for Dysport in 93% of comparisons.[38] As expected, the larger conversion ratio (4:1) had a larger field effect than 2.5:1, inferring the positive association between increasing dosage and increasing rate of diffusion.

The evidence for these assertions is far from definitive, however. Previously mentioned studies are relatively small, and their results are not contingent upon diffusion alone; the differential field effects may also be a result of injection technique and dosing used.

In vivo studies suggest that differences in molecular weights are not responsible for differences in diffusion. In one such study, the dissociation of Botox was analyzed using ion-exchange chromatography under various physiologic pHs. At more acidic pHs (such as those that would be encountered in the gut), Botox remained bound to its complexing proteins. However, at higher pHs, such as those encountered when injected to muscle, it dissociated from complexing proteins in less than a minute.[39] This may suggest that complexing proteins have little impact when using the toxin for aesthetic, injectable purposes.

There are multiple clinical studies, which also assert there is no difference in diffusion.[18] Carli et al. compared the diffusion rates of Botox, Dysport, and Xeomin by measuring neural cell adhesion molecule (N-CAM) in a mouse model. N-CAM is nearly absent from adult muscle in the mice model but reappears when muscle is denervated; subsequently, they used N-CAM expression to determine the extent of diffusion. When they injected 0.25 units of Botox, 1 unit Dysport, or 0.25 units of Xeomin into the tibialis anterior of mice, they found no significant difference between the products in respect to diffusion.[40] In humans, similar results could be seen. In a clinical study of 59 female patients, a forehead anhidrosis model was used to determine extent of diffusion, similarly to previous studies. Patients were randomized as to which side of the forehead received which toxin as well as the conversion ratio either 2:1 or 2.5:1 Dysport to Botox. Similar effects were seen at the lower dose equivalence (2:1) with a larger area seen at the higher dosage (2.5:1).

This underscores how crucial the chosen dosing equivalents are when designing these studies.[38] Given the small samples, variation with technique, and lack of consensus dosage equivalents, there is not conclusive evidence to state that there is a difference in diffusion rates of the different toxins. All these studies support a few key facts: diffusion varies by anatomic location and diffusion is dose dependent.[18]

Although the relative protein load may not necessarily impact the rate of diffusion, it does have potential implications for antigenicity. If the immune system develops neutralizing antibodies (NAbs) against the toxin, then the toxin can be neutralized, which ultimately results in treatment failure.[36] This was especially a problem with the original formulation of Botox used before 1998, which contained five times the amount of associated complexing proteins (25 ng per 100 units, vs. 5 ng). In a study by Jankovic et al. analyzing Botox use for cervical dystonia, the old formulation was six times more likely to elicit antibody formation.[41]

Risk factors for development of NAbs include large doses per injection, large cumulative doses, shorter intervals between injections, and use of "booster" injections 1 to 2 weeks after treatment.[42,43] In particular, it appears more common with use of botulinum toxin B (commercially available as Myobloc), which is used for cervical dystonia but not FDA approved for aesthetic purposes. Up to 44% of patients receiving Myobloc for cervical dystonia develop antibodies.[44]

Thankfully, the development of NAbs with BTA appears far rarer and infrequently leads to a loss of treatment efficacy. Naumann et al. analyzed the relative incidence of NAbs formation in a meta-analysis of 2240 patients in 16 clinical studies receiving Botox for five different indications. Subjects received an average of 3.8 treatments (range 1–15) with total doses varying from 10–20 units in glabellar lines to 20–500 in cervical dystonia. Development of NAbs were 1.28% in cervical dystonia (4/312), 0.46% in primary axillary hyperhidrosis (4/871), 0.32% in poststroke spasticity (1/317), 0.28% in glabellar lines (2/718), and 0% in overactive bladder (0/22). Of the 11 patients that developed NAbs, only three became clinically unresponsive to BTA.[45]

Reported rates of NAb formation with Dysport and Xeomin also appear to be low. The rates with Dysport range from 0% in glabellar lines to 1.2% in cervical dystonia.[46] Reported rates of Xeomin are less clear. In theory, Xeomin should be less antigenic since it has been formulated to exclude complexing proteins. Several studies support this premise. In a comparison of New Zealand white rabbits with Xeomin, Dysport, and Botox, Xeomin was the only toxin, which did not induce NAb formation.[47] In humans, similar results were seen. Patients with upper limb spasticity were injected with Xeomin followed by either five repeat Xeomin injections or five placebo injections. At 89 weeks after Xeomin injections, no patient developed NAbs.[48] However, during the clinical development program of Xeomin in the United States, 12 out of 1080 patients developed NAbs (1.1%).[49] This rate may not reflect the true antigenicity, though. The 12 patients who developed NAbs were previously treated with a different BTA formulation and subsequently, their immune systems may have already been primed against the toxin. Although rigorous clinical studies comparing NAb formation rates between the formulations are lacking, existing studies suggest that NAb formation is generally a rare event, especially for patients receiving aesthetic dosing of BTA.[18]

STORAGE AND RECONSTITUTION

BTA is commercially available as a desiccated powder, which must be reconstituted before administration. Manufacturer guidelines recommend reconstitution with preservative-free saline rather than preserved saline, which contains benzyl alcohol, a bacteriostatic agent.[50,51] Although a seemingly innocuous difference, it has important applications for the shelf life. To minimize the risk of bacterial contamination, use of preservative-free saline necessitates the use of the entire quantity in a single day, rather than any excess for future use, which has economic implications for the manufacturer versus the provider.[52]

However, there are several studies suggesting that same-day reconstitution is not the only method of effective administration. Several studies suggest BTA remains stable and equally efficacious with preservative-containing normal saline up to 5 weeks later.[53-56] Other studies suggest that the contamination risk to patients is actually minimal. In one such study, 127 consecutive reconstituted vials were used to treat one to three patients for an average of four to five procedures, each within the course of the week. Each vial was refrigerated then reaccessed by different personnel using individual, single-use sterile syringes to draw aliquots for each patient. At the end of the study, each vial was cultured, and no microbial growth was detected in any of the 127 vials.[57] Moreover, some studies assert preservative-containing normal saline is less painful to patients. In a prospective randomized control trial of 15 patients, Alam et al. found that 100% of patients reported less pain on their hemiface that was injected with preservative-containing reconstituted BTA versus the side with preservative-free BTA; the reported pain was on average 54% less.[52] These results have been corroborated by other randomized, controlled trials in subsequent years.[58-61]

Recognizing this data, the American Society for Dermatologic Surgery set forth guidelines in 2015 to specifically address the discrepancy between clinical data and suggested manufacturer's guidelines.[62] Consensus recommendations had two key findings for facial aesthetic use of BTA: (1) the same vial may be refrigerated or refrozen at least 4 weeks before efficacy is compromised and (2) a single vial can be used to treat multiple patients, assuming appropriate technique is used.[62]

The manner of reconstitution may also impact the efficacy of BTA. Swirling without inversion can potentially lead to loss of potential product.[63] Overly vigorous mixing can yield this result as well. In a study by Dressler et al., the impact of mechanical stress on BTA reconstitution was investigated. Ten vials of 100 units Botox were reconstituted with 2 mL normal saline using either a gentle or an aggressive reconstitution method. Potency was then analyzed using the time to diaphragm paralysis in a mouse model; the result was a 42% loss in potency, suggesting that mechanical stress may partially inactivate reconstituted BTA.[64]

The volume used for reconstitution is yet another area under debate. In management of spastic conditions, large volume dilution appears advantageous. Animal models suggest that higher volume of a low concentration may better relax skeletal muscles, likely since the greater volumes allow for more distribution of the product within the target muscle.[65,66] In a randomized, control trial of children with spastic hemiparesis resulting in elbow flexion contractures, children's biceps were injected with either a more dilute (5 mL per 100 units) or more concentrated solution of BTA (1 mL per 100 units). Children who received the higher volume, dilute BTA injection demonstrated a greater improvement in spasticity and range of motion.[67]

In aesthetic applications, most clinical studies do not show a relationship between dilution and efficacy, even with up to a fivefold dilution.[68-70] Other studies similarly show no difference in terms of efficacy, but instead suggest that dilution may be impacting other clinical factors, including patient pain and the degree of product spread. In one study, Hankins et al. injected the glabellar wrinkles of 46 patients with Botox at different concentrations ranging from 10 to 100 U/mL and followed the patients on a monthly basis. They found no difference in efficacy but noted larger volumes were associated with greater patient discomfort.[71] In a prospective, randomized control trial, Hsu et al. injected the crow's feet of 10 volunteers with 5 units of Botox, diluted to 100 U/mL on one side and diluted fivefold to 20 U/mL on the contralateral side. They found the area affected by BTA to be 50% greater in 9 of the 10 test subjects in the more dilute group.[72] In another randomized control study by Carruthers et al., 89 women were randomized to receive glabellar Botox, diluted to either 100, 22.2, 20, or 10 U/mL.

They found no statistically significant difference between dilution and response, although the six cases of eyebrow ptosis were all reported in the more dilute concentrations.[73] Lastly, Abbasi et al. injected two concentrations of Dysport (6 units in 0.1 mL or 6 units in 0.3 mL) into the first prominent horizontal crease 2.5 to 3 cm above the orbital rim. They found that the more dilute BTA had a significantly greater area of effect compared to the more concentrated BTA (794.1 mm^2 vs. 476.6 mm^2), although the study was limited because of the marked interpatient variation.[74]

There is no consensus opinion about the proper dilution of BTA for aesthetic purposes. Even an expert panel published in 2016 by the Global Aesthetics Consensus Group offered no clear guidelines. Instead, they acknowledged the difference in opinions, mentioning some panelists use more dilute concentrations when trying to achieve greater product spread while others feel it is associated with greater pain.[75]

ADMINISTRATION AND OPTIMIZING THE PATIENT EXPERIENCE

Minimizing patient discomfort is an essential to patient satisfaction. To minimize pain, multiple authors have tried to optimize administration techniques. Some authors have advocated for use of topical anesthetic cream (EMLA) to reduce patient discomfort.[76,77] Others have advocated for use of ice or ethyl chloride to cool the area, stating that this pretreatment can improve pain scores.[78-80] In one prospective study of 40 patients receiving periocular BTA for blepharospasm or wrinkle reduction, the impact of ice versus EMLA was directly compared. Patients had half their faces pretreated with EMLA, ice, or both on separate sides. Reported pain scores on a scale of 1 to 10 were significantly lower with EMLA (3.25) or with ice (3.0) than the control (5.85). In patients who received both EMLA and skin cooling, 56.2% (9/16) preferred the experience of EMLA.[81] Not every study has shown this positive effect, however. In a randomized control trial of 22 patients by Chorney et al., unilateral vibration, unilateral ice, and ice and vibration on either side were compared, finding no statistically significant difference in reported pain scores.[82] Furthermore, ice may impact the efficacy and spread of the toxin itself, especially since protein efficacy and diffusion is impacted by temperature.[80] Pirazzi et al. looked at the time of botulinum toxin to translocate across the plasma membrane in neurons in a rat model. At physiologic temperatures, this occurred in minutes; at 20 °C, the toxin could not translocate and enter neurons.[83] This suggests that further studies are needed to determine what, if any, impact cooling before or after treatment may have on the clinical outcome of the toxin.[18]

There is no recommended syringe type or needle to use with administration. In general, higher gauge needles should be used whenever possible to minimize discomfort.[84] There is no consensus on syringe type, but a study by Foglietti et al. attempted to quantify how much BTA product was being wasted when using different types of syringes. The group compared 1-mL tuberculin Luer slip (TB) syringes with detachable 25-gauge needles to 1-mL ultrafine insulin syringes with 31-gauge needles. TB syringes had 0.05 mL product or the equivalent of 2 units leftover, which the authors estimate could cost a busy injectable clinic up to $155,500 in lost product over the course of a year.[85]

Product may be injected either subcutaneously or intramuscularly. In one split-face comparison by Godin et al., 19 patients underwent BTA for forehead rhytids and were randomized to either intramuscular or subcutaneous injection. Both groups demonstrated similar efficacy as determined by eyebrow position and satisfaction surveys, but with less pain reported by the subcutaneous group.[86] In addition, intradermal injections may lower sebum production, which can result in patient-reported improvement of skin oiliness and pores.[87,88] Some evidence also suggests it may increase collagen production, promoting improved skin quality.[89] In a recent split-face randomized pilot study of 10 women by Sapra et al., no significant reduction was seen in terms of pore size or sebum production, but women with intradermal injections had significant improvement in skin texture and a relative midface lift at the end of 16 weeks.[90] Although larger studies are needed, these preliminary results suggest that intradermal aesthetic injection may provide added benefits beyond selective paralysis.

Postinjection care is another widespread component believed to optimize the patient's results. However, there is minimal evidence to support many protocols. Some advocate patients should keep their head elevated to minimize unwanted spread of the product, despite the lack of evidence that position changes can lead to lid ptosis.[91] Others claim increased muscle use postinjection may facilitate toxin spread. This is supported by a randomized control trial by Wei et al., where 98 patients were injected with BTA into their masseters and the subsequent duration of muscle atrophy was measured; they found that in patients asked to strengthen their chewing effort, postinjection had a prolonged period of atrophy, suggesting more effective spread and deactivation of the muscle.[92] There is limited information about the potential impact of postinjection massage but many caution against it, fearing it could facilitate undesired spread into adjacent facial mimetic muscles.[18]

INDICATIONS AND PATIENT EVALUATION

BTA treatment selectively weakens facial mimetic muscles, reducing rhytids that occur as a result of animation (see Figure 1). Some rhytids are static and will only respond to skin resurfacing procedures. For most facial rhytids, however, animation makes them worse to some degree; this degree determines the relative efficacy of BTA treatment.[16] Subsequently, comparison of the patient's static and dynamic rhytids is key to determining which areas would benefit from treatment. An understanding of facial anatomy is paramount for maximizing outcomes while minimizing risk of complications (see Figures 2–4).

Currently, all four formulations of BTA are approved by the FDA only for treatment of glabellar region in patients under 65 years; Botox is also approved for treatment of lateral periorbital lines and forehead lines.[93-95] Despite these relatively narrow indications, BTA is routinely used off-label with good success in a variety of diverse applications in patients of all ages.[4]

BTA is a class C medication for pregnant and breastfeeding patients.[93-95] It should be avoided in patients with neuromuscular diseases (such as myasthenia gravis or Eaton-Lambert syndrome).[4] In addition, BTA should be avoided in certain patients on medications, which could potentiate the toxin's effects (such as aminoglycosides or calcium channel blockers) or those with allergies to its components (including albumin or cow's milk protein).[4,93-95]

UPPER FACE

Glabellar Region

The glabellar region is made of several medial brow depressors including the corrugators supercilia, procerus, depressor supercili, and medial aspect of the orbicularis oculi.[96] The relative hyperactivity of these muscles to each other can result in the different configurations of vertical and horizontal rhytids. The procerus muscle is oriented vertically, originating from soft tissue over the nasal root inserting onto the central forehead. Hyperactivity leads to a bulge over the nasal root and an associated transverse rhytid.[4] Hyperactivity of the corrugators result in vertical glabellar rhytids. The corrugators often have an oblique head medially that depresses the medial

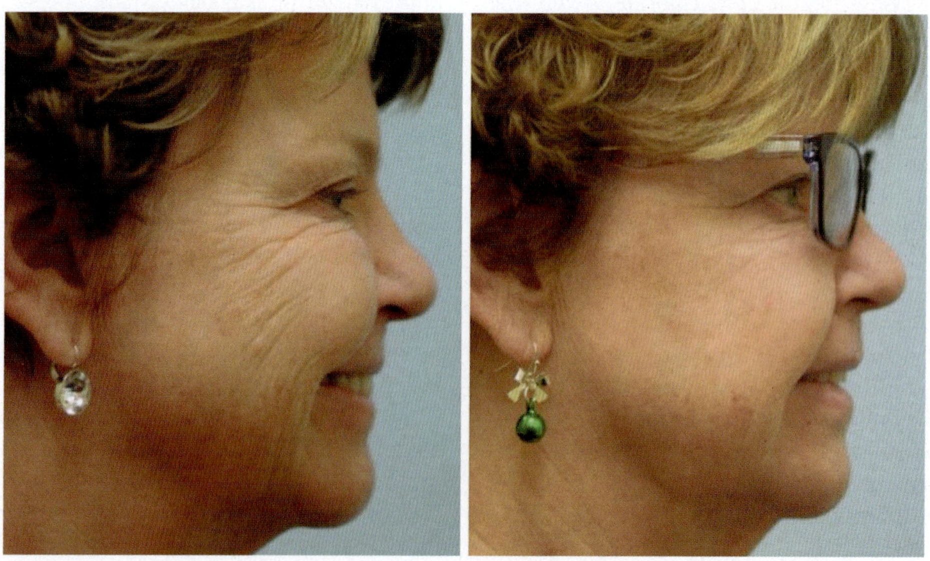

Fig. 3.1 Facial Rhytids showing the dynamic rhytids before and after (From Cosmetic Facial Surgery. Niamtu, Joe; Fagien, Steve; Lam, Sam. Published December 31, 2022. © 2023.)

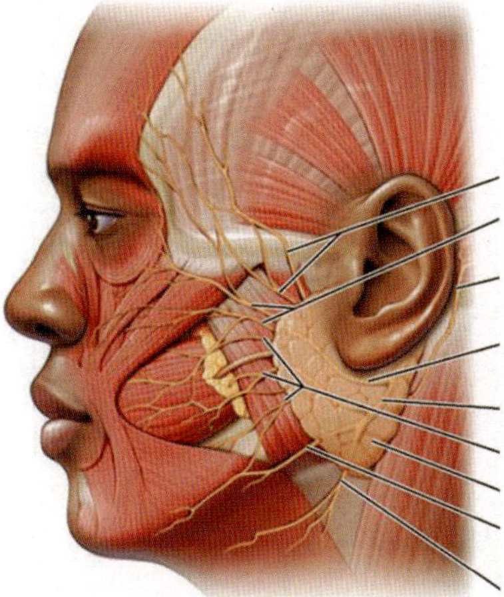

Fig. 3.2 Facial anatomy (From Cosmetic Facial Surgery. Niamtu, Joe; Nayak, Mike; Bharti, Gaurav; Willis, Zachary; Cuzalina, Angelo, Dr. Gentile, Richard, Dr. Published January 1, 2023. Pages 52-271. © 2023.)

brow and creates an oblique frown line as well. The corrugators are thickest medially, where they originate on average 2.9 mm lateral to the nasion. They arch cephalically anteriorly and slightly cephalad to the trochlea of the extraocular superior oblique, at a position usually 3.3 cm lateral to the nasion and 3.2 cm above the horizontal plane between the nasion and the lateral canthus.[97] The muscle then tapers laterally, with the lateral aspect of their tail usually 7.6 mm medial to the lateral orbital rim, roughly at the midpupillary line.[16,97] The fibers medially lie deep to the frontalis before interdigitating and passing "through" the frontalis and orbicularis oculi muscles before inserting into the brow skin.[98]

The glabella is most commonly injected in a 5-point "V" pattern, targeting the procerus and the corrugators' heads and tails bilaterally.[96] Typically 20 to 25 units (Botox equivalents) total are injected, with modifications made based on the relative hyperactivity of each muscle.[96] To treat the procerus, the injector pinches the

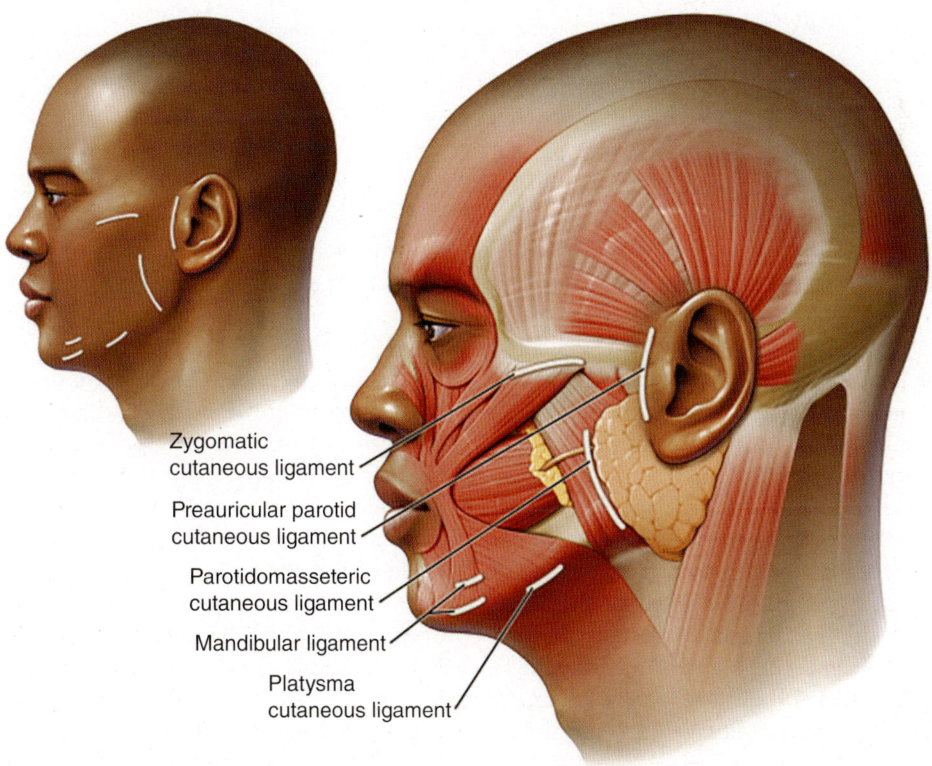

Fig. 3.3 Retaining ligaments of the face relevant to facelift surgery. [From Niamtu, J. Cosmetic Facial Surgery, 2nd ed. (2018). Philadelphia, PA: Elsevier. Fig. 3.15. Page 42)]

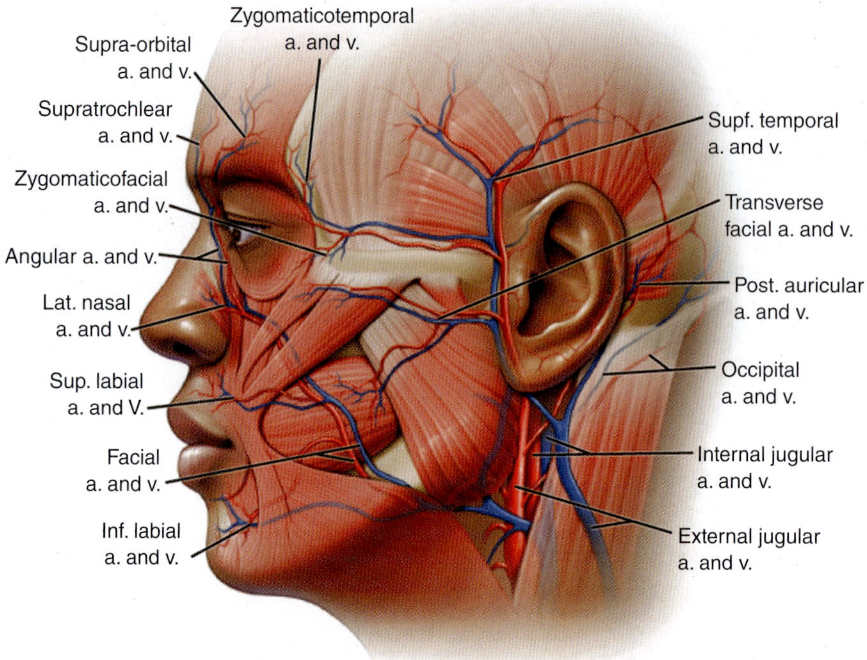

Fig. 3.4 Facial anatomy (From Cosmetic Facial Surgery. Niamtu, Joe; Nayak, Mike; Bharti, Gaurav; Willis, Zachary; Cuzalina, Angelo, Dr. Gentile, Richard, Dr. Published January 1, 2023. Pages 52-271. © 2023.)

muscle together and angles the needle upwards into the bulk of the muscle belly. The head and the tail of the corrugators are typically injected separately, at different depths given the tail's more superficial termination in the dermis. The corrugator is pinched and the needle is advanced in a superolateral direction, deep medially, and just subdermal laterally.[99] Deep placement laterally could result in injection deep to the supraorbital rim or potential diffusion of the product. This could ultimately result in weakening of the levator palpebrae superioris and ultimately eyelid ptosis.[100]

For this same reason, injection of the corrugators should be done at least 1 cm above the supraorbital rim to minimize the risk of ptosis. Other important strategies to minimize the risk of ptosis include orienting the needle away from the supraorbital rim during injection and digital pressure over the supraorbital rim to limit diffusion.[101]

If ptosis occurs despite these best efforts, treatment with 0.5% apraclonidine at a dosage of 1 to 2 drops, three times a day, can offer symptomatic relief for these patients. Apraclonidine acts on the alpha-adrenergic receptors of Müller's muscle, slightly lifting the lid correcting the ptosis. Thorough ophthalmologic history must be taken before apraclonidine as this medication poses a risk of closed angle glaucoma in at-risk individuals. Fortunately, most cases of BTA-induced ptosis are short-lived, lasting on average 4 weeks or less.

Frontalis Region

The frontalis serves an antagonist to the glabellar muscles, raising eyebrow position and, in doing so, causing the formation of horizontal forehead rhytids. Since the frontalis is the only muscle capable of brow elevation, treatment of the frontalis has a significant effect on brow position and function; therefore, treatment of the forehead will both smooth the rhytids and shape the brow. The muscle is often injected as a coordinated treatment with glabella and lateral orbicularis.[102]

The frontalis lacks all bony attachments; instead, it is contiguous with the superficial musculoaponeurotic system and the galea. Four major anatomic variants exist, as classified by Abramo et al. in an anatomic dissection of 20 fresh cadavers. Type I, or full form, is characterized by a continuous frontalis muscle spanning the entirety of the forehead. This type was most common (45%) and resulted in horizontal, straight line rhytids. Type II (30% of cadavers), or V-shaped, had an inverted projection of galea centrally across a single muscle belly. Thirty percent of cadavers had this subtype with their cutaneous rhytids taking the form of gull wings spanning the forehead. Type III, or central form, is a variation on Type I with a single spanning muscle belly but no lateral extension. Ten percent cadavers exhibited this subtype; their cutaneous rhytids were horizontal like Type I but limited laterally. Type IV, or lateral form, also has a V-shaped inverted projection. Unlike Type II, the galea extended in such a manner that it split the frontalis into two distinct lateral muscle bellies. Fifteen percent of cadavers displayed this muscle subtype with cutaneous rhytids that resembled a column of short, horizontal rhytids on either side, located over the brow.[103]

Understanding patient-specific anatomy is key to maximizing impact and avoiding complications. Most patients have a broad frontalis that extends past the temporal ridge. Failure to inject laterally into the frontalis can retain brow elevation laterally, resulting in a quizzical look. This is sometimes called a "Spock" or "Mephisto" appearance.[104] In addition, understanding patient-specific anatomy helps maximize product use. If patients have a Type II or Type IV frontalis muscle with a large, central galeal attachment, then central injections are of little benefit.[105] Lastly, the eyelid position of the patient must be inspected before injection. Certain patients compensate for eyelid malposition with activation of frontalis, subconsciously raising their eyebrows to increase the vertical aperture of their eyes. In these patients, if the frontalis is selectively weakened, secondary eyelid ptosis can be revealed.[100]

The frontalis is typically injected with 15 to 25 units spread among four to six injection locations. Men who typically have a larger, more robust frontalis muscle require a higher dosage to achieve the same effect.[16] Multiple injection patterns to the forehead have been described, with the most common being either a horizontal line of injections versus a V shape.[16] In a randomized control trial of 45 patients by Jabbour et al., the impact of injection pattern on brow position was investigated. Three patterns of five injection points were compared: a horizontal line 1 cm below the hairline, a horizontal line midforehead, and a "V shaped" pattern with the central injection point just above the eyebrows with the lateral injection points at the lateral canthi, 1 cm inferior to the hair line. The V-shaped pattern was found most effective in the treatment of forehead lines but with greater risk of brow depression; conversely, the upper horizontal forehead pattern was found to be less effective than the other two in terms of rhytid reduction but posed the least risk of brow ptosis.[102]

MIDFACE

Crow's Feet and Chemical Brow Lift

Laterally, the orbicularis oculi acts as a depressor of the lateral brow and creates lateral canthal rhytids, or "crow's feet." Injection of this area not only eliminates lateral canthal lines but helps open this area and create a chemical browlift. Injection of superolateral orbicularis oculi with to 4 units (Botox equivalents) has been found to raise the brow up to 3 mm.[106]

For most people, 7.5 U is adequate but 6 to 12 units may be injected per side based on the patient's anatomy.[107] In a randomized control trial by Lowe et al., dosages of 3, 6, 12, and 18 units per side were compared. The degree and duration of the impact on orbicularis oculi was found to increase incrementally up to 12 units.[108] Typically, the dosage is divided equally among three injection points (see Figure 5). Since the muscle lies superficially, injections should be raised as a subdermal wheal. Injections should lie 1.5 cm lateral to the lateral canthus to minimize potential medial spread to

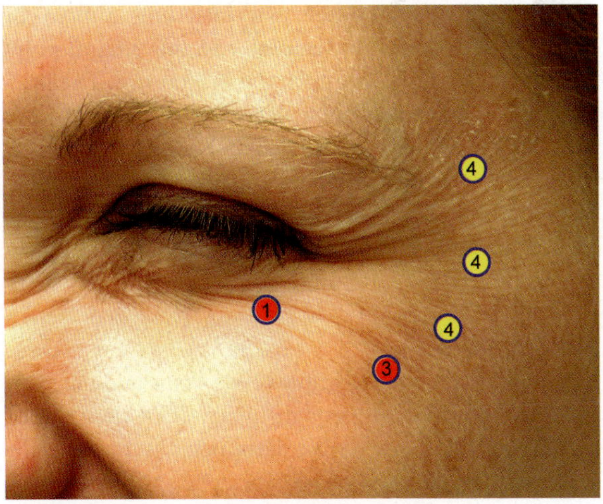

Fig. 3.5 Typical injection points for treating lateral canthal wrinkles (From Cosmetic Facial Surgery, Third Edition; Copyright © 2023 by Elsevier Inc. All rights reserved.)

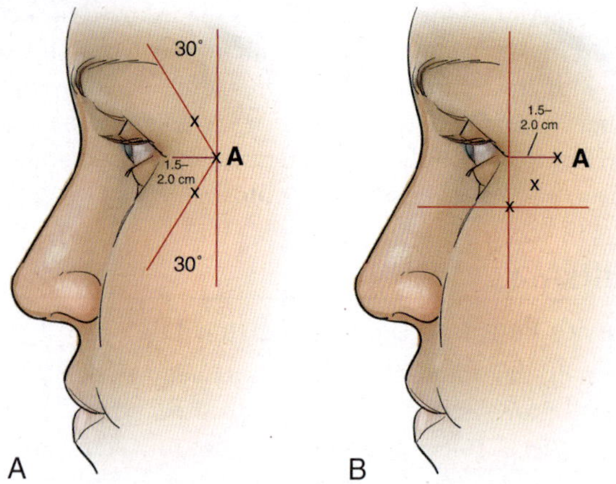

Fig. 3.6 Botox treatment for FDA-approved lateral canthal lines (crow's feet/CF) indication: 4 Units/0.1 mL of reconstituted Botox Cosmetic is injected into three sites per side (six total injection points) in the lateral orbicularis oculi muscle for a total of 24 Units/0.6 mL (12 Units per side). A, Standard CF injection pattern—the first injection (A) should be approximately 1.5 to 2.0 cm temporal to the lateral canthus and just temporal to the orbital rim, with the second and third injection (X) above and below the lateral canthus. B, Modified CF injection pattern—the first injection (A) should be approximately 1.5 to 2.0 cm temporal to the lateral canthus and just temporal to the orbital rim, with the second and third injection (X) below the lateral canthus. (Adapted from Botox package insert, Allergan, Inc.)

the extraocular muscles, which could yield diplopia (see Figure 6). The middle injection is placed in line with the lateral canthus; the other two injections should be spaced 1 cm inferior and superior to this central point and always at least 1 cm from the orbital rim. The inferior injection should not be placed below the zygomatic arch to minimize potential spread to the zygomatic major and potential weakening of the patient's smile.[107] If lateral brow lift is desired, this configuration may be shifted upwards slightly, so the superior injection is immediately under the brow.[105]

Eye Shaping

BTA may also be used to improve eye shape and the position of the lower lid through injection of the inferior orbicularis oculi. The orbicularis oculi is functionally separated into the pretarsal, preseptal, and preorbital muscle. The preseptal aspect of the muscle causes lower eyelid rhytids and can narrow the vertical palpebral aperture. The pretarsal orbicularis can create the "jelly roll" appearance under the lid margin during a smile. Before injection, any ptosis, lower lid laxity, or dry eye should be noted since BTA treatment could potentially worsen these. The toxin should be administered conservatively to the preseptal muscle to avoid weakening lower eyelid tone, which could result in impaired blink or epiphora. Preseptal injection with 2 to 4 U, 3 to 5 mm below the lash margin, just lateral to the midpupillary line can result in a more-open appearing eye with an increase in vertical aperture up to 0.5 mm at rest and 1.3 cm when smiling.[100,109] Pretarsal injection with 1 to 3 U can soften the "jelly roll" and flatten the bulge under the lid margin. Conservative injection in this area is of utmost importance to avoid lid malposition.

Transverse Nasal Rhytids

Animation of the periocular region can also result in activation of the nasalis muscle, resulting in nasal sidewall lines, also known as "*bunny lines.*" The nasalis is a paired muscle overlying the nasal sidewall. They can be injected with 2 to 5 U per side into the bulk of the muscle, placed high on the nose and superficially to prevent spread to the upper lip elevators, levator labii superioris, and levator labii alaeque.[110]

LOWER FACE

Gummy Smile

BTA can be used to improve "gummy smiles" or smiles with >2 mm gingival show above the dental line when smiling. Although some gummy smiles are skeletal or gingival in origin, hyperactivity of the levator labii superioris, levator labii superioris alaeque nasi, zygomaticus minor, and zygomaticus major muscle also contribute to the excessive gingival show.

Multiple injection patterns for this condition have been described. Hwang et al. studied 25 cadavers and described the "Yonsei Point," or a common point of the convergence points between the levator labii superioris, levator labii superioris, alaeque nasi, and the zygomaticus minor, located 1 cm lateral to the ala and 3 cm superior to the commissure. This group advocates for treatment with 3 U administered to this point on each side.[111] Alternatively, Sucupira et al. targeted only the levator labii superioris alaeque nasi by injecting 2 U 3 to 5 mm lateral to the ala. This group also reported good results with a reduced gingival show on average of 3 mm.

Nasal Tip Ptosis

The depressor septi nasi originates at the incisive fossa of the maxilla and inserts into the medial crus of the alar cartilage, just caudal to the septum.[112] Hyperactivity of this muscle results in nasal tip drooping while smiling.[113] To minimize this dynamic ptosis, 1 to 5 U may be injected at the nasal base or the nasal tip.

Depressor Anguli Oris

The depressor anguli oris (DAO) are fan-shaped muscles originating at the mandibular border and inserting into the oral commissure, interdigitating with modiolus complex, orbicularis oris, and risorius muscles. They serve to depress the lateral commissures of the mouth, with overactivity accentuating the melomental fold (marionette lines) and a downturn of the oral commissures.[16]

There are several methods to isolating this muscle. One such method proposed by Choi et al. following a cadaveric study of 42 hemifaces suggests the muscle can be easily located, drawing a vertical line directly from the modiolus to serve as a central reference point. From there, the DAO lies between an oblique line 30 degrees medial from this vertical to 45 degrees lateral to this vertical modiolus line and can be safely injected between these points.[114] In terms of the actual injection to this muscle, various patterns have been described. Some advocate for a single injection of 4 U (Botox equivalents), 1 cm lateral to the oral commissure along the mandibular border.[115] Others prefer multiple injections, namely two inferior and/or superior injection. The superior injection point is just lateral to the marionette line and 0.5 mm below the labial commissure in a superficial plane. The inferior injection points are positioned anterior to the jowl, 2 to 3 mm apart and each 3 to 4 mm from the mandibular border, in a deep plane just above bone. Typically 5 U (Botox equivalents) is injected superiorly, and 2 U inferiorly.[116]

Anatomic placement is paramount with this injection to avoid complications. Superiorly, the modiolus shares a common insertion with several other muscles of facial expression; injections too close to the modiolus can result in facial asymmetry or weakening of the orbicularis oris resulting in oral incompetence.[115] Inferiorly, diffusion of the product medially can result in weaking of the depressor labii inferioris (DLI) and ultimately result in an asymmetric smile and potential issues with phonation.[116]

Mentalis

The mentalis is a paired muscle of the lower lip, which serves as the primary evertor of the lower lip, originating from the anterior mandible below the incisor roots and inserting more superficially into the soft tissue of the chin below the labiomental sulcus. Centrally, the two muscle bellies are separated by a firm septum.[117] Laterally, the mentalis muscle connects with the DLI muscle and superiorly with the orbicularis ori. Hyperactivity of this muscle leads to chin rhytids and a "peau d'orange" appearance to the chin.[116] A superficial intradermal injection in this case is often very effective for dimpling.

Similar to injection of the DAO, treatment of the mentalis demands anatomic precision with preferential medial placement to avoid spread into the DLI, which could result in asymmetry.[115] Carruthers et al. advocated for a single injection in the midline muscle bulk, at or just below the prominence of the chin of 5 to 10 U (Botox equivalents), angled upward and then massaged laterally.[110] Others have recommended splitting this midline injection into two aliquots, delivered separately to each muscle belly by injecting 5 mm lateral to the midline on either side. With these bilateral injections, some have advocated for deep placement 2 mm above the mandibular border to target the muscle's origin while others have championed an injection 1 cm above the tip of the chin placed superficially, closer to its insertion near the skin.[16,116]

Masseter

The masseter, a thick rectangular muscle, spans from the zygomatic arch and the coronoid process of the mandible to the mandibular angle, acting as one of the muscles of mastication. It is comprised of two components: the pars superficialis and pars profunda. The pars superficialis originates from the tendinous aponeurosis of the maxillary process of the zygoma and from the anterior three-fourths of the inferior border of the zygomatic arch. It spans back and down to insert on the mandibular angle and inferior aspect of the lateral ramus. The pars profunda arises from the more medial aspect of the maxillary process of the zygoma and the posterior inferior border of the zygomatic arch. It spans downward and medially to insert on the lateral portion of the lateral mandibular ramus and the lateral coronoid process.[116]

The masseter lies in close vicinity to several other structures, which must be considered when injecting this muscle. A study of Hu et al. analyzed 40 hemifaces to map the topography of these structures relative to the muscle. They found the majority of the posterior muscle was covered by parotid gland.[118] Given this relationship, parotid gland hypertrophy must be ruled out as a cause of facial widening before masseteric injection.[4] The facial vein lies on the anterior surface of the muscle or anterior to the entirety of the muscle with the artery more anterior relative to the vein. The marginal mandibular branch lies inferior to the mandibular margin 7.9 mm posteriorly and 4.6 mm at the anterior aspect of the muscle. The parotid gland can be found using an imaginary line connecting the ear lobe to the angle of the mouth. Seventy-nine percent of cadavers had the parotid gland crossing or above this line.[118]

This thick, broad muscle can hypertrophy over time as a result of genetics, mastication habits, and bruxism, leading to a wide, square-angled jaw that can appear masculine. This particular issue is commonly identified in females ages 20 to 40 years of Asian descent.[119] BTA treatment offers symptomatic relief from clenching and grinding habits but can also promote reduction of masseter volume ranging from 18% to 30% at 3 months, helping to recontour the lower facial third and create a more heart-shaped face.[120-124] This reduction in volume is isolated to the muscle only without impacting the surrounding soft tissues.[125] Results last up to 9 to 10 months for lower facial recontouring and 6 to 7 months for functional improvement in bruxism.[126] Successful treatment of the masseter is also associated with a reduction in temporomandibular joint pain should it also be present pretreatment.

Several techniques for injection have been described. Hui et al. recommended drawing a line from the tragus to chelion and then dividing the muscle below into eight equal parts. From there, the muscle should be preferentially injected 7.4 mm above the angle of the mandible.[118] Kaya et al. described two injections, determined by connecting the tragus to the lateral palpebral fissure and then drawing a vertical line from this landmark. Roughly 5 cm (halfway down) one injection can be made on either side, 1 cm anterior and 1 cm posterior.[127] Trevedic advocated for three points to be injected in a triangular pattern. The two inferior points are spaced 1.5 cm each, 0.5 cm above the inferior border of the mandible. The third point is placed 2 cm above this point.[116] Dosing varies widely based on sex and ethnicity. White women may require only 15 to 25 U (Botox equivalents) per side whereas Asian women may require up to 50 U. Men require up to 10 U more per side given increased muscle bulk.[4]

Platysma

The platysma is a thin, flat, broad muscle that extends obliquely from its origin at the anterior thorax, clavicle, and acromion toward the mandible and oral commissure. Superficial platysmal fibers insert directly on the masseter, risorius, and DAO. Together, they act with the platysma and pull the oral commissures laterally and downward.[128] As the platysma ages, the anterior platysma can separate, creating diverging vertical bands with horizontal rhytids, accentuated with muscle contraction. This process is distinct from lipodystrophy and static rhytids, which do not benefit from BTA.[129] Targeting of these platysmal bands in select patients can lead to a more refined jaw line and smoother appearing neck.[130]

To treat these areas, the vertical band is grasped between the index finger and the thumb of the nondominant hand and injected with 2 to 5 U (Botox equivalents) injected intradermally and tangentially in five places spaced equidistantly spanning the length of the vertical band. Horizontal neck fold may also be injected with 1 to 2 U in a superficial wheal.[130] Grasping of the bands and direct injection is key to avoiding unwanted complications such as dysphagia, dysphonia, and neck weakness that could occur if deep injection spread to other neck muscles.[110]

If a sharper jawline is desired, the patient may benefit from simultaneous injections along the mandibular border and down the vertical bands, termed a "*Nefertiti Lift*" after the Egyptian queen renowned for her sharp jawline and graceful neck.[130] Patients are likely to benefit from BTA treatment if the mandibular border disappears with platysmal contraction and vertical bands are evident. The anterior platysmal band is injected intradermally with 2 to 5 U, in four points each, 1 to 2 cm apart. A second series of injections of 2 to 2.5 U is administered in four equidistant points along the mandible just above the bone. The most anterior injection a "double dose," administered at the same site as the most superior site of the first set of injections. This double dose point must be set 1 cm posterior to the hypothetical intersection point of where the nasolabial fold and the mandible would meet. This positioning helps avoid spread to the depressor labia inferioris muscle, which could result in smile asymmetry.[130]

Microbotox is an alternative technique where multiple, dilute droplets of BTA are injected into the dermis or immediately subdermal. This selectively weakens the muscle fibers, which tether the muscle to the dermis to improve rhytids and acts on the sebaceous glands to reduce oil, improving skin texture. Although technique may be applied anywhere in the body, the technique's originator argues in particular that use in the neck can cause better apposition of the platysma compared to a muscular injection.[131] The zone injected is defined by a line three finger breadths above and parallel to the mandible, one finger breadth posterior to the DAO down the cervicomental angle and anterior neck, the clavicle, and the border of the sternocleidomastoid. This area is injected 50 to 60 times with dilute Botox (reconstituted to 20 U/mL), delivering a total of 20 to 28 U per side. They report some smile asymmetry, presumably from spread to the depressor labii inferioris but no serious complications.[131]

No more than 50 U total should be used in this region because of risk of neck weakness, dysphagia, or dysphonia.[116,130,132] Injections above 75 to 100 U have been associated with dysphagia and weakness of neck flexors.[133] Even with as little as 60 U, cases of dysphagia requiring nasogastric tubes have been reported.[134]

CONCLUSIONS

Botulinum toxin A is the most common aesthetic procedure in the United States and a powerful tool of facial rejuvenation. For patients, this procedure offers a perceived low-risk way to improve dynamic rhytids and improve skin texture. For clinicians, this procedure affords the ability to form long-lasting connections with patients that can often lead to more invasive procedures in the future.[2] As the importance of neuromodulators in clinical practice continues to grow, mastery of this skill becomes essential practice for any aesthetic surgeon.

REFERENCES

1. American Society of Plastic Surgeons. *Plastic Surgery Statistics Reports*. ASPS National Clearinghouse of Plastic Surgery Procedural Statistics. Author; 2019. https://www.plasticsurgery.org/news/plastic-surgery-statistics?sub=2019+Plastic+Surgery+Statistics
2. Richards BG, Schleicher WF, D'Souza GF, Isakov R, Zins JE. The role of injectables in aesthetic surgery: financial implications. *Aesthet Surg J*. 2017;37(9):1039-1043.
3. Cooper L, Lui M, Nduka C. Botulinum toxin treatment for facial palsy: a systematic review. *J Plast Reconstruct Aesthet Surg*. 2017;70(6):833-841.
4. Janes LE, Connor LM, Moradi A, Alghoul M. Current use of cosmetic toxins to improve facial aesthetics. *Plast Reconstruct Surg*. 2021;147(4):644e-657e.
5. Winter L, Spiegel J. Botulinum toxin type-A in the treatment of glabellar lines. Clin Cosmet Investig Dermatol. 2009;3:1-4.
6. Scott AB. Botulinum toxin injection into extraocular muscles as an alternative to strabismus surgery. *Ophthalmology*. 1980;87(10):1044-1049.
7. Scott AB. Botulinum toxin injection of eye muscles to correct strabismus. *Trans Am Ophthalmol Soc*. 1981;79:734-770.
8. Scott AB, Rosenbaum A, Collins CC. Pharmacologic weakening of extraocular muscles. *Invest Ophthalmol*. 1973;12(12):924-927.
9. Ababneh OH, Cetinkaya A, Kulwin DR. Long-term efficacy and safety of botulinum toxin A injections to treat blepharospasm and hemifacial spasm. *Clin Exp Ophthalmol*. 2014;42(3):254-261.
10. Tsoy EA, Buckley EG, Dutton JJ. Treatment of blepharospasm with botulinum toxin. *Am J Ophthalmol*. 1985;99(2):176-179.
11. Scott AB, Kennedy RA, Stubbs HA. Botulinum A toxin injection as a treatment for blepharospasm. *Arch Ophthalmol*. 1985;103(3):347-350.
12. Elston JS. Botulinum toxin treatment of hemifacial spasm. *J Neurol Neurosurg Psychiatry*. 1986;49(7):827-829.
13. Chen S. Clinical uses of botulinum neurotoxins: current indications, limitations and future developments. *Toxins*. 2012;4(10):913-939.
14. Carruthers JD, Carruthers JA. Treatment of glabellar frown lines with C. botulinum-A exotoxin. *J Dermatol Surg Oncol*. 1992;18(1):17-21.
15. Administration, U.S.F.a.D. *BOTOX Cosmetic (OnabotulinumtoxinA) for Injection*, for Intramuscular Use. 2017. Accessed at: https://www.accessdata.fda.gov/drugsatfda_docs/label/2017/103000s5302lbl.pdf
16. Gart MS, Gutowski KA. Overview of botulinum toxins for aesthetic uses. *Clin Plast Surg*. 2016;43(3):459-471.

17. Park J, Lee MS, Harrison AR. Profile of Xeomin® (incobotulinumtoxinA) for the treatment of blepharospasm. *Clin Ophthalmol.* 2011;5:725-732.
18. Dover JS, Monheit G, Greener M, Pickett A. Botulinum toxin in aesthetic medicine: myths and realities. *Dermatol Surg.* 2018;44(2):249-260.
19. Brodsky MA, Swope DM, Grimes D. Diffusion of botulinum toxins. *Tremor Other Hyperkinet Mov (N Y).* 2012;2:tre-02-85-417-1.
20. Dorizas A, Krueger N, Sadick NS. Aesthetic uses of the botulinum toxin. *Dermatol Clin.* 2014;32(1):23-36.
21. Hambleton P, Pickett AM. Potency equivalence of botulinum toxin preparations. *J R Soc Med.* 1994;87(11):719.
22. Karsai S, Raulin C. Current evidence on the unit equivalence of different botulinum neurotoxin A formulations and recommendations for clinical practice in dermatology. *Dermatol Surg.* 2009;35(1):1-8.
23. Dressler D, Mander G, Fink K. Measuring the potency labelling of onabotulinumtoxinA (Botox(®)) and incobotulinumtoxinA (Xeomin (®)) in an LD50 assay. *J Neural Transm (Vienna).* 2012;119(1):13-15.
24. Hexsel D, Brum C, do Prado DZ, et al. Field effect of two commercial preparations of botulinum toxin type A: a prospective, double-blind, randomized clinical trial. *J Am Acad Dermatol.* 2012;67(2):226-232.
25. Marchetti A, Magar R, Findley L, et al. Retrospective evaluation of the dose of Dysport and BOTOX in the management of cervical dystonia and blepharospasm: the REAL DOSE study. *Mov Disord.* 2005;20(8):937-944.
26. Scaglione F. Conversion Ratio between Botox®, Dysport®, and Xeomin® in Clinical Practice. *Toxins (Basel).* 2016;8(3):65.
27. Kranz G, Haubenberger D, Voller B, et al. Respective potencies of Botox and Dysport in a human skin model: a randomized, double-blind study. *Mov Disord.* 2009;24(2):231-236.
28. Aoki KR, Ranoux D, Wissel J. Using translational medicine to understand clinical differences between botulinum toxin formulations. *Eur J Neurol.* 2006;13(suppl 4):10-19.
29. Lowe PL, Patnaik R, Lowe NJ. A comparison of two botulinum type a toxin preparations for the treatment of glabellar lines: double-blind, randomized, pilot study. *Dermatol Surg.* 2005;31(12):1651-1654.
30. Lowe P, Patnaik R, Lowe N. Comparison of two formulations of botulinum toxin type A for the treatment of glabellar lines: a double-blind, randomized study. *J Am Acad Dermatol.* 2006;55(6):975-980.
31. Lowe NJ, Shah A, Lowe PL, Patnaik R. Dosing, efficacy and safety plus the use of computerized photography for botulinum toxins type A for upper facial lines. *J Cosmet Laser Ther.* 2010;12(2):106-111.
32. Karsai S, Adrian R, Hammes S, Thimm J, Raulin C. A randomized double-blind study of the effect of Botox and Dysport/Reloxin on forehead wrinkles and electromyographic activity. *Arch Dermatol.* 2007;143(11): 1447-1449.
33. Pickett A. Dysport: pharmacological properties and factors that influence toxin action. *Toxicon.* 2009;54(5):683-689.
34. Hexsel DM, Soirefmann M, Rodrigues TC, do Prado DZ. Increasing the field effects of similar doses of Clostridium botulinum type A toxin-hemagglutinin complex in the treatment of compensatory hyperhidrosis. *Arch Dermatol.* 2009;145(7):837-840.
35. Benefield DA, Dessain SK, Shine N, Ohi MD, Lacy DB. Molecular assembly of botulinum neurotoxin progenitor complexes. *Proc Natl Acad Sci U S A.* 2013;110(14): 5630-5635.
36. Frevert J, Dressler D. Complexing proteins in botulinum toxin type A drugs: a help or a hindrance? *Biologics.* 2010;4:325-332.
37. Cliff SH, Judodihardjo H, Eltringham E. Different formulations of botulinum toxin type A have different migration characteristics: a double-blind, randomized study. *J Cosmet Dermatol.* 2008;7(1):50-54.
38. Trindade de Almeida AR, Marques E, de Almeida J, Cunha T, Boraso R. Pilot study comparing the diffusion of two formulations of botulinum toxin type A in patients with forehead hyperhidrosis. *Dermatol Surg.* 2007;33(1 Spec No.):S37-S43.
39. Karl-Heinz E, Taylor HV. Dissociation of the 900kDa neurotoxin complex from C. botulinum under physiological conditions. *Toxicon.* 2008;51:10.
40. Carli L, Montecucco C, Rossetto O. Assay of diffusion of different botulinum neurotoxin type a formulations injected in the mouse leg. *Muscle Nerve.* 2009;40(3): 374-380.
41. Jankovic J, Vuong KD, Ahsan J. Comparison of efficacy and immunogenicity of original versus current botulinum toxin in cervical dystonia. *Neurology.* 2003;60(7): 1186-1188.
42. Naumann M, Boo LM, Ackerman AH, Gallagher CJ. Immunogenicity of botulinum toxins. *J Neural Transm (Vienna).* 2013;120(2):275-290.
43. Bellows S, Jankovic J. Immunogenicity associated with botulinum toxin treatment. *Toxins.* 2019;11(9):491.
44. Jankovic J, Hunter C, Dolimbek BZ, et al. Clinico-immunologic aspects of botulinum toxin type B treatment of cervical dystonia. *Neurology.* 2006;67(12):2233-2235.
45. Naumann M, Carruthers A, Carruthers J, et al. Meta-analysis of neutralizing antibody conversion with onabotulinumtoxinA (BOTOX®) across multiple indications. *Mov Disord.* 2010;25(13):2211-2218.
46. Brin MF, James C, Maltman J. Botulinum toxin type A products are not interchangeable: a review of the evidence. *Biologics.* 2014;8:227-241.

47. Blümel J, Frevert J, Schwaier A. Comparative antigenicity of three preparations of botulinum neurotoxin type A in the rabbit. *Neurotox Res.* 2006;9:238.
48. Kanovsky P, Platz T, Comes G, Grafe SK, Sassin I. FP12MO03 NT 201, botulinum neurotoxin free from complexing proteins, Xeomin(c) provided sustained efficacy and was safe in spasticity: 89 weeks long-term data. *J Neurol Sci.* 2009;285.
49. Greensboro, N.M.P., Xeomin: Summary of product characteristics.
50. Dysport [package insert]. Berkshire (united Kingtom): Ipsen Ltd.
51. Botox cosmetic [package insert]. Irvine (CA): Allergan, Inc.
52. Alam M, Dover JS, Arndt KA. Pain associated with injection of botulinum A exotoxin reconstituted using isotonic sodium chloride with and without preservative: a double-blind, randomized controlled trial. *Arch Dermatol.* 2002;138(4):510-514.
53. Klein AW. Dilution and storage of botulinum toxin. *Dermatol Surg.* 1998;24(11):1179-1180.
54. Mclellan K, Das RE, Ekong TA, Sesardic D. Therapeutic botulinum type a toxin: factors affecting potency. *Toxicon.* 1996;34(9):975-985.
55. Huang W, Foster JA, Rogachefsky AS. Pharmacology of botulinum toxin. *J Am Acad Dermatol.* 2000;43(2): 249-259.
56. Garcia A, Fulton Jr JE. Cosmetic denervation of the muscles of facial expression with botulinum toxin A dose-response study. *Dermatol Surg.* 1996;22(1):39-43.
57. Alam M, Yoo SS, Wrone DA, White LE, Kim JY. Sterility assessment of multiple use botulinum A exotoxin vials: a prospective simulation. *J Am Acad Dermatol.* 2006;55(2):272-275.
58. Allen SB, Goldenberg NA. Pain difference associated with injection of abobotulinumtoxinA reconstituted with preserved saline and preservative-free saline: a prospective, randomized, side-by-side, double-blind study. *Dermatol Surg.* 2012;38(6):867-870.
59. Sarifakioglu N, Sarifakioglu E. Evaluating effects of preservative-containing saline solution on pain perception during botulinum toxin type-a injections at different locations: a prospective, single-blinded, randomized controlled trial. *Aesthetic Plast Surg.* 2005;29(2):113-115.
60. Kwiat DM, Bersani TA, Bersani A. Increased patient comfort utilizing botulinum toxin type a reconstituted with preserved versus nonpreserved saline. *Ophthalmic Plast Reconstr Surg.* 2004;20(3):186-189.
61. van Laborde S, Dover JS, Moore M, Stewart B, Arndt KA, Alam M. Reduction in injection pain with botulinum toxin type B further diluted using saline with preservative: a double-blind, randomized controlled trial. *J Am Acad Dermatol.* 2003;48(6):875-877.
62. Alam M, Bolotin D, Carruthers J, et al. Consensus statement regarding storage and reuse of previously reconstituted neuromodulators. *Dermatol Surg.* 2015; 41(3):321-326.
63. Carey WD. Incorrect reconstitution of incobotulinumtoxin A leads to loss of neurotoxin. *J Drugs Dermatol.* 2014;13(6):735-738.
64. Dressler D, Bigalke H. Reconstituting botulinum toxin drugs: shaking, stirring or what? *J Neural Transm (Vienna).* 2016;123(5):523-525.
65. Shaari CM, Sanders I. Quantifying how location and dose of botulinum toxin injections affect muscle paralysis. *Muscle Nerve.* 1993;16(9):964-969.
66. Kim HS, Hwang JH, Jeong ST, et al. Effect of muscle activity and botulinum toxin dilution volume on muscle paralysis. *Dev Med Child Neurol.* 2003;45(3):200-206.
67. Gracies JM, Lugassy M, Weisz DJ, Vecchio M, Flanagan S, Simpson DM. Botulinum toxin dilution and endplate targeting in spasticity: a double-blind controlled study. *Arch Phys Med Rehabil.* 2009;90(1):9-16.e2.
68. Carruthers A, Bogle M, Carruthers JD, et al. A randomized, evaluator-blinded, two-center study of the safety and effect of volume on the diffusion and efficacy of botulinum toxin type A in the treatment of lateral orbital rhytides. *Dermatol Surg.* 2007;33(5):567-571.
69. Prager W, Zschocke I, Reich C, Brocatti L, Henning K, Steinkraus V. [Does dilution have an impact on cosmetic results with BoNT/A? Complex-protein-free BoNT/A for treatment of glabella lines]. *Hautarzt.* 2009;60(10):815-820.
70. Rzany BJ, Ascher B, Avelar RL, et al. A multicenter, randomized, double-blind, placebo-controlled, single-dose, phase III, non-inferiority study comparing prabotulinumtoxin A and onabotulinumtoxin A for the treatment of moderate to severe glabellar lines in adult patients. *Aesthet Surg J.* 2020;40(4):413-429.
71. Hankins CL, Strimling R, Rogers GS. Botulinum A toxin for glabellar wrinkles. Dose and response. *Dermatol Surg.* 1998;24(11):1181-1183.
72. Hsu TS, Dover JS, Arndt KA. Effect of volume and concentration on the diffusion of botulinum exotoxin A. *Arch Dermatol.* 2004;140(11):1351-1354.
73. Carruthers A, Carruthers J, Cohen J. Dilution volume of botulinum toxin type A for the treatment of glabellar rhytides: does it matter? *Dermatol Surg.* 2007;33 (1 Spec No):S97-S104.
74. Abbasi NR, Durfee MA, Petrell K, Dover JS, Arndt KA. A small study of the relationship between abobotulinum toxin A concentration and forehead wrinkle reduction. *Arch Dermatol.* 2012;148(1):119-121.
75. Sundaram H, Signorini M, Liew S, et al. Global Aesthetics Consensus: Botulinum toxin type A—evidence-based review, emerging concepts, and

consensus recommendations for aesthetic use, including updates on complications. *Plast Reconstr Surg.* 2016;137(3):518e-529e.
76. Carruthers A, Carruthers J. Single-center, double-blind, randomized study to evaluate the efficacy of 4% lidocaine cream versus vehicle cream during botulinum toxin type A treatments. *Dermatol Surg.* 2005;31(12):1655-1659.
77. Sami MS, Soparkar CN, Patrinely JR, Hollier LM, Hollier LH. Efficacy of botulinum toxin type A after topical anesthesia. *Ophthalmic Plast Reconstr Surg.* 2006;22(6):448-452.
78. Saeliw P, Preechawai P, Aui-aree N. Evaluating the effects of ice application on patient comfort before and after botulinum toxin type A injections. *J Med Assoc Thai.* 2010;93(10):1200-1204.
79. Sarifakioglu N, Sarifakioglu E. Evaluating the effects of ice application on the pain felt during botulinum toxin type-A injections: a prospective, randomized, single-blind controlled trial. *Ann Plast Surg.* 2004;53(6): 543-546.
80. Irkoren S, Ozkan HS, Karaca H. A clinical comparison of EMLA cream and ethyl chloride spray application for pain relief of forehead botulinum toxin injection. *Ann Plast Surg.* 2015;75(3):272-274.
81. Elibol O, Ozkan B, Hekimhan PK, Cağlar Y. Efficacy of skin cooling and EMLA cream application for pain relief of periocular botulinum toxin injection. *Ophthalmic Plast Reconstr Surg.* 2007;23(2):130-133.
82. Chorney SR, Villwock JA, Suryadevara AC. Vibration versus ice to reduce cosmetic botulinum toxin injection pain—a randomized controlled trial. *Ear Nose Throat J.* 2019;98(6):351–355.
83. Pirazzini M, Rossetto O, Bertasio C, et al. Time course and temperature dependence of the membrane translocation of tetanus and botulinum neurotoxins C and D in neurons. *Biochem Biophys Res Commun.* 2013;430(1):38-42.
84. Fouché JJ, Van Loghem JAJ, Thuis J, De Heer LM, van Oijen MGH. Left/right pain asymmetry with injectable cosmetic treatments for the face. *Aesthet Surg J.* 2017;37(6):708-714.
85. Foglietti MA, Wright L, Foglietti-Fostyk A. Botulinum toxin therapy: is syringe type related to cost-effectiveness? *Ann Plast Surg.* 2018;80(3):287-289.
86. Gordin EA, Luginbuhl AL, Ortlip T, Heffelfinger RN, Krein H. Subcutaneous vs intramuscular botulinum toxin: split-face randomized study. *JAMA Facial Plast Surg.* 2014;16(3):193-198.
87. Rose AE, Goldberg DJ. Safety and efficacy of intradermal injection of botulinum toxin for the treatment of oily skin. *Dermatol Surg.* 2013;39(3 Pt 1):443-448.
88. Shah AR. Use of intradermal botulinum toxin to reduce sebum production and facial pore size. *J Drugs Dermatol.* 2008;7(9):847-850.
89. Chang SP, Tsai HH, Chen WY, Lee WR, Chen PL, Tsai TH. The wrinkles soothing effect on the middle and lower face by intradermal injection of botulinum toxin type A. *Int J Dermatol.* 2008;47(12):1287-1294.
90. Sapra P, Demay S, Sapra S, Khanna J, Mraud K, Bonadonna J. A single-blind, split-face, randomized, pilot study comparing the effects of intradermal and intramuscular injection of two commercially available botulinum toxin A formulas to reduce signs of facial aging. *J Clin Aesthet Dermatol.* 2017;10(2):34-44.
91. de Sa Earp AP, Marmur ES. The five D's of botulinum toxin: doses, dilution, diffusion, duration and dogma. *J Cosmet Laser Ther.* 2008;10(2):93-102.
92. Wei J, Xu H, Dong J, Li Q, Dai C. Prolonging the duration of masseter muscle reduction by adjusting the masticatory movements after the treatment of masseter muscle hypertrophy with botulinum toxin type a injection. *Dermatol Surg.* 2015;41(suppl 1):S101-S109.
93. Dysport. *AbobotulainumtoxinA: Full Prescribing Information.* Available at: https://www.galderma.com/us/sites/g/files/jcdfhc341/files/2020-11/1066038%20Dysport%20PI.pdf?_ga=2.98258518.878584266.1614617021-1744198382.1614617021&_gac=1.128997502.1614617021.Cj0KCQiAvvKBBhCXARIsACTePW9eYUXazZJF-ZINacrkRDIUAIq57D5MleB6v1qo8-otBWEo8MylASIgaAsJ8EALw_wcB.
94. Xeomin. *IncobotulinumtoxinA: Full Prescribing Information.* Available at: https://www.xeomin.com/pdf/xeomin-medication-guide.pdf.
95. Allergan, I.B.C.A. *OnabotulinumtoxinA: Full prescribing Information.* Available at: https://media.allergan.com/actavis/actavis/media/allergan-pdf-documents/product-prescribing/20190626-BOTOX-Cosmetic-Insert-72715US10-Med-Guide-v2-0MG1145.pdf.
96. de Almeida AR, da Costa Marques ER, Banegas R, Kadunc BV. Glabellar contraction patterns: a tool to optimize botulinum toxin treatment. *Dermatol Surg.* 2012;38(9):1506-1515.
97. Janis JE, Ghavami A, Lemmon JA, Leedy JE, Guyuron B. Anatomy of the corrugator supercilii muscle: part I. Corrugator topography. *Plast Reconstr Surg.* 2007;120(6): 1647-1653.
98. Knize DM. An anatomically based study of the mechanism of eyebrow ptosis. *Plast Reconstr Surg.* 1996;97(7): 1321-1333.
99. de Maio M, DeBoulle K, Braz A, Rohrich RJ. Facial assessment and injection guide for botulinum toxin and injectable hyaluronic acid fillers: focus on the upper face. *Plast Reconstruct Surg.* 2017;140(4):540e-550e.
100. Fagien S. Temporary management of upper lid ptosis, lid malposition, and eyelid fissure asymmetry with botulinum toxin type A. *Plast Reconstruct Surg.* 2004; 114(7):1892-1902.

101. King M. Management of ptosis. *J Clin Aesthet Dermatol.* 2016;9(12):E1-E4.
102. Jabbour SF, Awaida CJ, ElKhoury JS, et al. The impact of upper face botulinum toxin injections on eyebrow height and forehead lines: a randomized controlled trial and an algorithmic approach to forehead injection. *Plast Reconstruct Surg.* 2018;142(5):1212-1217.
103. Abramo AC, Do Amaral TP, Lessio BP, De Lima GA. Anatomy of forehead, glabellar, nasal and orbital muscles, and their correlation with distinctive patterns of skin lines on the upper third of the face: reviewing concepts. *Aesthetic Plast Surg.* 2016;40(6):962-971.
104. Jaspers GW, Pijpe J, Jansma J. The use of botulinum toxin type A in cosmetic facial procedures. *Int J Oral Maxillofac Surg.* 2011;40(2):127-133.
105. Qaqish C. Botulinum toxin use in the upper face. *Atlas Oral Maxillofac Surg Clin North Am.* 2016;24(2):95-103.
106. Huang W, Rogachefsky AS, Foster JA. Browlift with botulinum toxin. *Dermatol Surg.* 2000;26(1):55-60.
107. Matarasso SL, Matarasso A. Treatment guidelines for botulinum toxin type A for the periocular region and a report on partial upper lip ptosis following injections to the lateral canthal rhytids. *Plast Reconstruct Surg.* 2001;108(1): 208-217.
108. Lowe NJ, Ascher B, Heckmann M, et al. Double-blind, randomized, placebo-controlled, dose-response study of the safety and efficacy of botulinum toxin type A in subjects with crow's feet. *Dermatol Surg.* 2005;31(3):257-262.
109. Flynn TC, Carruthers JA, Carruthers JA. Botulinum-A toxin treatment of the lower eyelid improves infraorbital rhytides and widens the eye. *Dermatol Surg.* 2001; 27(8):703-708.
110. Carruthers J, Fagien S, Matarasso SL. Consensus recommendations on the use of botulinum toxin type A in facial aesthetics. *Plast Reconstruct Surg.* 2004;114(6): 1S-22S.
111. Hwang WS, Hur MS, Hu KS, et al. Surface anatomy of the lip elevator muscles for the treatment of gummy smile using botulinum toxin. *Angle Orthod.* 2009;79(1):70-77.
112. Sinno S, Chang JB, Saadeh PB, Lee MR. Anatomy and surgical treatment of the depressor septi nasi muscle: a systematic review. *Plast Reconstruct Surg.* 2015;135(5): 838e-848e.
113. Rohrich RJ, Huynh B, Muzaffar AR, Adams Jr WP, Robinson Jr JB. Importance of the depressor septi nasi muscle in rhinoplasty: anatomic study and clinical application. *Plast Reconstr Surg.* 2000;105(1):376-388.
114. Choi YJ, Kim JS, Gil YC, et al. Anatomical considerations regarding the location and boundary of the depressor anguli oris muscle with reference to botulinum toxin injection. *Plast Reconstruct Surg.* 2014;134(5): 917-921.
115. Wu DC, Fabi SG, Goldman MP. Neurotoxins: current concepts in cosmetic use on the face and neck—lower face. *Plast Reconstruct Surg.* 2015;136(suppl 5):76S-79S.
116. Trévidic P, Sykes J, Criollo-Lamilla G. Anatomy of the lower face and botulinum toxin injections. *Plast Reconstruct Surg.* 2015;136(suppl 5):84S-91S.
117. Zide BM, McCarthy J. The mentalis muscle: an essential component of chin and lower lip position. *Plast Reconstruct Surg.* 1989;83(3):413-420.
118. Hu KS, Kim ST, Hur MS, et al. Topography of the masseter muscle in relation to treatment with botulinum toxin type A. *Oral Surg Oral Med Oral Pathol Oral Radiol Endod.* 2010;110(2):167-171.
119. Shome D, Khare S, Kapoor R. Efficacy of botulinum toxin in treating Asian Indian patients with Masseter hypertrophy: a 4-year follow-up study. *Plast Reconstruct Surg.* 2019;144(3):390e-396e.
120. Yu CC, Chen PK, Chen YR. Botulinum toxin A for lower facial contouring: A prospective study. *Aesthetic Plast Surg.* 2007;31(5):445-453.
121. Kim JH, Shin JH, Kim ST, Kim CY. Effects of two different units of botulinum toxin type a evaluated by computed tomography and electromyographic measurements of human masseter muscle. *Plast Reconstr Surg.* 2007;119(2):711-717.
122. Kim NH, Chung JH, Park RH, Park JB. The use of botulinum toxin type A in aesthetic mandibular contouring. *Plast Reconstr Surg.* 2005;115(3):919-930.
123. Shim WH, Yoon SH, Park JH, Choi YC, Kim ST. Effect of botulinum toxin type A injection on lower facial contouring evaluated using a three-dimensional laser scan. *Dermatol Surg.* 2010;36(suppl 4):2161-2166.
124. Park MY, Ahn KY, Jung DS. Botulinum toxin type A treatment for contouring of the lower face. *Dermatol Surg.* 2003;29(5):477-483.
125. Park G, Choi YC, Bae JH, Kim ST. Does botulinum toxin injection into masseter muscles affect subcutaneous thickness? *Aesthet Surg J.* 2018;38(2): 192-198.
126. Liew S, Dart A. Nonsurgical reshaping of the lower face. *Aesthet Surg J.* 2008;28(3):251-257.
127. Kaya B, Apaydin N, Loukas M, Tubbs RS. The topographic anatomy of the masseteric nerve: a cadaveric study with an emphasis on the effective zone of botulinum toxin A injections in masseter. *J Plast Reconstr Aesthet Surg.* 2014;67(12):1663-1668.
128. Goldman A, Wollina U. Elevation of the corner of the mouth using botulinum toxin type A. *J Cutan Med Surg.* 2010;3(3):145-150.
129. Rohrich RJ, Rios JL, Smith PD, Gutowski KA. Neck rejuvenation revisited. *Plast Reconstruct Surg.* 2006; 118(5):1251-1263.

130. Levy PM. Neurotoxins: current concepts in cosmetic use on the face and neck jawline contouring/platysma bands/necklace lines. *Plast Reconstruct Surg*. 2015; 136(suppl 5):80S-83S.
131. Wu WTL. Microbotox of the lower face and neck: evolution of a personal technique and its clinical effects. *Plast Reconstruct Surg*. 2015;136(suppl 5):92S-100S.
132. Raspaldo H, Niforos FR, Gassia V, et al. Lower-face and neck antiaging treatment and prevention using onabotulinumtoxin A: the 2010 multidisciplinary French consensus – part 2. *J Cosmet Dermatol*. 2011; 10(2):131-149.
133. Carruthers A, Carruthers J. Clinical indications and injection technique for the cosmetic use of botulinum A exotoxin. *Dermatol Surg*. 1998;24(11): 1189-1194.
134. Carruthers J, Carruthers A. Practical cosmetic botox techniques. *J Cutan Med Surg*. 1999;3(4_suppl):S49-S52.

4

Soft Tissue Fillers

Brayann O. Aleman, Jonathan Cabin, and Babak Azizzadeh

BRIEF INTRODUCTION

- Anatomic neurovascular, muscular, and anatomy of each region is imperative.
- Soft tissue fillers can refer to a multitude of substances that are injected into the skin or subdermal area for cosmetic or therapeutic use.
- Cosmetically, soft tissue fillers are best used to volumize areas of hollowness, camouflage areas of gravitational changes of aging, or improve anatomic harmony by changing the relationships and proportions of various anatomic features.
- There are many different types of soft tissue fillers; the most ubiquitous being those made from hyaluronic acid, which is temporary, reversible, and inert.
- In assessing a patient for soft tissue filler application, it is crucial to perform a targeted history and physical examination and evaluate the patient as to their expectations and understanding of the risks involved.
- As soft tissue filler is an invasive medical procedure, it is crucial that patients understand the risks, benefits, and alternative treatments for their concerns and sign a consent form that formally indicates that they have this understanding.
- In choosing a soft tissue filler, it is important to consider the target area and the goals to ensure that the filler is appropriate for that application.
- Soft tissue fillers can be injected via a traditional needle or through a cannula approach. Although arguably requiring more skill and time, a cannula approach is safer and leads to more natural results with less downtime and potential bruising and swelling.
- All practitioners performing soft tissue filler should be fluent in the potential risks and side effects they may encounter.
- All practitioners should have an emergency plan, including available products and referral pathways, for devastating vascular consequences such as tissue necrosis, blindness, or stroke.

BACKGROUND INFORMATION/ ANATOMIC PEARLS

Introduction

"Soft tissue fillers" is an umbrella term for a wide array of substances intended for dermal or subdermal injection, with the goal of antiaging, cosmetic enhancement, functional improvement, or correction of medical, surgical, or trauma-related defects. The therapeutic effect of soft tissue fillers is through direct volume replenishment of the treated areas and/or in the biostimulation of volumizing/skin-strengthening byproducts such as collagen and elastin.

Recently, studies have revealed an increase in patients seeking minimally invasive treatments to correct aging changes and as a "rejuvenation" procedure to delay the appearance of facial aging or enhance their existing facial features.

Although commonly regarded by the lay public as a treatment for "wrinkles," the major value of soft tissue fillers is not necessarily in filling the superficial dermal and cuticular divots related to the integrity of the skin—the cause of true wrinkling—but instead in restoring volume to areas of age-, disease-, or trauma-related volume deficits. In addition—especially in younger patients—fillers can provide additional volumetric augmentation to change the proportionality of cosmetic features to balance and harmonize overall facial/body structure.

History

The concept of soft tissue filler dates back to the 19th century when autologous fat grafting was first attempted. Autologous fat grafting—or the transfer of fat from one part of the body to another as a living transplant—persists to this day as a well-regarded permanent volumization technique, especially as an adjunct to other plastic surgery procedures such as rhytidectomy (facelift) or mastopexy (breast lift) procedures. A detailed discussion of the techniques and use cases of fat grafting is beyond the scope of this chapter and textbook.

Paraffin wax—a white or colorless solid wax made from saturated hydrocarbons—was the first reported nonautologous dermal filler. Its first documented use was in the mid-1890s, yet some form of paraffin wax injection was continued into the mid-20th century. Paraffin wax injection fell out of favor because of the high migration rates, vascular occlusion, and granuloma formation.[1]

Purified bovine dermal collagen was the first U.S. Food and Drug Administration (FDA)-approved filler substance, developed in the 1970s as a xenogenic soft tissue filler and first approved in 1981 under the brand name Zyderm for correction of contour irregularities in the dermis. Although highly effective, given its xenogenic origin, it required two rounds of preapplication sensitivity testing, which made its application more complex. In addition, its irreversibility led to difficult complications.

Clinical Use of Injectable Dermal Fillers: A Decade of Experience

A turning point for dermal fillers was in the development and approval of a hyaluronic acid (HA) filler in 2003. Relatively nonreactive and reversible, it ushered in a new era of safe and effective nonsurgical filling.[1] This also served to popularize and normalize soft tissue filler as a reasonable treatment for aging and volume disproportionalities (see Figure 4.1).

In general, HA is a glycosaminoglycan disaccharide found in all human tissue but predominantly in the vitreous, skin, and synovial fluid. The skin comprises approximately 50% of the total body hyaluronic acid.[1]

HA for fillers is extracted from bacterial fermentation and lacks animal-derived proteins. Later, the HA undergoes stabilization to prevent enzymatically or oxidative degradation once injected into the body. In addition, cross-linking with 1,4-butanediol diglycidyl ether creates a polymer.[2] The degree of cross-link will modify the rheology properties and longevity of the filler Table 4.1.

Rheology is the science that studies the consistency, compression, and elasticity properties of liquids and gels. As of the writing of this chapter, HA is by far-and-away the most used type of filler globally.

Aside from various modifications of HA—both in manufacturing processes and additives (like lidocaine)—three additional synthetic filler substances entered the market after the first HA: poly-L-lactic acid (PLLA) (Sculptra), calcium hydroxyl-apatite (CaHA) (Radiesse), and polymethyl methacrylate (Bellafill). Unlike HA, all three of these additional filler substances have biostimulator properties and thus prompt the body to self-volumize by creating more collagen. Biostimulating fillers are considered "semi-permanent": although collagen is not predictably broken down by the body, over time, it is subject to the same aging degradation that all collagen sustains (Table 4.2).

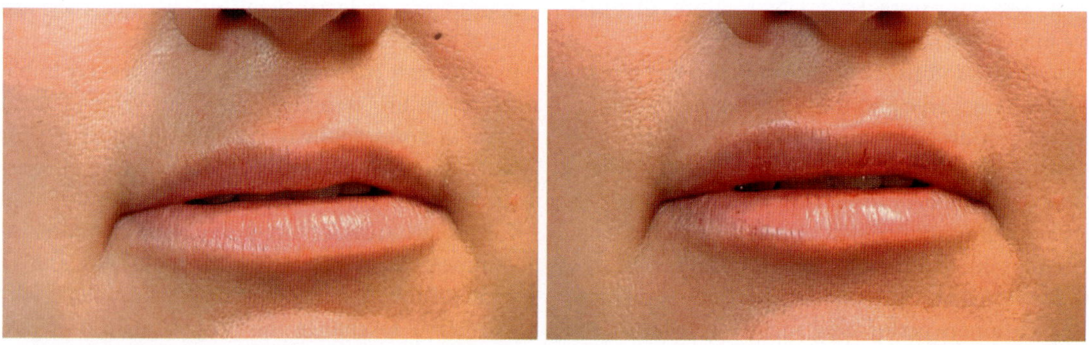

Fig. 4.1 Before and after one syringe of hyaluronic acid filler. (From Atlas of Oral and Maxillofacial Surgery. Caplin, Courtney. Published December 31, 2023. © 2024.)

TABLE 4.1 Biodegradable Synthetic Fillers

Product	HA Concentration mg/mL	% Cross-Linked
Restylane	20	1.20%
Restylane Lyft	20	1.20%
Restylane Silk	20	1.20%
Restylane Kysse	20	7%
Restylane Contour	20	7%
Restylane Defyne	20	8%
RHA 2	23	3%
RHA 3	23	3.50%
RHA 4	23	4%
Juvederm Ultra	24	6%
Juvederm Ultra Plus	24	8%
Juvederm Voluma	20	Highly (proprietary)
Juvederm Volbella	15	Highly (proprietary)
Juvederm Vollure	17.5	Highly (proprietary)
Revanesse Versa	25	7%
Belotero	22.5	Cannot be measured

HA, Hyaluronic acid; *RHA*, resilient hyaluronic acid.

TABLE 4.2 Nonbiodegradable Synthetic Fillers

Product	Brand Name
Polymethyl-methacrylate microspheres	Artefill, Belafill
Calcium hydroxylapatite	Radiesse
Polyalylimide	Aquamid

TABLE 4.3 Allogenic Fillers

Product	Brand Name
Human Tissue Collagen Matrix	Dermalogen, Dermaplant
Acellular Human Dermal Matrix	Alloderm

In addition to the synthetic fillers discussed earlier, a newer category of filler comes from donated fat that is purified to a cell-less allograft adipose matrix (Renuva). A combination of collagen, proteins, and growth factors, it is thought to provide a targeted scaffolding for the patient's own body to build fat. It is commonly used to create permanent volumetric changes and in cases where fat grafting is required but the patient does not have adequate donor fat (Table 4.3).

As technology will surely continue to develop, research and development will continue to expand on our understanding of soft tissue fillers.

Types of Soft Tissue Fillers

Fillers can be categorized in countless ways according to clinical applications, molecular structure, or scientific properties. We find it most helpful to organize soft tissue fillers into four general categories, each with their own benefits and potential risks and drawbacks (Table 4.4):

1. biodegradable synthetic (e.g., HA, CHA, and PLLA)
2. nonbiodegradable synthetic (e.g., polymethylmethacrylate microspheres, polyacrylamide hydrogel polymers, and silicone)
3. allogenic biologic (e.g., collagen, allogenic purified fat)
4. autologous biologic (e.g., fat transfer)

There are several other materials that have been used outside of the United States which currently do not have FDA approval for distribution in North America, and these are briefly discussed below.

Aquamid (Contura, Soeborg, Denmark) is a polyacrylamide gel which is biocompatible, stable, and nonresorbable. It consists of 2.5% cross-linked polyacrylamide

TABLE 4.4 General Soft Tissue Filler Categories

Category	Substances	Common Brand Names	Pros	Cons
Nonbiodegradable	Calcium hydroxylapatite	Radiesse	Expensive Excellent results for bony augmentation Biocompatible Collagen stimulation Minimal migration Easy to mold	Nonreversible Nonsuitable for thin skin, mucosa, and superficial layers Dyschromia, skin color changes when is placed too superficial
Nonbiodegradable	Polymethyl-methacrylate microspheres	Artefill, Belafill	Contains collagen	Nonreversible Reported granuloma formation
Biodegradable	PLLA	Sculptra	Long-lasting results Stimulate collagen production	Nonreversible
Biodegradable	Hyaluronic acid	Aptique, Esthélis, Elevess, Hylaform, Juvederm, Perlane, Prevelle, Puragen, Restylane	Reversible	Cost Nonpermanent
Nonbiodegradable	Polyalkylimide	Aquamid	Semi-permanent Collagen stimulation	Inflammatory reaction, nodule formation, granuloma formation

PLLA, Poly-L-lactic acid.

and nonpyrogenic water. It has been commerically used in Europe for decades.

Ellansé (Sinclair Pharmaceuticals, London, UK) is a biodegradable, collagen-type I biostimulant consisting of polycaprolactone microspheres in carboxymethyl cellulose gel. Ellansé was introduced in Europe in 2009. Its biodegradation occurs by hydrolysis of ester linkages, with CO_2 and H_2O as end products that are ultimately eliminated from the body. Ellansé has four presentations with different in vivo longevity of 1 to 4 years, respectively (Ellansé-S, Ellansé-M, Ellansé-L, Ellansé-E).

Other important subjective and objective considerations for soft tissue fillers are:

- Duration—how long does the product create change in the tissues? While each product has a certain duration profile as specified by the manufacturer and based upon clinical trials, this has also been found to vary based on placement and the patient's own, non-quantifiable ability to break down filler. Officially quoted filler duration is somewhat biased and based upon clinical study endpoints in the filler approval process, and many practitioners agree that even HA fillers can last many years past their stated duration.
- Affinity for water (hydrophilic properties)—all fillers, especially HA fillers, have a particular affinity for water, which is naturally occurring in human tissue. Depending on a particular filler's hydrophilic nature, a certain amount of water will incorporate itself within the filler. This affinity for water is important to consider depending on the intended effect and injection area. For example, particularly, hydrophilic fillers should never be injected in the area underneath the eyes, an area that is associated with a significant amount of efflux and influx of water. This can create fluctuating infraorbital puffiness that is not aesthetically desireable.
- Amount of Cross-linking—quantifies the cross-linking molecules per every 100 units of HA. The extent of cross-linking results in fillers that feel firmer and leads to enhanced longevity of fillers. Nevertheless, as cross-linking is a non-organic modification of HA, excessive cross-linking may lead to biocompatibility

issues and higher risk of complications such as swelling. The physiologic reason is that alterations increase the risk of foreign body reaction. This immune response may lead to delayed inflammatory reactions such as swelling, granulomas, and nodules.[2,3]

- G-Prime—this refers to the "rheology" of the filler, or its viscosity, flexibility, and elasticity. In other words, it is a value that indicates the runniness and pliability of a filler. A higher G-prime filler tends to be more appropriate in areas where structure and "lifting" are required, whereas a lower G-prime filler is more appropriate in areas where there is more movement or the filler is injected more superficially.
- Reversibility—this refers to the ability to deactivate or dissolve a filler. This is an important factor to consider, as filler that is reversible can be considered safer, given the practitioner's ability to dissolve it should any issues occur. Reversability also tends to be reassuring, as patients are comforted to know that they can have the filler easily removed. The only reversible fillers that are currently available are those that are constructed of HA.
- Biostimulatory properties—fillers that result in biostimulation create lasting, more permanent change by encouraging the body to create more collagen.
- Approved areas of use—depending on the particular location, all available soft tissue fillers have approved techniques and areas of use. Although fillers are frequently used "off-label," it may be important to consider where and how they are approved for injection. Injecting "off-label"—while common—poses some additional liability concerns for the practitioner.
- Risk profile—soft tissue fillers can vary in terms of the potential risks.

PREPROCEDURE CONSIDERATIONS

Introduction

Over the past 20 years, soft tissue fillers have become ubiquitous. Especially with the advent of social media and the newfound focus on photography and online presence, fillers are viewed as a panacea for antiaging.

Although soft tissue fillers can be profound in their ability to reduce signs of aging and positively change anatomic proportionality, they have significant potential side effects and, if not used correctly and in the appropriate patient, can have a range of consequences from relatively harmless to serious and even life-threatening.

As such, it is important to understand the indications for treatment in patient selection, how to guide the patient, and to plan for injection.

Tissue augmentation occurs in a three-dimensional pattern. As such, a complete understanding of the anatomy, tissue resilience, elasticity, and resistance is important to predict the filler's behavior once injected.

Indications

Cosmetic Augmentation

The best-known and most popular application for dermal fillers is cosmetic augmentation. Cosmetic augmentation falls into three main categories; however, these categories are not mutually exclusive.

More traditionally, dermal fillers restore volume to areas where age-related volume loss has occurred. An example of this is a patient who has age-related volume loss in their lateral cheeks and would like the volume restored to where it once was (see Figure 4.2).

A different but overlapping category is the use of dermal filler to camouflage the stigmata of aging related to gravitational changes. The classic example of this is the patient who has jowling along their anterior jawline, in which filler is placed on either side of the jowl to reduce the transitional contour irregularities and shadowing caused by the jowl.

The third broad category of cosmetic augmentation is the use of filler to augment areas of the face or body that have not necessarily lost volume or are suffering from age-related changes, but instead to alter the proportions amongst various related anatomic features. As a younger and younger audience seeks out fillers, this use case comprises a larger percentage of filler patients. An example is nonsurgical rhinoplasty, which uses filler to reshape the nose to a more aesthetically pleasing shape, one that has a better relationship to the surrounding facial features.

Common areas of soft tissue filler augmentation are:

FACE

1. Upper and lower mucosal lip
2. Chin
3. Lateral cheeks
4. Medial cheek
5. Prejowl sulcus (anterior jawline)
6. Posterior jawline
7. Marionette folds

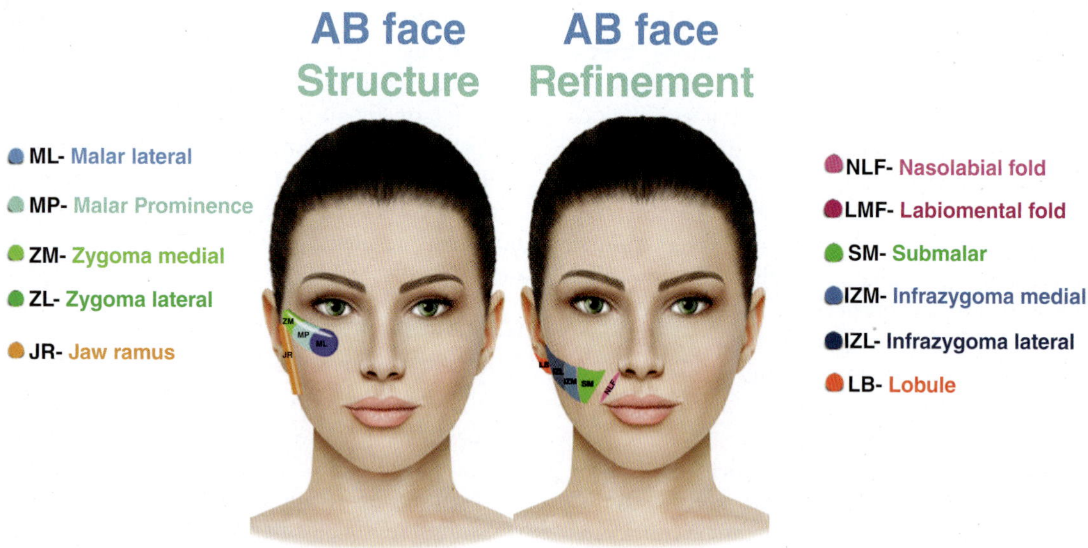

Fig. 4.2 Midface anatomical facial areas that can be treated with fillers. (From Procedures in Cosmetic Dermatology: Soft Tissue Augmentation. Trindade de Almeida, Ada Regina; de Abreu, Luciana; Braz, André Vieira. Published December 31, 2023. © 2024.)

8. Nasolabial folds
9. Brow
10. Superorbital hollows (A-frame deformity)
11. Temples
12. Earlobe rejuvenation
13. Nose
14. Neck and chest
15. Superficial skin wrinkling
16. Periorbital

BODY
1. Buttocks
2. Breasts
3. Hands

Rhytid Correction

Many patients seek dermal fillers to correct skin rhytids. Rhytids are folds/lines within the skin itself, related to generalized skin aging—called *static wrinkles*—or connected to movement in the area that creates a stereotypical pattern of wrinkling—called *dynamic wrinkles*. As a person ages, the dynamic wrinkling of the face corresponds to what eventually develops as the "relaxed skin tension lines" (RSTLs), which are stereotypical patterns of wrinkling that corresponds to natural facial movement patterns.

Dermal fillers can be used to correct rhytids—however, rhytid correction with filler is fraught with complexity and risk and should be cautiously approached. In particular, dynamic wrinkling can create challenges, as the area inherently moves, and filler—being a static gel—can look unnatural. In addition, true rhytids exist in the skin organ itself. Volumizing these lines can pose a challenge, as it requires the placement of filler into an inherently dense dermis. In the author's experience, even the term "dermal fillers" is a misnomer, as fillers are best utilized to volumize when placed in sub-dermal locations.

Disease- or Trauma-Related Revolumization

Some of the first FDA-approvals for dermal fillers were in treating volume loss related to disease. The most well known of these examples is PLLA (Sculptra), which was first FDA-approved for use in patients who suffered facial lipodystrophy (or loss of subdermal fat) usually as a consequence of HIV or AIDS.

Patients that have suffered from longstanding unilateral facial paralysis or paresis are another group that can benefit from the application of filler. In these patients, dramatic differences in movement from one side to the other of the face lead to differences in aging between the two sides, with the unaffected side having a greater amount of gravitational and volumetric aging changes than the affected side. In addition, total denervation of certain larger facial muscles—like the zygomaticus major—can result in significant muscle atrophy, leading to noticeable differences in side-to-side volume.

In patients with more aging on their unaffected side, dermal filler can be used—most commonly in the area of the midcheek and undereye—to restore a semblance of static symmetry to these patients. And in patients who have significant muscle atrophy on their affected side, the filler can be used on this site to restore symmetry as well. Many patients require bilateral filler—in varying areas—to create static symmetry.

Trauma can result in the permanent loss of volume because of tissue death and/or bony depression. In some cases, bones are reset, but in other cases, patients may be left with permanent volume defects from bones that were not reset—either because the risk of resetting these bones was too high or they did not receive the care that was required. In these patients, filler can be used to restore volume.

Congenital defects, such as Parry-Romberg syndrome, hemifacial microsomia, Goldenhar syndrome, and rheumatoid conditions affecting lower jaw growth, unilateral condylar hyperplasia, and so forth, may generate bony and soft tissue contour defects and deformities. Soft tissue augmentation is an essential tool in the cosmetic management of these conditions. Volumization of the affected areas may camouflage or enhance the cosmetic appearance of the patients, creating a significant positive socio-psychologic impact on the patient's life.

Depressed/Atrophic Scarring

Depressed or atrophic scarring is defined as a scar that sits below the normal surface of the skin, giving the skin a sunken or pitted look. The most common cause of this type of scarring is in the aftermath of trauma, severe acne, or a virus causing pox (most commonly varicella or chickenpox).

These scars can cosmetically upset the patient. In these cases, a filler can sometimes be used to successfully volumize within the dermal/subdermal area. This volumization tends to be most impactful after a subcision procedure, which uses a sharp instrument or needle to release any tethered scarring between the dermis and deeper tissues. Even with the use of filler and subcision, atrophic scarring remains a challenging problem, as volumization does not always fully compensate for the inherent thinning of the dermis.

Functional

A relatively newer and controversial use of dermal filler is in support of structure to improve function—particularly around the eye. In patients with ectropion or lax lower lid—whether or not related to disease—filler can be placed to create more structure to support the lid superiorly. Similarly, techniques have been described to use filler to create more support in the brow, thus helping to subtly lift the brow/lid complex and alleviate tissue ptosis in patients with heavy brows and/or lids.

Patient Evaluation

When a patient presents for soft tissue filler, a comprehensive evaluation must be performed.

With the social media boom, filters, and fisheye/zoom dysmorphia, patients increasingly present with misconceptions and unrealistic expectations regarding their aesthetic baseline and possible enhancements. The practitioner's first responsibility is to re-educate patients on the physiology of the facial aging process, and to provide surgical and nonsurgical recommendations within this realistic construct.

As with any invasive procedure, getting a complete medical history is important to ensure the patient's candidacy for safe and effective soft tissue fillers application.

In particular, the following areas of inquiry are particularly important:

- History of general cosmetic procedures and/or procedures in the intended treatment area. This will give the practitioner insight into the patient's exposure to cosmetic procedures and how the patient has tolerated these interventions previously.
- Surgical or nonsurgical interventions in the area of the intended treatment, as this could change the treatment plan. As an example—a patient who has previously had nasal surgery (rhinoplasty) will be at higher risk for nasal soft tissue fillers, given the rearranged vasculature of the nose. As another example—extreme caution must be taken in a patient with a previous implant or permanent filler in the area of intended soft tissue filler treatment, as this is a significant risk of infection with additional manipulation.[4-6]
- Bleeding disorders—as is true with any invasive surgical or nonsurgical procedure, patients with any coagulopathic condition are considered at high risk for complications, including excessive bleeding, bruising, and swelling. In particular, a patient with a

procoagulopathic, proclotting medical condition may be more prone to having severe complications related to blood flow restriction, including skin necrosis or blindness.[7-10]

- Immunosuppression—soft tissue fillers are technically categorized as implants, as they are foreign materials placed into the cutaneous or subcutaneous, deeper tissues. As such, any patient with native, medication- or disease-based immunosuppression is at a higher risk of acute or delayed infection because of bacterial contamination of the filler from skin bacteria. For these reasons, practitioners should use their best judgment in proceeding with injecting immunosuppressed patients.
- Current medications and supplementation—the most important medications and supplements for which to screen are anticoagulants. In addition to prescribed anticoagulants, such as warfarin (Coumadin) and clopidogrel (Plavix), over-the-counter medications that contain ibuprofen or aspirin, and certain herbal supplementation, can create significant anticoagulation.
- Allergies and history of anaphylaxis—allergies to the components within the dermal fillers are rare. In 2017, a retrospective study based on the manufacturer and user facility device experience (MAUDE) revealed 594 (11.82%) cases of allergic reactions from 2007 to 2017.[11] Management of allergic reactions can be treated with antihistaminic medications and dissolving the dermal filler to surgical excision, depending on the type of filler used. A true allergic reaction can be confirmed with an allergy test on the forearm of the patient with an observation period of at least 72 hours.[12]
- Infections near the injection site—active injection on the site is a complete contraindication for the procedure. The procedure must be aborted until full resolution of the infectious process is resolved. Any inflammatory or infective cutaneous conditions such as dermatitis, rosacea, and Herpes virus should be treated and enable enough healing time to restore natural skin protective function.[13]
- Infectious complications are the leading cause of adverse events. Meticulous skin disinfection and field preparation are essential to decrease bacterial inosculation to deep tissues.[12] Bacterial biofilm growth is associated with late inflammatory reactions and nodule formation. In vitro studies revealed that repeated passes significantly increase *Streptococcus epidermidis* biofilm growth through a contaminated area. In addition, microbiome analysis detected predominance in *Pseudomonas*, *Staphylococcus*, and *Propionibacterium*, regardless of filler type.[12,14]
- Psychologic stability and ability to follow directions—as with any other surgical procedure, patient screening and psychologic evaluation before cosmetic procedures is a crucial step. The prevalence of psychiatric disorders in cosmetic surgery patients, such as body dysmorphic disease, ranges from 4% to 57%. It is essential to evaluate the motivation and expectations of the patient. In addition, cooperation with preoperative and postoperative instructions is essential for treatment success and complications avoidance.[15,16]
- Oral and sinus evaluation—complete oral health history will give the practitioner a perspective on the patient's oral health habits and possible subclinical infections. Cases with facial odontogenic cellulitis after recent filler injections have been published, where the actual etiology of the cellulitis was an infected tooth. In addition, a complicated sinus infection diagnosis may challenge the diagnosis and mimic postoperative filler complications.[5]
- COVID vaccination—delayed inflammatory response on the injected areas associated with covid vaccination has been well documented. Inflammatory reactions take place on average after 2 to 10 days postvaccination. The mechanism of action of delayed inflammatory responses is not well understood. Still, it is thought to be caused by the binding and blockade of angiotensin-2 converting enzyme receptors, which are targeted by the SARS-CoV-2 virus spike protein for access into the cells. Clinically, it can be presented as diffuse or localized edema with symptomatic and inflammatory erythematous papules and nodules.[17,18]
- The inflammatory reaction is usually self-limiting with a resolution time of approximately 1 to 7 days, but it can be mitigated by high-dose steroid therapy, angiotensin-converting enzyme inhibitors, or dissolution of the filler by intralesional hyaluronidase injection.[19]

A systematic physical evaluation of the skin, muscle, deep and superficial fat compartments, facial bones, and the regional aging changes of each anatomic area and layer will define the optimal treatment and outcome expectations.

There are facial physical phenotipic characteristics that distinguish feminine from masculine features.

Generally, females have a more oval shape with wider intermalar distance than intergonial distance. In counterpart, males tend to have a similar intermalar and gonial distance, with a strong jawline definition. In addition, the concept of beauty also varies between ethnicities.

More subjectively, it is critical that a practitioner use their best judgment regarding the psychologic and emotional readiness of any patient who presents for soft tissue fillers. Particularly with patients who present for cosmetic enhancement, close attention must be paid to the patient's motives and expectations in receiving these fillers. Practitioners should use extra care in patients who seem to be generally unhappy or depressed or otherwise seem to be trying to solve baseline emotional problems with cosmetic procedures. Similarly, patients with unrealistic expectations about the anticipated change should be counseled extensively regarding the appropriate expectations. If the physician has any suspicion on the practitioner's part of excessive expectations or inappropriate motivation, it is always best to counsel the patient to receive a psychologic evaluation before following up on possible procedures.

PROCEDURAL TECHNIQUES

Informed Consent

Before injection of any soft tissue filler, a discussion must be held with the patient that reviews the relevant risks and expectations of the fillers. A document must be signed by the patient (or their guardian) indicating that these risks were discussed and understood. It is beyond the scope to describe the content of informed consent. Nevertheless, a comprehensive description of possible complications must be described in layman's terminology.

Mirror

Providing a mirror to the patient and direct identification of the concerned anatomic area by the patient is a powerful method to determine the patient desires and expectations objectively. Understanding the patient aesthetic and beauty concepts is key to success.

Nowadays, computed aid simulation is an instrument that allows the physician to recreate a three-dimensional virtual surface of the existing patient soft tissue anatomy. This technology consists of optical facial scanning of the treating area. Then the document is transported into a virtual platform where a three-dimensional model is created.

TABLE 4.5 Filler Selection According to the Anatomic Area

Location	Filler
Brow augmentation	Restylane-L Belotero balance
Tear through and A-frame deformity	Restylane-L Belotero balance
Malar augmentation	Restylane lyft Restylane contour, RHA-4, Juvederm Volluma
Lip augmentation	Restylane Kysse Restylane Refyne Versa lips Juvederm Ultra
Nasolabial folds	Juverderm Ultra Juvederm Ultra Plus Juvederm Vollure Restylane Refyne Restylane Defyne RHA-3
Fine lines	RHA-2 Belotero Balance
Nonsurgical rhinoplasty	Restylane Lyft Restylane-L

RHA, Resilient hyaluronic acid.

The virtual model can be analyzed, including texture, color, pigmentations, contours, and volumes. The soft tissues can be modified, allowing the physician to measure the soft tissue transformation objectively. The virtual transformation is shared with the patient, allowing them to visualize and communicate the expected outcome. The disadvantage is the cost of the software and optical scanner.

Preparation and Set-Up

Choose the right filler. The selection of the dermal filler with the optimal rheology properties for each anatomic area and desired treatment is crucial for optimal results and avoidance of complications (Table 4.5).

The preoperative photograph is an essential part of the treatment. The clinical photographs should be taken with a consistent and systematic approach with high-quality cameras and studio lighting. The practitioner should avoid taking photos for medical purposes with phone cameras because of the high degree of facial deformation and fish-eye effect.

High-quality photographs will allow the practitioner to appreciate contour changes, shadows, fine lines and creases, vascularity, and colors.

Recommended photographs are:

1. Frontal
   a. Rest
   b. Smile

c. Raised brows
d. Frowning
e. Eyes (at rest and sextants)
f. Smiling
g. Bunny lines
h. Clenching
i. Platysma activation (depressing the corners of the mouth).

2. Oblique 3/4 (bilateral)
3. Lateral (at rest and smiling)
4. Bird view
5. Worm's view.

In general, clinical photography will:

1. Demonstrate and guide the patient on the diagnosis, treatment, and expectations.
2. Decrease misunderstandings and patient disappointment.
3. Demonstrate subtle changes after the treatment.
4. Provide objective and critical practitioner observation of their results.
5. Provide medico-legal evidence.

The only photos you will regret are those you never took.

Patient Prep and Drape

As with any surgical procedure, adequate skin disinfection is imperative. The patient must be instructed not to wear any cosmetic products.

The skin must be cleaned and disinfected. Disinfection agents such as isopropyl alcohol, chlorhexidine gluconate, povidone-iodine, chloroxylenol, and benzalkonium chloride can be used.

An aseptic technique will significantly minimize the risk of cross-contamination. Similarly, the needle or cannula must be treated with a sterile technique to avoid contamination and bacterial inoculation into the tissues. If the cannula or needle gets contaminated, immediate replacement is advised.[13]

Different Mixtures

The temples, perioral, and undereye areas are the most frequently treated areas with fillers mixed with different substances.

In 2019, Libby et al. realized a survey demonstrating the prevalence of mixing fillers among American Society for Dermatologic Surgery members.[20]

Among the essential factors when mixing the fillers with different substances, the rheologic properties modification, precisely the viscosity, is highly important. Decreasing the viscosity will decrease the extraction force for volume augmentation.

Filler blending is used for deep filler placement to soften volume augmentation and decrease the risk of lumps and bumps secondary to filler conglomeration. Sterile water, normal saline, lidocaine, or lidocaine with epinephrine are the most frequently used.[20,21]

One main characteristic of HA fillers is biologic reabsorption and secondary volume loss. Many practitioners compensate for this by adding CaHA filler into the HA filler.[20,22,23]

Procedural Steps

Cannula versus needle—in general, the two injection methods have been studied in matters of safety, soft tissue plane precision, and recommended anatomic area of injection.

Cannula injection has increased the precision of the intended plane of implantation. This has been confirmed in cadaveric and ultrasound-guided studies where filler injection was compared, and cannulas resulted in a more precise injection of material than needles.[24,25]

Furthermore, in a retrospective cohort study, 370 dermatologists with a mean practice of 20 years reported 1.7 million dermal filler syringes injected from August 2018 to 2019.[26]

The risk of occlusion with dermal filler using a needle was 1 occlusion per 6410 per 1-mL syringe and 1 per 40,882 with cannulas, with a total of 77.1% lower odds for vascular compromise.

Vascular occlusion and significant complications are potentially decreased with the use of microcannulas. Moreover, the gauge of the needles and cannulas also plays an essential factor in the risk of vascular penetration. The smaller the gauge, the less force is needed to injure a vessel wall. Interestingly, there is no significant difference in arterial penetration comparing 27-gauge needles and cannulas.[27]

Types of injection techniques (see Figure 4.3):

1. Linear threading.
2. Depot/serial puncture
3. Fanning
4. Cross-hatching
5. Tower technique

Comfort measures:

a. Icing

Icing the injection will reduce blood flow by vasoconstriction. Tissue reduction decreases

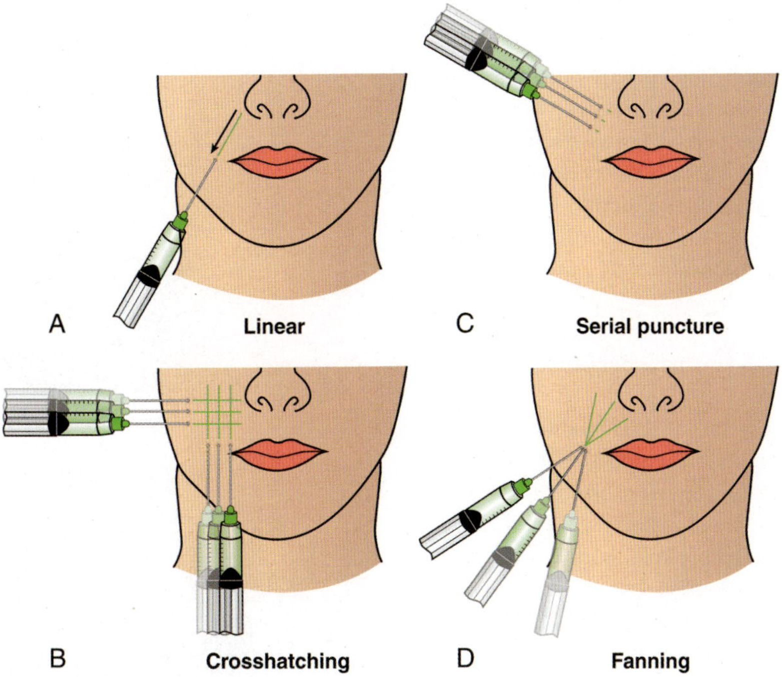

Fig. 4.3 Illustration of injection techniques. (From ENT Secrets. Fairmont, Isabel, MD, MS; Ferril, Geoffrey, MD. Published December 31, 2022. © 2023.)

cellular metabolism and catecholamine levels and increases endorphin concentrations. This will lead to delayed pain signal transmission to the central nervous system.[28-31]

Moreover, multiple studies demonstrate decreased pain perception upon injection. In addition, comparative studies have proved a significant decrease in bruising within the two groups.[30]

b. Vibrational therapy and stress ball

Vibrational analgesia, first described in 1965 by Melzack, is a nondrug stimulation to reduce pain associated with injections. Continuous vibration stimulates A-β fibers decreasing the conduction of pain through the C fibers into the central nervous system.[32-34]

c. Numbing

Local anesthesia can substantially decrease pain and discomfort. Anesthetics agents can be applied locally on creams, ointments, and gels. One con of topical anesthesia is the risk of contact dermatitis and allergic reactions to the conservatives and other components of anesthetic agents.

It is paramount to eliminate any residual topical agent and perform thorough facial disinfection before the injection to avoid, as mentioned earlier, complications such as bacterial inosculation, filler contamination, and delayed inflammatory responses.

Local anesthesia infiltration is another analgesic option. Unfortunately, tissue distortion is the highest disadvantage. Regional facial blocks with minimal infiltration are recommended to decrease soft tissue distortion. In addition, if local anesthesia with vasoconstriction is used, it can obscure the diagnosis of one of the most disastrous complications, vascular obstruction.

POSTPROCEDURE CONSIDERATIONS

General recommendations are:

Immediate:

1. Avoid touching the area
2. Avoid cosmetic products for at least 24 hours
3. Avoid nonsteroidal antiinflammatory drugs and anticoagulants for 24 hours
4. No facial waxing, peels, or any skin treatment
5. Do not massage in the area

6. Avoid sun exposure
7. Avoid intense exercise
8. In case of soreness, the patient can take a mild analgesic such as acetaminophen
9. Patients with history of herpes simplex virus must start antiviral prophylaxis 2 days before the procedure and continue antiviral therapy for 5 to 7 days
10. Keep your face clean and wash with a gentle soap
11. Avoid high-sodium food

After 24 hours

1. Apply sunblock
2. In case of bruising, you may apply arnica ointment/pills
3. The patient can restart anticoagulants

It is highly recommended and emphasized to the patient the presence of postinjection swelling, bruising, and asymmetries. Early reintervention to correct pseudoasymmetries secondary to residual swelling may lead to unfavorable outcomes and patient displeasure.

The follow-up appointments should take place after 2 weeks to allow sufficient healing time.

COMPLICATIONS AND OUTCOMES

Introduction

The overarching goal of any cosmetic treatment—soft tissue fillers included—is to create a cosmetic change perceived as positive by the patient (with the assumption that the patient has reasonable, nondistorted expectations) (see Figure 4.4). As discussed throughout this chapter, there is a multitude of soft tissue filler options from which to choose and countless potential applications throughout the human body.

Although the allure of soft tissue fillers is the ability to quickly, sometimes instantaneously, make a change—as with any medical treatment, there are side effects, risks, and potentially severe complications that need to be appreciated and for which the practitioner must mitigate.

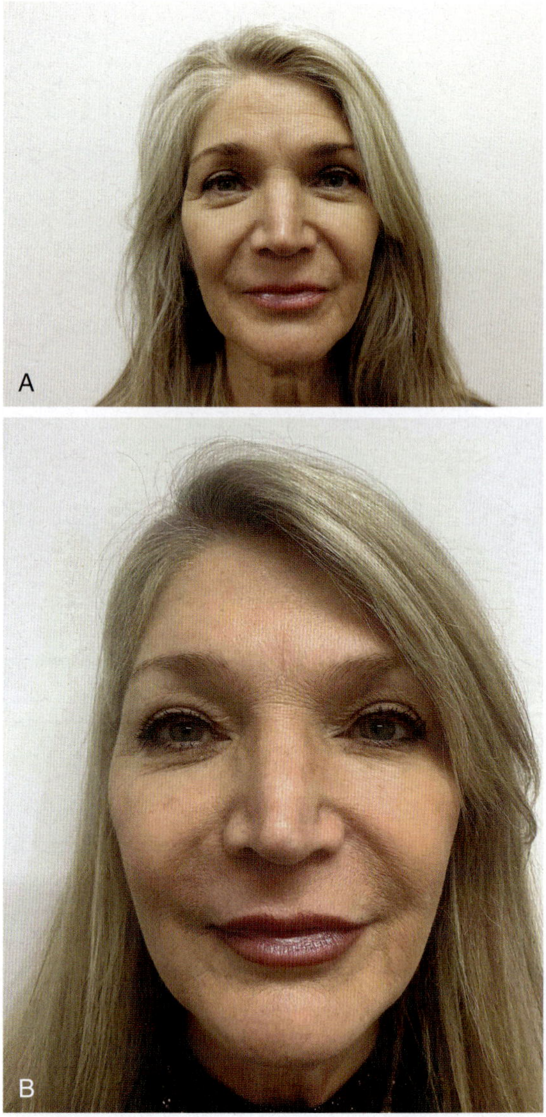

Fig. 4.4 Combination of higher G-prime hyaluronic acid (HA) fillers along the malar cheeks and lateral jawline with lower G-prime HA fillers in the nasolabial folds and marionettes to achieve a global aesthetic improvement. (A) Patient's baseline. (B) Two weeks after combination of higher G-prime hyaluronic acid (HA) fillers along the malar cheeks and lateral jawline with lower G-prime HA fillers in the nasolabial folds and marionettes. (Copyright Omer Ibrahim, MD)

PATIENT DISTASTE

Mitigation—do less and titrate up. It is wise to perform soft augmentation progressively and with small doses. Immediate inflammatory response after the injection may cause tissue deformation, camouflaging irregularities, or obscuring contour transitions during the treatment. In these circumstances, and if any uncertainty, a conservative treatment allows the practitioner to reevaluate the contours after the postoperative swelling resolves and retreats if necessary.

Furthermore, patients that want conservative and subtle changes should be treated cautiously. Thorough communication with the patient is vital. It is essential to understand the patient's expectations and guide the patient on possible outcomes, treatment plans, the possibility of undertreatment, and how it will be managed. In order words, good practitioner-patient communication is the key to safe and satisfied patients.

With the inclusion of new materials and techniques and perception shifting either from the patient, practitioner, or both, there is a predisposition to overfilled and unaesthetic outcomes.

It is better to err and undertreat than overfill and have a displeased patient who does not trust the practitioner anymore. The main goal is a natural, pleasant result.

DISCOMFORT/PAIN

Nowadays, most HA filler contains lidocaine within their formulation, diminishing discomfort and injection pain. It has been proven that lidocaine does not affect the efficiency and longevity of the filler but may affect its viscosity.[3]

Other maneuvers may include the application of topical anesthesia, local anesthesia injection, and icing the injection site before the procedure.

Furthermore, removing all traces of topical anesthesia and performing meticulous facial disinfection before the injection is vital. Suppose the practitioner decides to inject local anesthesia. In that case, performing regional facial blocks and keeping the dose as minimum as possible to avoid soft tissue distortion by infiltrating the surrounding tissues is recommended.

DISCOLORATIONS

The Tyndall effect or Tyndall phenomenon was described in the 19th century by the Irish physicist John Tyndall. It is defined by the scattering of a light beam when it passes through a colloidal medium. A colloid can be either aerosols, emulsions, sols, or gels. The light deviated from its original trajectory, creating a characteristic blue hue.[35]

This phenomenon can be observed when fillers are injected in a superficial layer or large boluses are injected into a thin skin area, allowing daylight to go across the skin into the filler and then scatter. These visible discolorations can be significantly upsetting and distressing for the patients.

Preoperatively, evaluation of the skin thickness of the injected area is fundamental to adequately inject into deeper layers and avoid this complication. The most frequent site is the tear trough, perioral regions, and hands.[36]

The treatment is limited to massaging, hyaluronidase injections, or direct excision.

BRUISING AND SWELLING

Postinjection bruising and swelling will depend on the injection technique, vasculature of the injection site, the anatomic area, injected, and the patient natural inflammatory response. Fortunately, postinjection bruising and swelling are self-limiting and usually resolve within 2 to 5 days.

Delayed swelling and edema can be associated with the type of filler used. HA fillers are hydrophilic. Fillers with higher concentrations of HA recruit higher amounts of water to reach homeostasis.

In addition, HA fillers with cross-linked and higher HA concentrations placed in deeper layers have been reported to cause a late-onset inflammatory reaction.

The disadvantage with high cross-linked concentrations is that enzymatic dissolution by hyaluronidase could be insufficient, leaving subclinical residues of HA and, if necessary, requiring repeated injections to dissolve the filler fully.

MIGRATION

In general, HA fillers are biodegradable and designed to last 12 to 18 months. Multiple studies have demonstrated higher longevity rates, up to 12 years. Furthermore, this longer life span is not only associated with the type of filler injected but also with the anatomic area where it was injected.[37,38]

There are three types of migration:

1. Immediate migration. Injection of large volumes, inadequate filler selection, excessive injection force, repeated injections on an anatomic site, excessive postinjection massage, and poor injection technique will promote the migration of the filler into adjacent tissues through the path of less resistance.
2. Pseudomigration (not a real migration). As we know, soft tissue aging is accompanied by positional and volumetric tissue changes into an inferior-medial vector. In addition, physiologic aging changes include loss of skin elasticity, muscle atrophy, bone resorption, volume shifting, panfacial fat atrophy, etc. These slow and dynamic changes may contribute to spatial position alterations compared to its original

injection location. If the facial tissues change and relocate by nature, why would the filler stay static in a determined position?

3. Delayed migration. There is not enough scientific evidence that confirms delayed migration. Muscle dynamics may contribute to the displacement of the fillers into a more static facial space. Most published studies suspect migration without a systematic methodology that objectively confirms this phenomenon in a long-term observational study. In 2022, Robert Master, based on MRI studies, showed evidence of different filler longevity on different anatomic sites and stable dimensional and topographic location of the filler after 27 months of the initial treatment.[38]

ALLERGIC REACTIONS

Allergic reactions are possible but extremely rare. Type I hypersensitivity reactions to the components within the dermal fillers are rare. In 2017, a retrospective study based on MAUDE revealed 594 (11.82%) cases of allergic reactions from 2007 to 2017.[11] Most publications with HA fillers hypersensitive reactions do not report direct skin allergy test confirmation of a genuine allergic reaction.

Local urticaria, swelling, and angioedema are signs of an allergic reaction. The treatment includes antihistaminic medications, steroids, allergy skin tests, hyaluronidase injections, and direct excision.

SKIN NECROSIS

This disastrous complication may lead to complex scarring and advanced surgical reconstruction techniques. In general, the incidence of vascular occlusion with fillers is 3 in 1000 injections and 3–9 in 10,000 injections.[10,39,40] The higher incidence of vascular complications is the nose and nasolabial fold (52%), forehead and eyebrows (12.1%), glabella (8.2%), lower eyelid and tear through (7.1%), cheeks (7.1%), lips (6.2%), temporal region (16%), perioral (2.7%), and lastly the chin (2.5%).[8]

Immediate signs of vascular compromise include ischemia, blanching, numbness, pain, mottling, and blistering in delayed cases.

Different protocols have been published:[41]

1. Early detection
2. Treat within 90 minutes
3. Warm compress and massage 5 to 10 minutes every 30 to 60 minutes (avoid burning the skin)
4. High-dose hyaluronidase injections of 500 to 1500 IU and repeat every 24 hours as needed
5. Aspirin two pills of 325 mg daily for 1 week
6. Nitroglycerin pastes two to three times daily until improvement noted
7. Hyperbaric oxygen
8. Daily follow-up
9. Routine wound care (daily dressings, antibiotic ointment)
10. Adequate wound and patient hydration
11. Wound debridement as needed

Recommendations before any injections include:

1. Injection of <0.1 cc per injection
2. Retrograde injection
3. Aspiration
4. Low injection pressure
5. Use of cannulas
6. Knowledge of the anatomic area
7. Possible use of lidocaine with epinephrine

BLINDNESS

Blindness is one of the most catastrophic complications. With the increased use worldwide, serious complications with permanent sequela are increasing in prevalence. In 2019, in a study of prevalence of blindness, the associated filler was used, the anatomic areas where injected.[42]

Filler Type	Number of Cases	Percentage
Autologous fat	90	47
Hyaluronic acid	53	28
Others (PLLA, Polyalkylimide, Polymethyl-metracrylate microspheres)	40	21
Calcium hydroxylapatite	7	4

The areas with a higher risk of postfiller injection blindness are the glabellar complex, nose, nasolabial fold, forehead, and temple.[42]

It has been noted that the prevalence of diffuse occlusion of the ophthalmic artery constriction is more prevalent with autologous fat injection. The rationale is the bigger particle size compared to HA. HA fillers particles have a 400-μm size particle.[42-44]

HA seems to show a higher prevalence of central retinal artery blockage, which has a caliber of approximately

160 μm. In addition, some studies demonstrated a poorer prognosis when blindness occurs secondary to fat graft injections.[42,44]

Recommended management:[45]

- Abort the procedure immediately
- Hyaluronidase injection (retrobulbar) 300 to 600 units (27–30 gauge 1.5-inch needle)
- Aspirin 325 mg two tabs chewed
- Hot pads
- Nitropaste gel
- Ocular massage
- Emergency room transportation
- Ophthalmology consultation within 90 minutes (retina specialist)
- Continuous assessment to rule out a cerebrovascular accident

Unfortunately, cadaveric studies have not demonstrated the ability to cross the dural sheath of the optic bundle, suggesting that retrobulbar injection of hyaluronidase would be ineffective in case of cerebrovascular accident. Immediate neurosurgical, neurology, and interventional radiology consultation would be advised.[46]

Preventive measurements:

1. Injection of <0.1 cc per injection
2. Retrograde injection
3. Aspiration
4. Low injection pressure
5. Use of cannulas
6. Knowledge of the anatomic area
7. Possible use of lidocaine with epinephrine

LYMPHATIC DISRUPTION

Anatomically, the lymphatic capillaries and precollectors are located in the dermis. Later, the drainage continues into the fat layer and the deep lymphatic vessels located within the musculoaponeurotic system.[47]

In the midface, three main lymphatic drainage paths exist. The medial portion of the lower eyelid creates a superficial system than runs inferiorly into the nasolabial junction and drains into the submandibular lymph nodes, and the lateral portion forms both superficial and deep systems, which fuse and drain into the preauricular and parotid lymph nodes. The third system runs deep into the orbicularis oculi muscle and drains to the lateral system.[47]

Fillers cause volumetric tridimensional displacement of the tissues. Volumetric changes may displace and cause partial or total occlusion of the lymphatic precollector lymphatic vessels.

Other risk factors for persistent edema are:[48]

1. Female
2. A previous surgical procedure in the affected area
3. History of previous filler injections
4. History of allergies
5. History of eyelid edema
6. Juvéderm HA fillers (higher water affinity)
7. Large volumes of filler injected
8. Age (50–60 years old)

The management of this complication can be frustrating for the patient and the physician. Persistent edema can last up to 6 months without significant improvement. Definitive management includes hyaluronidase injections in the case of HA fillers, direct excision, and radiofrequency therapy.

REFERENCES

1. Kontis TC, Rivkin A. The history of injectable facial fillers. *Facial Plast Surg*. 2009;25(2):67-72.
2. *Hyaluronan: Structure and Physical Properties*. Available at: https://www.glycoforum.gr.jp/article/01A2.html. Accessed October 8, 2022.
3. Tezel A, Fredrickson GH. The science of hyaluronic acid dermal fillers. *J Cosmet Laser Ther*. 2008;10(1):35-42.
4. Yu JTS, Peng L, Ataullah S. Chronic eyelid edema following periocular hyaluronic acid filler treatment. *Ophthalmic Plast Reconstr Surg*. 2017;33(6):e139-e140.
5. Decates TS, Kruijt Spanjer EC, Saini R, Velthuis PJ, Niessen FM. Unilateral facial edema after filler injection of the lower eyelid. *Dermatol Ther*. 2020;33(4):e13539.
6. Iverson SM, Patel RM. Dermal filler-associated malar edema: treatment of a persistent adverse effect. *Orbit (London)*. 2017;36(6):473-475.
7. Abduljabbar MH, Basendwh MA. Complications of hyaluronic acid fillers and their managements. *J Dermatol Dermatol Surg*. 2016;20(2):100-106.
8. Oranges CM, Brucato D, Schaefer DJ, Kalbermatten DF, Harder Y. Complications of nonpermanent facial fillers: a systematic review. *Plast Reconstr Surg Glob Open*. 2021;9(10):e3851.
9. Guthrie A, Kadakia S, Cranford J, Sawhney R, Ducic Y. A review of complications and their treatments in facial aesthetic surgery. *Am J Cosmet Surg*. 2017;34(2):73-80.
10. Hwang CJ. Periorbital injectables: understanding and avoiding complications. *J Cutan Aesthet Surg*. 2016;9(2):73-79.

11. Povolotskiy R, Oleck NC, Hatzis CM, Paskhover B. Adverse events associated with aesthetic dermal fillers: a 10-year retrospective study of FDA data. *Am J Cosmet Surg*. 2018;35(3):143-151.
12. Marusza W, Olszanski R, Sierdzinski J, et al. Treatment of late bacterial infections resulting from soft-tissue filler injections. *Infect Drug Resist*. 2019;12:469-480.
13. Murthy R, Eccleston D, Mckeown D, Parikh A, Shotter S. Improving aseptic injection standards in aesthetic clinical practice. *Dermatol Ther*. 2021;34(1):e14416.
14. Saththianathan M, Johani K, Taylor A, et al. The role of bacterial biofilm in adverse soft-tissue filler reactions: a combined laboratory and clinical study. *Plast Reconstr Surg*. 2017;139(3):613-621.
15. Bascarane S, Kuppili PP, Menon V. Psychiatric Assessment in Cosmetic Surgery Bascarane Psychiatric assessment and management of clients undergoing cosmetic surgery: overview and need for an integrated approach. *Indian J Plast Surg*. 2021;54(1):8-19.
16. *Psychological Assessment of Cosmetic Surgery Patients*. Plastic Surgery Key. Available at: https://plasticsurgerykey.com/psychological-assessment-of-cosmetic-surgery-patients/. Accessed October 15, 2022.
17. Munavalli GG, Guthridge R, Knutsen-Larson S, Brodsky A, Matthew E, Landau M. COVID-19/SARS-CoV-2 virus spike protein-related delayed inflammatory reaction to hyaluronic acid dermal fillers: a challenging clinical conundrum in diagnosis and treatment. *Arch Dermatol Res*. 2022;314(1):1-15.
18. Funt DK. Treatment of delayed-onset inflammatory reactions to hyaluronic acid filler: an algorithmic approach. *Plast Reconstr Surg Glob Open*. 2022;10(6):e4362.
19. Funt DK. Treatment of delayed-onset inflammatory reactions to hyaluronic acid filler: an algorithmic approach. *Plast Reconstr Surg Glob Open*. 2022;10(6):e4362.
20. Libby TJ, Williams RF, el Habr C, Tinklepaugh A, Ciocon D. Mixing of injectable fillers: a national survey. *Dermatol Surg*. 2019;45(1):117-123.
21. Raspaldo H, de Boulle K, Levy PM. Longevity of effects of hyaluronic acid plus lidocaine facial filler. *J Cosmet Dermatol*. 2010;9(1):11-15.
22. Chang JW, Koo WY, Kim EK, Lee SW, Lee JH. Facial rejuvenation using a mixture of calcium hydroxylapatite filler and hyaluronic acid filler. *J Craniofac Surg*. 2020;31(1):e18-e21.
23. de Almeida AT, Figueredo V, da Cunha ALG, et al. Consensus recommendations for the use of hyperdiluted calcium hydroxyapatite (Radiesse) as a face and body biostimulatory agent. *Plast Reconstr Surg Glob Open*. 2019;7(3):e2160.
24. van Loghem JAJ, Humzah D, Kerscher M. Cannula versus sharp needle for placement of soft tissue fillers: an observational cadaver study. *Aesthet Surg J*. 2017;38(1):73-88.
25. Iwayama T, Hashikawa K, Osaki T, Yamashiro K, Horita N, Fukumoto T. Ultrasonography-guided cannula method for hyaluronic acid filler injection with evaluation using laser speckle flowgraphy. *Plast Reconstr Surg Glob Open*. 2018;6(4):e1776.
26. Alam M, Kakar R, Dover JS, et al. Rates of vascular occlusion associated with using needles vs cannulas for filler injection. *JAMA Dermatol*. 2021;157(2):174-180.
27. Pavicic T, Webb KL, Frank K, Gotkin RH, Tamura B, Cotofana S. Arterial wall penetration forces in needles versus cannulas. *Plast Reconstr Surg*. 2019;143(3):504E-512E.
28. Wang H, Guan J, Zhang X, et al. Effect of cold application on pain and bruising in patients with subcutaneous injection of low-molecular-weight heparin: a meta-analysis. *Clin Appl Thromb Hemost*. 2020;26:1076029620905349.
29. Algafly AA, George KP. The effect of cryotherapy on nerve conduction velocity, pain threshold and pain tolerance. *Br J Sports Med*. 2007;41(6):365-369.
30. Kuzu N, Ucar H. The effect of cold on the occurrence of bruising, haematoma and pain at the injection site in subcutaneous low molecular weight heparin. *Int J Nurs Stud*. 2001;38(1):51-59.
31. Smith KC, Comite SL, Storwick GS. Ice minimizes discomfort associated with injection of botulinum toxin type A for the treatment of palmar and plantar hyperhidrosis. *Dermatol Surg*. 2007;33(suppl 1):S88-S91.
32. Kuwahara H, Ogawa R. Using a vibration device to ease pain during facial needling and injection. *Eplasty*. 2016;16:e9.
33. Mally P, Czyz CN, Chan NJ, Wulc AE. Vibration anesthesia for the reduction of pain with facial dermal filler injections. *Aesthetic Plast Surg*. 2014;38(2):413-418.
34. Sharma P, Czyz CN, Wulc AE. Investigating the efficacy of vibration anesthesia to reduce pain from cosmetic botulinum toxin injections. *Aesthet Surg J*. 2011;31(8):966-971.
35. King M. Management of Tyndall effect. *J Clin Aesthet Dermatol*. 2016;9(11):E6. Accessed October 16, 2022.
36. Delorenzi C. Complications of injectable fillers, part I. *Aesthet Surg J*. 2013;33(4):561-575.
37. Master M. Hyaluronic acid filler longevity and localization: magnetic resonance imaging evidence. *Plast Reconstr Surg*. 2021:147:50E-53E.
38. Master M, Roberts S. Long-term MRI follow-up of hyaluronic acid dermal filler. *Plast Reconstr Surg Glob Open*. 2022;10(4):E4252.
39. Halepas S, Peters SM, Goldsmith JL, Ferneini EM. Vascular compromise after soft tissue facial fillers: case

report and review of current treatment protocols. *J Oral Maxillofac Surg*. 2020;78(3):440-445.

40. Beleznay K, Humphrey S, Carruthers JD, Carruthers A. Vascular compromise from soft tissue augmentation: experience with 12 cases and recommendations for optimal outcomes. *J Clin Aesthet Dermatol*. 2014;7(9):37-43. Available at: https://pubmed.ncbi.nlm.nih.gov/25276276/. Accessed October 18, 2022.
41. Cohen JL, Biesman BS, Dayan SH, et al. Treatment of hyaluronic acid filler-induced impending necrosis with hyaluronidase: consensus recommendations. *Aesthet Surg J*. 2015;35(7):844-849.
42. Chatrath V, Banerjee PS, Goodman GJ, Rahman E. Soft-tissue filler-associated blindness: a systematic review of case reports and case series. *Plast Reconstr Surg Glob Open*. 2019;7(4):e2173.
43. Kim YK, Jung C, Woo SJ, Park KH. Cerebral angiographic findings of cosmetic facial filler-related ophthalmic and retinal artery occlusion. *J Korean Med Sci*. 2015;30(12):1847-1855.
44. Chen Y, Wang W, Li J, Yu Y, Li L, Lu N. Fundus artery occlusion caused by cosmetic facial injections. *Chin Med J (Engl)*. 2014;127(8):1434-1437. Available at: https://pubmed.ncbi.nlm.nih.gov/24762584/. Accessed October 18, 2022.
45. Chesnut C. Restoration of visual loss with retrobulbar hyaluronidase injection after hyaluronic acid filler. *Dermatol Surg*. 2018;44(3):435-437.
46. Paap MK, Milman T, Ugradar S, Silkiss RZ. Assessing retrobulbar hyaluronidase as a treatment for filler-induced blindness in a cadaver model. *Plast Reconstr Surg*. 2019; 144(2):315-320.
47. Lamb JP, Surek CC, eds. Chapter 2: The Lymphatic Anatomy of the Lower Eyelid and the Malar Region of the Face. In: *Facial Volumization: An Anatomic Approach*. New York: Thieme Medical Publishers; 2017.
48. Griepentrog GJ, Lucarelli MJ, Burkat CN, Lemke BN, Rose JG. Periorbital edema following hyaluronic acid gel injection: a retrospective review. *Am J Cosmet Surg*. 2011;28(4):251-254.

5

Laser Resurfacing*

Steven R. Cohen, Ahmad N. Saad, Tracy Leong, and E. Victor Ross

BRIEF INTRODUCTION

A logical approach to rejuvenation follows an understanding of skin anatomy and physiology, as they relate to skin aging. Any assessment of the face should include the surface, where sun and aging result in pigment inhomogeneities, wrinkles, and telangiectasia. Epidermal changes include basilar hyperpigmentation, hyperkeratosis, and thinning of the "living" portion of the epidermis. Another component of skin aging derives from changes in the dermis, where decreased glycosaminoglycans (GAGs), decreased elastin fibers, and changes in the character of collagen result in fine lines, sallowness, and eventually in cobblestoning of the skin. Microscopically, the changes present as solar elastosis. Also, weakened blood vessels dilate and present as telangiectasia. In some patients, hyperpigmentation results from both dermal and epidermal pigment dyschromias. The third component of aging skin results from bone regression, weakening of connections from the hypodermis to the surface, and volume loss.[1,2]

Most energy-based interventions address one or more of these components of skin aging.

Epidermal pigmentation can be addressed by pigment-specific lasers or laser peels. In the first case, visible light is used to selectively heat the epidermis. Proper parameter selection allows for preferential targeting of the hyperpigmented lesion, whereas the normal background "innocent" bystander skin is unharmed. Traditional "nonfractional" laser peels, on the other hand, target water and therefore heat a confluent "slab" of the uppermost skin. The depths of ablation of heating are determined by wavelength, power density, fluence, and pulse-width.[1]

Blood vessels are heated by three broad categories of devices: (a) visible light technologies (520–600 nm); (b) near-infrared I (NIR I) technologies (755, 800 nm); and (c) NIR II (940, 980, 1064 nm). The former is associated with very strong hemoglobin (HgB) and melanin heating, the second by moderate HgB and melanin heating, and the third by moderate HgB heating but relatively weak melanin heating. Deep-heating devices have included laser, halogen lamps, xenon flash lamps with long wavelength cut-off filters, radiofrequency (RF), ultrasound (US), and combination technologies.[3]

The word "laser" is an acronym for the term light amplification by stimulated emission of radiation. The device itself consists of an energy source, a laser medium, and a resonating tube. The medium can be a gas, liquid, or solid, and this will often be used to name the type of laser (e.g., ruby laser and CO_2 laser). The light emitted is composed of photons that travel in the same direction, making laser light highly directional. Laser light is monochromatic, which means that all photons have the same wavelength. By contrast, intense pulsed light (IPL) consists of many different wavelengths. The specific wavelength of each laser will determine how the laser beam interacts with tissue. The light can be reflected by tissue, scattered by the tissue, or transmitted through tissue. The intention is that the laser light be absorbed by a specific target tissue (the "chromophore"). The mechanism by which lasers are used to target specific tissue is called *selective photothermolysis* (SPT; photo = light; thermolysis = decomposition by heat).[4]

*Adapted from: Steven R. Cohen, Ahmad N. Saad, Tracy Leong, and E. Victor Ross; Plastic Surgery, Volume 2: Aesthetic Surgery, Fourth Edition

Lasers can be broadly broken into two categories, ablative and nonablative. Until recently, ablative (meaning "to remove") lasers have been the "gold standard" of care for wrinkle reduction. The carbon dioxide laser with a wavelength of 10,600 nm and the Er : YAG (erbium-doped yttrium aluminum garnet) with a wavelength of 2940 nm are mainstays of ablative laser treatment. A relative newcomer is Er : YSGG (erbium: yttrium–scandium–gallium–garnet) (at 2790 nm).[5] With each of these lasers, an intense burst of energy is delivered onto the skin. The energy heats water in the skin and causes both the water and tissues to vaporize. With each pass of the laser, a controlled depth of skin is vaporized and/or coagulated. In response to the injury and subsequent healing, new layers of collagen are produced. While ablative nonfractional lasers can be very effective and have a firm place in laser skin rejuvenation, each can be associated with risks of infection, scarring, hypopigmentation, and unnatural alterations in the texture and sheen of the skin. Moreover, complex aftercare is required until the skin is fully healed. Resolution of erythema may take months.

Nonablative nonfractional treatments are safer than their ablative counterparts but require epidermal cooling, which may reduce efficacy of the treatment. In general, small therapeutic windows are associated with nonablative treatments and, outside of dyschromia reduction with visible light approaches, only modest cosmetic enhancement is achieved. The Nd : YAG (neodymium-doped yttrium aluminum garnet) 1320 nm pulsed laser is an example of a nonablative laser in wide clinical use. IPL, monopolar RF skin tightening, light-heat energy (LHE), and light-emitting diode (LED) are all examples of nonablative treatments.[1-3]

Skin rejuvenation with fractional photothermolysis represents a newer class of therapy (Fig. 5.1). Thousands of microscopic wounds surrounded by viable tissue permit rapid healing and are made with a variety of laser wavelengths and delivery systems. Immediate and delayed therapeutic results are seen through a combination of epidermal coagulation for surface enhancement and dermal heating for deeper remodeling. Unlike SPT, in which targets are damaged based on color contrast, fractional photothermolysis only damages specific zones based on the pattern of the microbeams, leaving other zones completely intact. Fractional laser techniques began with a 1550 nm wavelength. The concept of a fractional laser can be applied, however, to almost any wavelength of light and can be used with both ablative

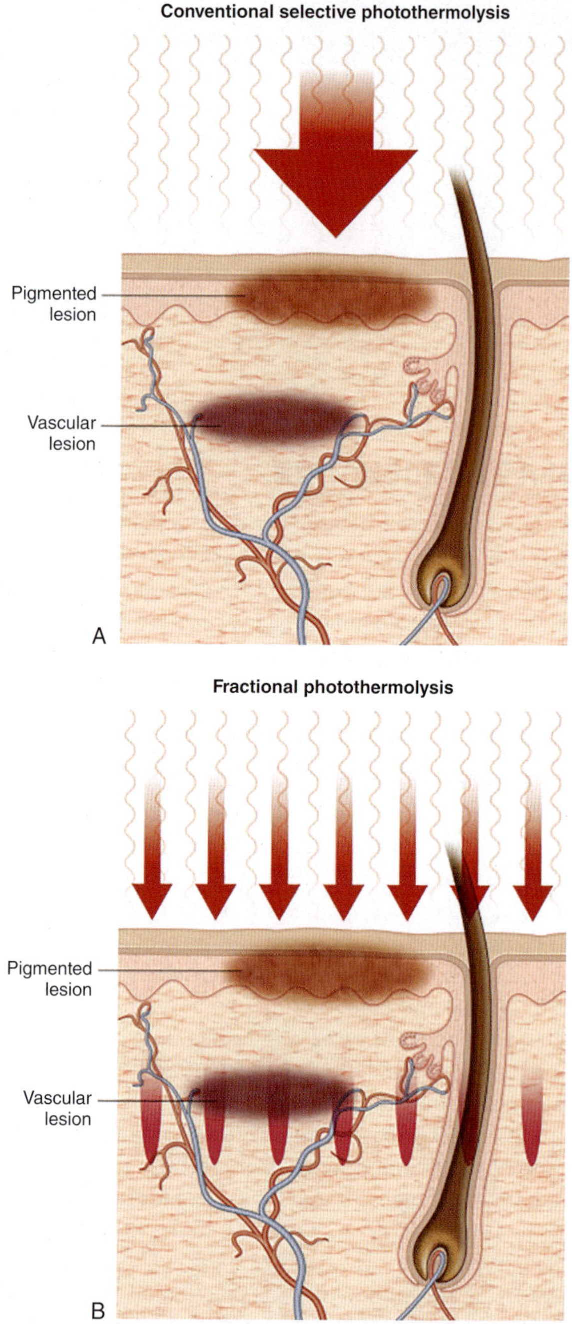

Fig. 5.1 Conventional (A) versus fractional (B) photothermolysis.

laser resurfacing and nonablative laser rejuvenation. With increasingly aggressive densities and depths of injury, the fractional approach may achieve comparable results to nonfractional approaches, without the associated side effects.[4]

BACKGROUND INFORMATION/ ANATOMIC PEARLS

Biology of Wound Healing

The three main stages of wound healing include reepithelialization, scar formation, and wound contraction.[6]

In superficial insults to the skin, the basal layer of epidermis is intact and is capable of proliferating and repopulating the epidermis. This form involves minimal involvement of the underlying dermis, and thus no scar formation ensues. Following deeper injuries to skin, wound healing relies on keratinocytes from the wound edge and skin adnexa to migrate and proliferate. Collagen within the dermis is affected and undergoes some change. The migration of keratinocytes from the wound edge begins within hours of injury and involves four phases: (1) *Mobilization:* epithelial cells immediately adjacent to the wound enlarge, flatten, and detach from neighboring cells and the basement membrane; (2) *Migration:* as marginal cells migrate, the cells immediately behind them also tend to flatten, break connections, and drift along. The epithelial stream continues until advancing cells contact cells from the other side, whereupon motion stops abruptly—a process called *contact inhibition*; (3) *Proliferation/mitosis:* fixed basal cells away from the wound edge begin mitosis to replace the migrating cells. The cells that have migrated in turn start to divide and multiply; (4) *Differentiation:* once the wound gap is bridged by advancing cells from the perimeter, normal differentiation of basal cells occurs. The stimuli for keratinocyte migration and proliferation include loss of cell-to-cell contact, growth factors (epidermal growth factor, transforming growth factor alpha [TGF-α], keratinocyte growth factor, TGF-β), loss of contact with normal components of a basement membrane (type IV collagen and laminin), and contact with proteins of the provisional matrix (fibrin, fibronectin, type I collagen).[6,7]

Reepithelialization is facilitated by a moist environment (the proper dressing), debridement of scabs (fibrin, dead neutrophils, and other debris), growth factors, and high concentration of skin adnexa (the face and scalp).[6,7]

Once contact of keratinocytes occurs and contact inhibition is achieved, hemidesmosomes re-form, cells become more basaloid, and cellular proliferation generates a multilaminated neoepidermis that is slightly thinner.[6,7]

Wound healing that occurs following deeper insults to the skin (deeper chemical peels) results in the scar formation pathway of wound healing. The phases of this process include inflammation, proliferation, and remodeling.

LASER-TISSUE INTERACTIONS AND PROPERTIES OF LASERS

An understanding of light-tissue and electrical-tissue interactions allows physicians to expand their laser repertoire and optimize outcomes. Lasers as light sources are useful because they allow for exquisite control of where and how much one heats.[8] However, tissue reactions are not intrinsically specific to the heating source. In principle, a large number of nonlaser devices (i.e., IPL) can be used for heating skin.[8] In many cases, laser is simply a way to convert lamplight to a more powerful monochromatic form. With respect to lasing media, there are diode lasers, solid-state lasers, and gas lasers.[1] An example of a solid-state laser is the erbium : glass laser. These lasers have a solid rod that is pumped by a flash lamp. Miniaturized diode lasers have become popular. Some diode lasers are housed separately from the handpiece and delivered by fiberoptics. Others are configured with the laser diodes in the handpiece. IPL devices are increasingly comparable to lasers that emit millisecond (ms) domain pulses. Absorption spectra of skin chromophores are broad, and therefore a broadband light source is a logical approach for certain cosmetic applications.[1]

Basic parameters for any procedure using light are power, time, and spot size, for continuous wave lasers; and for pulsed lasers, the energy per pulse, pulse duration, spot size, fluence, and repetition rate.[9] All of these parameters should be considered in characterizing a laser procedure. Energy is measured in joules (J). The amount of energy delivered per unit area is the fluence, sometimes called the *dose* or *radiant exposure*, given usually in J/cm^2. The rate of energy delivery is called *power*, measured in watts (W). One watt is 1 joule per second (W = J/s). The power delivered per unit area is called the *irradiance* or *power density*, usually given in W/cm^2. Laser exposure duration (called *pulse-width* for pulsed lasers) is the time over which energy is delivered.[1]

Fluence is equal to the irradiance times the exposure duration.[10] Other important factors are the laser exposure spot size (which for wavelengths from 400–1200 nm greatly affects intensity inside the skin), whether the incident light is convergent, divergent, or diffuse, and the uniformity of irradiance over the exposure area (spatial beam profile). The pulse profile, that is, the character of the pulse shape in time (instantaneous power vs. time), is another feature that can impact the tissue response.[9-11]

Molecular Basis of Light-Tissue Interaction

In any light-tissue interaction, the thermal or photochemical effects depend on the local absorbed energy density at the target. Spatial localization of temperature elevation is possible when: (1) the absorption coefficient of the target exceeds that of surrounding tissue (SPT); (2) when the "innocent bystander" tissues are cooled so that their peak temperatures do not exceed some damage threshold;[11] or (3) by applying very small (usually <500 μm in diameter) beamlets or microbeams (i.e., fractional methods—*vide supra*). Localized heating, for example, in telangiectases and lentigines, follows from the relative excess of HgB and melanin, respectively, in the lesions versus surrounding skin. In contrast, "nonfractional" mid-infrared (MIR) lasers spatially confine temperature elevation by using heating and cooling schemes that allow for selective dermal heating.[12]

Targeting discrete chromophores offers advantages over targeting tissue water, especially where the ratio of light absorption between the chromophore and surrounding tissue is large (i.e., >10).[11-13] For example, at least in lighter skinned patients, targeting dermal HgB can be achieved with minimal surface cooling. Whereas cooling is desirable, even in these cases, when the primary indication is analgesia rather than epidermal protection. Also, the risk of a severe injury to the skin is lessened, as there is no bulk heating. Lastly, because temperature elevations are localized, there is often less pain than with devices targeting ubiquitous tissue water. Thermal injury is determined by time/temperature combinations. Protein denaturation is dependent linearly on exposure time and exponentially on temperature. That is, cell death is more sensitive to temperature than time.[11] Most devices for rejuvenation are based on photothermal or "electrothermal" mechanisms, that is, the conversion of light or electrical energy to heat. More recently, US devices have been applied to tighten the skin.[14] Two processes govern all interactions of light with matter: absorption and scattering. The absorption spectra of major skin chromophores dominate laser-tissue interactions. If tissues were clear, then only absorption would be required to characterize light propagation in skin. However, the dermis is white because of light scatter (milk is a reasonable model for the dermis with regard to scattering). Scattering is responsible for much of the light's behavior in the skin (beam dispersion, spot size effects, etc.). The main scattering wavelengths are between 400 and 1200 nm (those where tissue water absorption is poor).[1]

There are three chromophores of interest in skin (water, blood, and melanin). Water makes up about 65% of the dermis and lower epidermis. There is some water absorption in the ultraviolet (UV). Between 400 and 800 nm, water absorption is quite small (which is consistent with our real-world experience that visible light propagates quite readily through a glass of water). Beyond 800 nm, there is a small peak at 980 nm, followed by larger peaks at 1480 and 10,600 nm. The water maximum is 2940 nm (Er : YAG).[1]

SELECTIVE PHOTOTHERMOLYSIS

With the exception of cases where water is heated, rejuvenation of the skin is based on discrete heating by chromophores of relatively low concentration (i.e., melanin, HgB). Anderson described the concept of SPT more than 25 years ago.[4] He noted that extreme localized heating achieved with SPT relies on: (1) a wavelength that reaches and is preferentially absorbed by the desired target structures; (2) an exposure duration less than or equal to the time necessary for cooling of the target structures; and (3) sufficient energy to damage the target.[4] The heterogeneity of the skin with respect to HgB and melanin allows for very selective injury in thousands of microscopic targets.

The *thermal relaxation time* is the time it takes for a target to cool to a certain percentage of its peak temperature (after laser exposure). Larger targets take longer to cool, and therefore spatial selectivity is preserved with a wider range of pulse durations. Even so, as a general rule, assuming adequate fluences are applied, longer pulse durations will result in greater collateral damage. In laser scenarios, we assume instantaneous heating of the target, so that τ is usually thought of as the time for cooling *after* the pulse.[4]

Reaction Types

Photothermal

Most laser applications rely on heating. Photothermal approaches depend on the type and degree of heating, from coagulation to vaporization. There is a range of effects on tissue based on temperature. Below 43 °C, the skin remains unharmed, even for exposures as long as 20 min. Thus, one can exceed body temperature by about 5 °C without a measurable change in the skin. The first change is a conformational change in the molecular structure. These typically occur at temperatures from 42 to 50 °C. At higher temperatures, very short times (seconds or in extreme cases [>100 °C] less than 1 ms) can induce cell death.[1,4]

Photochemical

Photochemical reactions are governed by specific reaction pathways, and the most common photosensitizer (PS) in skin is protoporphyrin IX. This PS is formed in skin cells by the prodrug, aminolevulinic acid (ALA).[1,4]

Biostimulation

Biostimulation (also called *low-level laser therapy*) belongs to the group of photochemical interactions. Most biostimulation studies involve low-power lasers, and this field continues to be a subject of controversy. Home-use devices that use LEDs are now available in a wide range of wavelength ranges. Typical fluences are in the range of 1 to 10 J/cm^2, and normally there is no acute temperature elevation, nor any clinical endpoint.[1,4]

Cooling

Before the addition of surface cooling, fluence thresholds for efficacy and epidermal damage were often close. Visible light technologies (especially green-yellow light sources such as IPL, potassium titanium oxide phosphate [KTP] laser, and pulsed dye laser [PDL]) are the wavelength ranges where epidermal damage is most likely. The epidermis is an innocent bystander in cutaneous laser applications where the intended targets, such as hair follicles or blood vessels, are located in the dermis.[1,4]

Beyond visible light (green, yellow, and red) sources, surface cooling also has been used in NIR and MIR lasers. With NIR lasers, surface cooling is important, but not only because of dermal/epidermal junction-derived epidermal heating. In addition, deep beam penetration may cause catastrophic bulk heating. With MIR lasers (1.32, 1.45, and 1.54 μm), the chromophore is water. It follows that with even very low fluences, surface cooling is imperative. Without cooling or a fractional design, water's ubiquitous nature in the skin causes a laser-induced top-to-bottom injury. All techniques are susceptible to operator error and device failure. It follows that as physicians rely more heavily on cooling devices, any lack of their proper deployment unveils the dark side of cooling. Fractured sapphire windows, disabled cryogen spray apparatus, and crimped forced air chiller tubes have all contributed to unintended epidermal injury.[1,4]

Nonablative Facial Skin Rejuvenation

The original concept of nonablative skin rejuvenation (NSR) was wrinkle reduction by selective dermal heating.[15,16] Deeply penetrating nonfractional mid-IR lasers coupled with surface cooling were designed to "bypass" the epidermis. A slab-like dermal injury was created. Unfortunately, "CO_2-like" results were never replicated because dermal heating was either too deep or too mild. Superficial severe dermal heating was almost always associated with epidermal damage. It followed that all of these devices "bypassed" the solar elastosis ultimately responsible for most static wrinkles of the face.[1,4]

The "nonablative" term has now evolved to include any electrical-, light-, RF-, or US-based intervention with "relative" epidermal preservation.[17] In addition to wrinkle reduction, new outcome measures include acne scar improvement, telangiectasia resolution, homogenization of pigment, pore size reduction, skin tightening (jowls, neck, and some extrafacial sites), and "improved" skin tone.[15-17]

RF- and US-based technologies have recently gained more popularity. RF energy uses the tissue's resistance within the skin to transform the RF into thermal energy. This modality can be used for patients of all skin types, promoting new collagen production and contraction. US-based technologies create "thermal coagulation points" in the skin, inducing new collagen production and skin tightening.

Sadick developed a classification scheme for NSR based on photodamage type. In his paper, type I photodamage consisted of surface irregularities, of which there were three subtypes. Type 1a included rosacea and telangiectases; 1b was comprised of pore size and skin roughness; and type 1c included pigmentation changes. Type II rejuvenation included deeper wrinkles and volume loss.[17]

Fractional Resurfacing

Resurfacing with fractional photothermolysis represents a newer class of therapy (see Fig. 5.1). The stratum corneum is left largely intact as thousands of microscopic

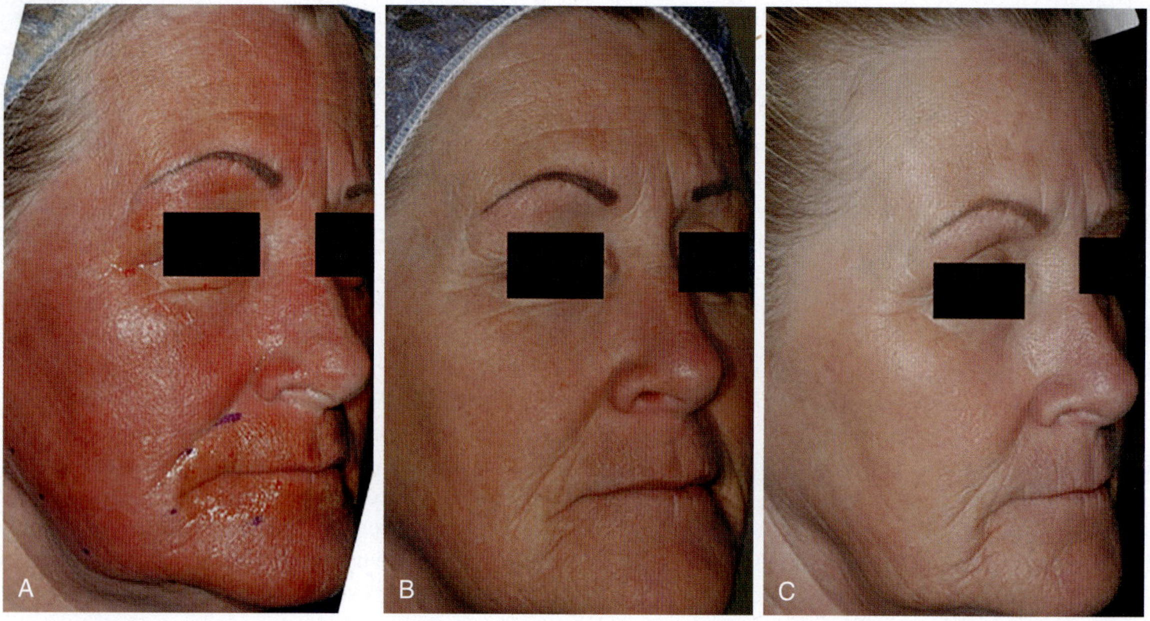

Fig. 5.2 Fractional resurfacing (2940 nm): (A) immediately after treatment, (B) before laser, and (C) 3 months after laser.

wounds surrounded by viable tissue are made with a variety of laser wavelengths and delivery systems. Immediate and delayed results are seen through a combination of epidermal coagulation for resurfacing effect and dermal heating for deeper remodeling.

As mentioned earlier, fractional laser resurfacing first became commercially available in 2003.[18] The initial fractional laser uses an erbium-doped fiber to deliver 3000 infrared (1550 nm) laser pulses per second and targets water as a chromophore. The original fractionated laser created an array of microthermal treatment zones (MTZs) measuring 50 to 150 μm in densities ranging from 400 to 6400 MTZ/cm^2.[18] Each MTZ forms a column of thermally denatured collagen from the epidermis to mid-dermis. In contrast to nonfractional lasers, fractional lasers coagulate only a portion of the treated area, sparing islands of viable epidermis and untreated dermis that maintain the skin's barrier function while speeding reepithelialization (Fig. 5.2).[1,18]

PREPROCEDURE CONSIDERATIONS

Diagnosis and Clinical Evaluation

Adequate evaluation and photographic documentation of the patient before laser treatment is essential.[18-20] This assessment includes consideration of the severity of actinic damage, depth and number of rhytides, and need for any additional resurfacing procedures. The patient with deep rhytides and excessive facial skin laxity is likely a better candidate for traditional rhytidectomy. The patient with moderate photodamage and medium rhytides may be a more optimal candidate for one of the many types of resurfacing procedures. Some patients may benefit from both procedures because rhytidectomy typically addresses skin quantity and soft-tissue malposition, whereas resurfacing addresses skin quality.[19,20] It should be noted, however, that great care should be undertaken when both rhytidectomy and resurfacing are performed concurrently. If rhytidectomy is performed, it is recommended to avoid any resurfacing of the undermined facial skin, as wound healing issues may ensue.[19,20]

An important tool of the evaluation of the patient for a resurfacing procedure is Fitzpatrick's scale of sun-reactive skin types. This scale describes patients' reactions to UV radiation and existing degree of pigmentation. Type I patients always burn and never tan. Type II patients tan only with difficulty and usually burn. Type III patients tan but sometimes burn. Type IV patients rarely burn and tan with ease. Type V patients tan very easily and very rarely burn. Type VI patients tan very easily and never burn.[21] Patients with lighter skin types can expect to undergo peeling or laser treatments with minimal concern for abnormal pigment changes, whereas individuals with darker skin are at higher risk for unwanted hyperpigmentation or hypopigmentation.[21] An often ignored rule is that patients tend to revert to their constitutive color after resurfacing (unless it is carried out very deeply). So, although there is a concern that constitutively dark patients might be at risk for temporary dyspigmentation, on a practical level, it is the severely photodamaged type II and type III patients that present the greatest challenges in moderate-depth resurfacing. This group of patients, once their bronzing is removed by the procedure, tend to remain "white" after the photodamage is reduced. This can result in conspicuous lines of demarcation between treated and untreated areas. Another helpful classification system is the Glogau[22] photodamage scale. Type 1 patients have little wrinkling, no keratoses, no scarring, and require no make-up. Type 2 patients have early wrinkling, early actinic changes, minimal scarring, and require a small amount of make-up. Type 3 patients have wrinkles present at rest, moderate actinic keratoses (AKs), moderate scarring, and always require make-up. Type 4 patients have severe wrinkling, AKs, and scarring that even large amounts of make-up do not cover.

A thorough medical history and review of systems should be completed in concert with the physical examination, as part of a thorough patient workup.[19,20] Preexisting cardiac, hepatic, and renal disease may influence the treatment decision and choice of chemical peel or alternative resurfacing method. The use of exogenous estrogens, oral contraceptives, and other photosensitizing medications have been shown to predispose patients to unpredictable pigment changes.[19,20] Therefore, such agents should be avoided several weeks before and after treatment. For any procedure that includes epidermal compromise, the physician should provide antiviral prophylaxis several days before and after the treatment for those patients with a history of herpes simplex infection. Prophylaxis will help minimize chances of unwanted viral reactivation as the reepithelialization process occurs. It is also advisable to allow any existing viral-type lesion to heal completely before proceeding with a resurfacing procedure.[19,20]

Patient cooperation and compliance with the posttreatment regimen is required to ensure normal wound healing and to avoid complications.[19,20] It is ill advised to treat patients likely to be noncompliant or unable to avoid sun exposure because of occupation. Men are considered less optimal candidates because of thicker, oilier skin that risks uneven penetration of the peeling agent or laser. Men are also less likely to be willing to use camouflage make-up in the event of pigmentary disturbances. Patients with a decreased number of epithelial appendages from prior radiation treatment or current isotretinoin (Accutane) use are also poor candidates because healing will proceed more slowly, and scarring is more likely. Consider recent use of Accutane an absolute contraindication to medium and deep peels, or certain types of laser resurfacing. One should wait at least 6 months after stopping Accutane to allow sufficient regeneration of epithelial appendages before treatment.[19,20] For nonablative treatments, the role of isotretinoin (Accutane) in wound healing is unclear. Most likely, healing will proceed unimpeded, and no special precautions are necessary. Still, treatments during an actual course of Accutane should only be undertaken if the benefits outweigh the potential risks.

CONTRAINDICATIONS

Laser and chemical resurfacing have common contraindications. These include active bacterial, viral, fungal, or herpetic infection; open wounds; history of drugs with photosensitizing potential; preexisting inflammatory dermatoses; uncooperative patients; patients with unrealistic expectations; history of abnormal or keloid-type scarring.[19,20]

PROCEDURAL CONSIDERATIONS

Patient Selection and Treatment

For wavelengths from 520 to 800 nm, the primary absorbers are HgB and melanin, so that improvement of pigmentation and vascularity is achieved by direct heating of melanosomes and HgB (either by a single wavelength or flash lamp).[23] While devices targeting HgB/vessels are confined to pulse-widths ranging from 0.45 to 100 ms, melanosome heating is achieved by either Q-switched nanosecond pulses, or gentler heating with millisecond-domain pulses. For discrete smaller (0.1–0.6 mm) telangiectases, PDL, KTP laser, or IPL can be applied (Fig. 5.3).[23] For larger vessels (>1 mm) and/or darker skin, the Nd : YAG laser is preferred, but care

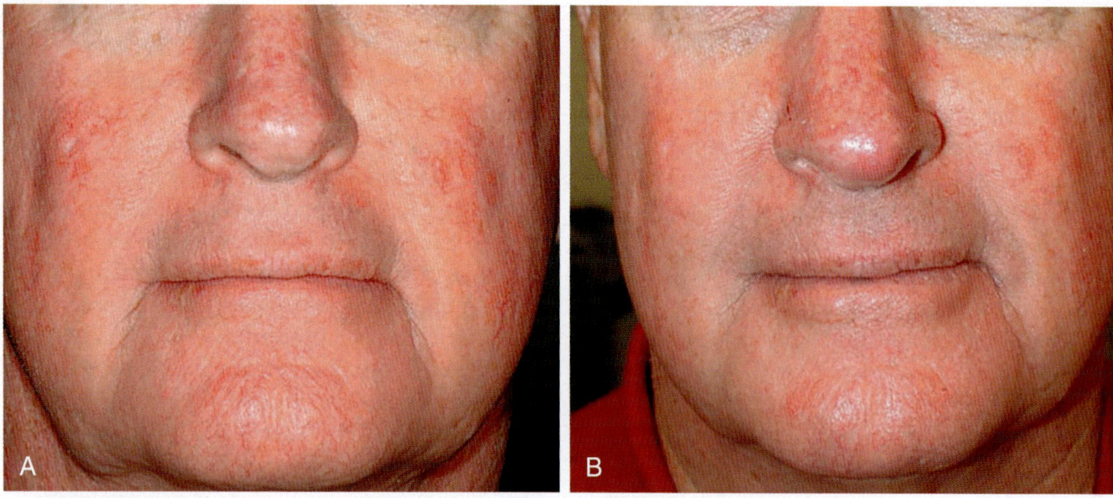

Fig. 5.3 (A) Pre- and (B) post-KTP (potassium titanium oxide phosphate) laser treatment (8 J/cm 2, 20 ms).

must be taken to apply the smallest fluence and smallest spot sufficient for closure. An alternative would be a combination of 595-nm and 1064-nm sequential pulses that can simultaneously address both smaller and larger telangiectases.[24]

If a patient presents with telangiectases confined to very small areas, we typically use a small spot size (1–4 mm) and the long pulsed KTP laser or PDL.[1,23] Alternatively, we use nonpurpuric settings with an IPL. The specific type of PDL determines the spot size, fluence range, and cooling type, and pulse-width. Modern PDLs can generate effective fluences with 10 to 12 mm spots; moreover, the macropulses (pulse envelopes) are comprised of 6 to 8 micropulses, allowing for greater efficacy without a high risk of purpura. However, the most popular modern PDL requires two passes for complete rejuvenation, one for treatment of pigmented lesions (with a dedicated pigmented lesion "compression" handpiece) or the cooling device disabled, and another for treatment of vascular lesions.[1,23] More recently, the alexandrite laser has been used for medium-diameter blood vessels. The depth of penetration permits coagulation of vessels as large as 1 to 2 mm, but the high melanin absorption limits its usefulness to lighter patients unless very aggressive cooling is applied.[25]

If a lighter patient presents with a few discrete lentigines, we use the Q-switched alexandrite laser. The endpoint is frosty whitening. The only exception to our Q-switched approach for isolated dyschromias is when a patient has a pressing engagement where "robust" crusting is intolerable. In these cases, despite the better one-time treatment clearance with nanosecond pulses, we apply millisecond devices, as the delayed "coffee-ground" crusts tend to be less obvious.[1,23,24]

On the other hand, in darker skinned groups, we usually observe some persistence of pigment after Q-switched 532-, 755-, and 694-nm applications. In this scenario, it is sometimes difficult to determine after a short interval whether the pigment represents residual melanin in the treated lesion or postinflammatory hyperpigmentation (PIH). As patients usually report almost complete clearance of the lesions after 3 to 7 days, we suggest, at least for thinner lentigines that most persistent pigmentation is postinflammatory. We therefore delay repeat treatments for 8 to 12 weeks, allowing for at least partial resolution of any PIH. Unfortunately, this period is poorly accepted by patients, who, with the exception of exophytic seborrheic keratoses (SKs), are disappointed or angry that the lesions are darker than on initial presentation. Clearing of PIH can be accelerated by use of creams containing hydroquinone, tretinoin, and/or topical steroids of various strengths and combinations. Pretreatment with these agents might decrease the risk of PIH. Sun protection is essential. For lighter, thinner SKs, one can apply multiple 532-nm nanosecond pulses. For some thicker, darker SKs, the long-pulsed diode laser or long-pulsed alexandrite can be used to clinical endpoint of graying. Care must be taken to mask any darker perilesional background skin.[1,26] A recent article suggests that longer pulse visible light technologies are less likely to cause PIH in darker patients.[27] However, for lighter lentigines or somewhat tanned skin, whether one applies PDL with compression, IPL, or KTP laser, selective lesional heating is compromised because there is often insufficient color contrast. For these so-called "*low-contrast*" lesions, the "therapeutic index" is dangerously small.

For diffuse hyperpigmentation (also called *actinic bronzing*), we apply the long-pulsed variable spot KTP laser with contact cooling as a first choice. This laser enjoys a low rate of side effects, will not damage the hair bulb (important for male patients), and the handpiece is light and maneuverable. When confronted with a combination of darker and lighter lentigines in Caucasian patients, we use the Q-switched alexandrite laser for the lighter lentigines first, followed by panfacial treatment with IPL or KTP laser in the same session. We use the pulsed CO_2 laser or Er : YAG laser for some lighter lentigines, particularly if they are evolving into an SK.[1,23-26] More exophytic, lighter SKs must be treated with ablative lasers, or as an alternative, so long as there is at least minimal color contrast. We focus the Q-switched alexandrite beam to a very small spot (1–2 mm) and vaporize smaller, flatter SKs by repeated pulses (the Q 532-nm laser can be used as well). Sometimes slight bleeding is observed, but this technique is associated with rapid healing. Alternatively, the long-pulsed diode laser (810 nm) or long-pulsed alexandrite laser can be used for some pigmented SKs.[1,6] High fluences must be applied, and in darker patients, one should mask the normal surrounding skin with a plastic "guard."[26]

We also use the long-pulse alexandrite laser for panfacial rejuvenation, both with and without cooling. With cooling, both vessels and pigment can be treated; however, only light-skinned patients are appropriate candidates, as the ratio for melanin : HgB heating is high for 755 nm. For treatment of exclusively pigmented lesions, no cooling is necessary. Like the IPL, one must be careful to avoid darker beard areas to decrease the risk of alopecia.[1,23-26]

For flash lamp systems, filters placed between the lamp and skin are configured to optimize heating of specific targets. In choosing a laser or IPL for panfacial rejuvenation of the face or neck, the pulse configuration should achieve maximal differential heating between the epidermis and the dermal vessels. Models show that longer pulses (or pulse trains) favor vessel heating over epidermal heating.[1,26]

Melasma is a challenging condition to treat with lasers, most likely because of its dynamic and inflammatory nature (compared with the static nature of lentigines).[28] Ablative lasers sometimes improve the condition; however, the ablation normally has to be carried out deeply (or *very* superficially—just involving the upper epidermis), or PIH may outweigh any achievement gains. On the other hand, longer pulsed visible light laser technologies, Q-switched Nd : YAG lasers, and fractional approaches can sometimes achieve gradual improvement in melasma, so long as the settings are not too high.[29,30] If the patient presents exclusively with melasma and no discrete "static" pigmented lesions (i.e., lentigines), we start with topical hydroquinone and retinoids before considering interventional therapy. Use of the Q-switched Nd : YAG laser, treating every 1 to 2 weeks for approximately eight sessions, often clears some of the pigment; however, there is a high relapse rate. Also, recently, guttate hypomelanosis has been reported after multiple treatments with Q-switch Nd: YAG laser.[31,32] We have not found Q-switched alexandrite, Q-switched ruby, or Q-switched 532-nm lasers helpful in melasma.[1,26] In all cases, although there is nice resolution within 1 week, worsening of the melasma usually follows.

Small nevi can be lightened by repeated Q-switched Nd : YAG and Q-switched alexandrite laser sessions; we reserve these treatments for Asian patients with small, discrete, uniformly colored lesions on the face. Long-pulsed alexandrite lasers can be used. Red scars and traumatic tattoos can be treated by a combination of PDL and Q-switched YAG laser.[1,23-30] Banal-appearing flesh-colored nevi in White patients can be treated by ablative CO_2 or Er : YAG lasers. Optimally, a shave of the lesions is performed to debulk the lesions (at least one of which should be submitted for pathologic interpretation as a representative sample if all of the lesions are clinically similar), after which the laser can be used with a small spot (1–2 mm) to vaporize the lesions "flush" with the surrounding skin. Recurrence is not uncommon; also, even in cases where flattening has been achieved, surface darkening can occur. Q-switched alexandrite or ruby laser treatments are then applied until the pigment remains clear.

Improvement in wrinkles can be performed by primary heating of vasculature (low-fluence PDL, low-fluence KTP, or low-fluence 1064 nm). These technologies depend solely on a cascade effect, that is, release of inflammatory mediators after capillary heating for wrinkle reduction. Short-pulsed (0.3–50 ms) low-fluence Nd : YAG lasers have been used for rejuvenation. The principle is that gentle sequential heating over a large volume (or either possibly through focal heating of microvessels) might stimulate new collagen deposition, tighten skin, reduce inflammation, and even reduce pore size.[33-35] One example is the "Genesis" procedure where 5000 to 12,000 pulses are painted over the face at 5 to 7 Hz with a 5-mm spot at 12 to 15 J/cm^2. The endpoint is localized transient skin warming just below the pain threshold. No anesthetic is applied, thus ensuring that the patient will provide feedback regarding excessive temperatures. A newer version of this laser includes a real-time temperature feedback option.[36]

Improvement in skin can be performed by heating of dermal tissue water (1.32-, 1.54-, and 1.45-μm devices). These lasers heat tissue water. It follows that, without surface cooling, unless very small fluences or microbeams (<0.4 mm) are applied, a top-to-bottom broad thermal injury is observed. All of these wavelengths can be made to heat the reticular dermis with the proper mixture of fluences, repetition rates, epidermal cooling, and pulse duration.[37-40]

Acne scars are common and can be improved via nonablative techniques. Jacob et al.[41] proposed a three-type scar system: ice pick, rolling, and boxcar. Ice pick scars are narrow, deep, sharply demarcated "holes" that extend into the deep dermis or subcutaneous layer. Rolling scars are usually wider than 4 to 5 mm and stem from the tethering of otherwise normal-looking skin. Boxcar scars are depressions with sharply demarcated vertical edges. Another classification scheme includes other scar designations, including macular scars (erythematous, white, or brown), elastolytic scars (like mini-striae), papular scars, and hypertrophic scars.[42]

A rational approach considers the microscopic anatomy of the scar. Rolling scars occur deep in the follicle and are the end-product of inflammation that causes destruction of the subcuticular fat. A number of "dedicated" skin-tightening procedures can be applied (RF- or US-based energy). Although sometimes helpful, predictable improvement is lacking, and the intervention should only be reserved for rolling scars or others with volume loss (atrophy). For boxcar scars, fractional technologies should be considered first (nonablative or ablative), depending on the patient's expectations and tolerance for downtime. The best results are achieved with high densities (20%–30% surface area per treatment) and "deeper" holes.[1,17,18]

Long-pulse and millisecond-domain Nd : YAG devices have been applied to acne scars.[43] The Q-switched Nd : YAG laser beam is typically delivered at 2 to 4 J/cm^2 with a 4 to 6 mm spot and three passes per region. The endpoint is erythema and, occasionally, petechiae. The treatments are only mildly uncomfortable, with the exception of male patients, where pulses over hair-bearing areas can be more painful. In applying the longer pulse systems, multiple passes (usually three) are delivered at 10 to 50 J/cm^2. Endpoints are mild erythema and edema.[43] Care should be taken to avoid black-haired areas in male patients to avoid potential hair reduction. Fillers can complement the aforementioned procedures, particularly when there is marked volume loss associated with rolling-type scars (Fig. 5.4).

First proposed as a means for treating individual AKs, photodynamic therapy (PDT) is now being used with blue and red light for "photo" peels. In one configuration, 20% liquid ALA solution is spread lightly over the skin for 0.5 to 2 h, after which the entire cosmetic unit is irradiated with a wide array of light sources (Fig. 5.5). ALA has been shown to enhance the pulsed light responses for dyschromias and vascular lesions.[44] We use ALA in the following manner: if a patient presents with AKs, telangiectases, and dyschromias, we combine ALA with a pulsed visible light source followed by 5 to 10 min of a continuous wave (CW) red light source. In this scenario, immediately after an acetone scrub, the solution is applied, and 30 min later a 5% lidocaine cream is applied. After an additional 30 min, the pulsed light source is used, immediately followed by the CW light source. Refrigerated air is applied for anesthesia. We shorten the ALA application period with numbing cream, as we have found it accelerates the ALA absorption and enhances the PDT effect. If the patient presents solely with AKs and few dyschromias and telangiectases (and if the patient desires insurance coverage for the entire procedure), we apply ALA (without anesthesia) for 1 to 2 h, followed by application of red CW light. Although ALA-PDT has been recommended for sebaceous hyperplasia,[45] we have only found it helpful with longer incubation times and CW red light.

More recently, the fractional 1927-nm laser has received U.S. Food and Drug Administration (FDA)

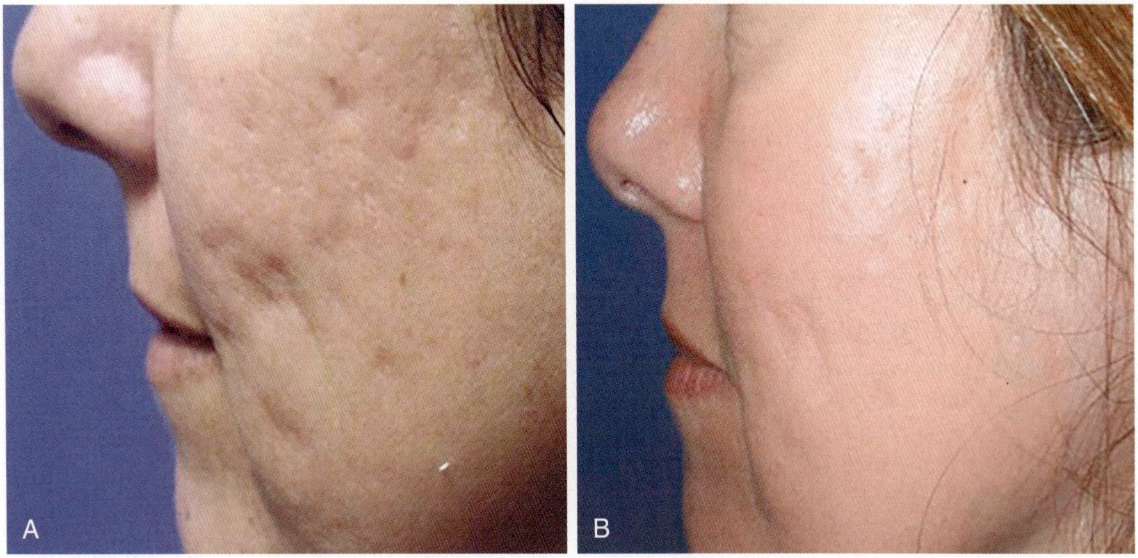

Fig. 5.4 Acne scar treatment with 1550-nm erbium : glass fractional laser: (A) before and (B) 6 months after these treatments.

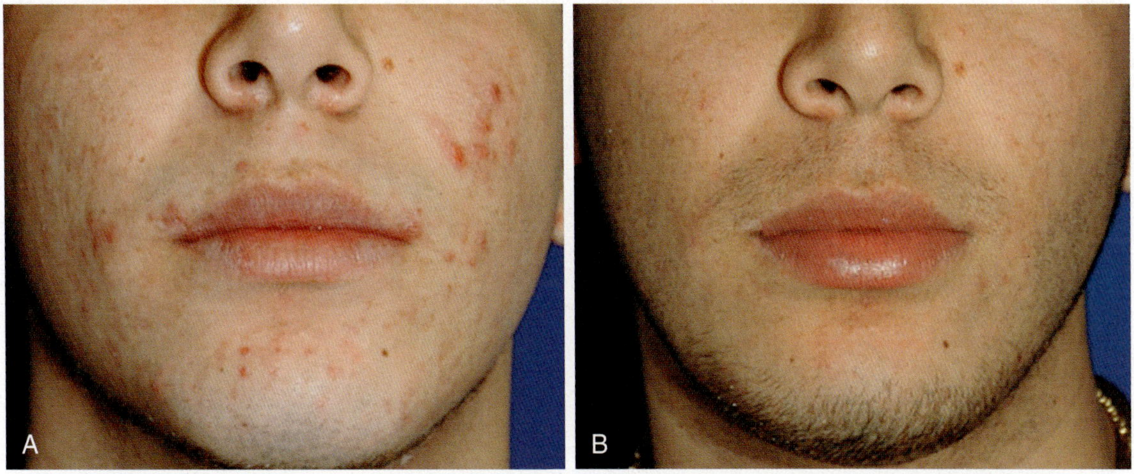

Fig. 5.5 Photodynamic therapy with aminolevulinic acid: **(A)** before and **(B)** after treatment.

clearance for AKs. The laser is used in a multiple-pass session until about 90% coverage is achieved. With this high-coverage mode, the entirety of the AK can be eliminated when the laser is applied in a full-face or segmental-face fashion as a field therapy. For tinker lesion, pretreatment curettage is sometimes applied.

DEEPER HEATING LONG-PULSE SKIN-TIGHTENING PROCEDURES

Recently, multimodal approaches for treatment of facial aging have become common practice. It is essential that the operator of laser devices becomes familiar with other available technologies to be able to deliver a more comprehensive approach to the aging face and achieve superior outcomes. There are a number of deep-heating handpieces for skin tightening. The main approaches include: (1) monopolar RF; (2) bipolar RF; (3) tripolar RF; (4) fractionated RF needles; (5) xenon flash lamp with rapid repetition rates and filtering that features 800 to 1200 nm portion of the output spectrum; (6) deep-heating halogen lamps; and (7) US. Most deep-heating strategies are based on time/temperature-dependent heating of collagen, which can produce focal "fractional" fibril damage.

Monopolar RF uses a controlled RF pulse to selectively heat zones of the lower dermis and subdermis while avoiding injury to the superficial dermis through use of a cryogen spray.[46] It was approved by the FDA in 2005 for full-body skin-tightening treatments. Some studies have revealed high patient satisfaction with the device when proper technique and patient selection are used.[46] Treatment typically involves between one and three applications of the RF to the affected areas, depending on the severity of the deformity. Pain and downtime are minimal. Most patients are able to resume all normal activities immediately after treatment. Appropriate patients include those with mild to moderate rhytids who understand the limitations of the device (Fig. 5.6).[46]

The new generation of "injectable" monopolar RF uses temperature-controlled RF by deploying an array of needles to a prescribed depth in the skin. This device allows the operator to "inject" the RF energy while at the same time regulate the tissue temperature through sensitive probes and provide a more controlled therapy. One such device achieves skin tightening by coagulating deeper dermal zones (2–3 mm deep) by deploying five pairs of needle electrodes into the skin for each "pulse." Temperatures of about 70 °C are sustained for about 4 s, 1 to 3 mm beneath the skin surface in the most common application.

Bipolar and tripolar RF technologies are also available and effectively treat rhytids, skin laxity, acne, vascular and pigmented lesions.[47-53]

Deeper penetration halogen lamps heat the upper 1 to 2 mm of the dermis. Pulses typically last 2 to 6 s and are accompanied by surface cooling. Xenon flash lamp devices have been electronically modulated to deliver rapid pulse trains with surface cooling. Like their halogen counterparts, the goal is sustained elevation of the dermal temperature. Low-cost IR (temperature) meters are used during treatment to maintain surface temperatures of 38 to 41 °C. A newly introduced US system (Ultherapy, Ulthera Inc., Mesa, AZ) coagulates small

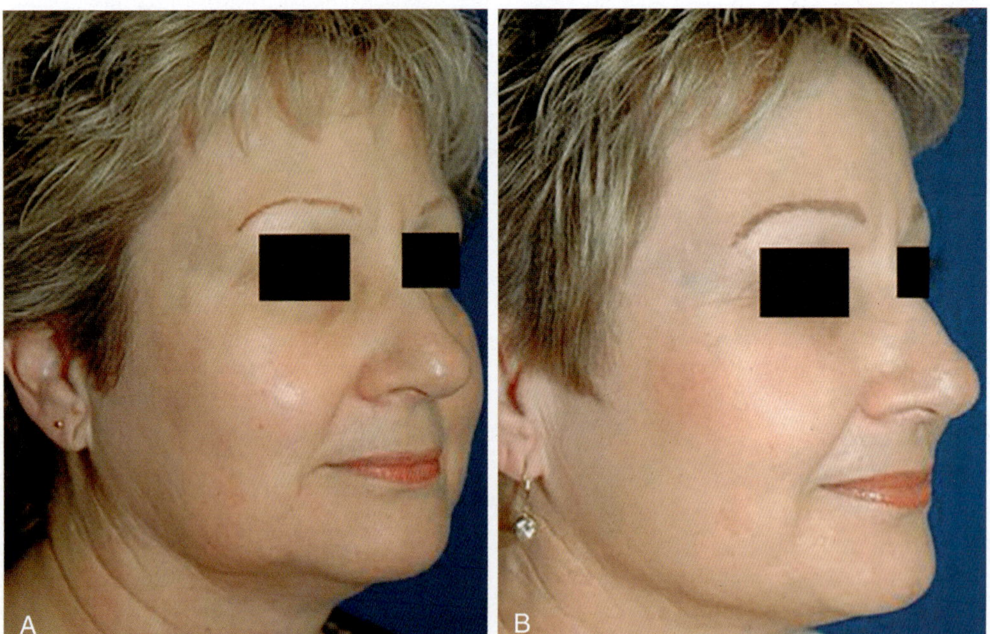

Fig. 5.6 (A) Pre- and (B) 6 months posttreatment with monopolar radiofrequency.

dermal zones about 3 to 5 mm deep in the dermis. The depth is dependent on the transducer configuration. The goal is brow, cheek, and neck elevation/tightening.

FRACTIONAL PHOTOTHERMOLYSIS

A broad array of fractional lasers has appeared on the market since the introduction of the technology. In general, the critical determinant for long-term skin resurfacing results is not the degree of immediate skin tightening, but the production of new collagen—a biologic process that is highly dependent upon the depth of damage.[1,54,55]

Fractional lasers penetrate deeply into the skin dermis with thousands of tiny MTZs, using a technique called *fractional photothermolysis*.[18,54,55] Treating the skin fractionally with patterns of microscopic laser spots, each of which is 70 to 100 μm in diameter, results in a unique wound healing process. This is aided by the fact that each laser spot (MTZ) is surrounded by healthy tissue. Many of the stem cells and melanocytes in the papillary dermis are spared. Fractional wound healing results in both rapid reepithelialization of the epidermis as well as collagen remodeling to depths of 400 to 700 μm.[18,54,55]

Clinical studies[4,5,56] suggest that four to six treatments spaced about 1 week apart produce a gradual remodeling of dermal matrix components, firming collagen and elastin. A topical anesthetic and a blue dye were used before treatment, which takes about 60 min. Laser treatment itself takes another 45 min. With the newer lasers, the blue dye is no longer needed.

Side effects are generally minimal. A mild sunburn sensation occurs for approximately 1 h after the treatment. The skin has a pinkish tone for 1 to 3 days (see Fig. 5.5). This is a normal sign of healing. Swelling is minimal. Within 24 h, new epidermal skin begins to emerge. This process of skin repair involves flaking and bronzing. The use of sunscreen throughout the process is absolutely necessary. Optimal improvement may take 3 to 6 months.[4,5,56]

Fractional laser treatment appears to be effective in reduction of fine wrinkles; rejuvenation of sun-damaged skin on the face, neck, chest, shoulders, hands, and arms; reduction of age spots, blotches, and dyschromia; acne scars; hyperpigmentation; and in some patients, coarse and deeper wrinkles may demonstrate considerable improvement.[18,54,55]

In 2004, fractional laser was introduced to the market (Fraxel Re:store 1500, Solta Medical, Pleasanton, CA). It is a 1550-nm fractionated erbium : glass laser. This version combines proprietary advancements in optical technology with medical software, offering physicians a treatment option that penetrates up to 30% deeper than the previous version laser, delivering consistent dosage control and optimizing lesion depths. This leap in technology provides patients a safe and effective, noninvasive treatment option for skin conditions ranging from mild sun damage to severe acne scarring.[18,54,55]

With the newly designed optical zoom hand control system, physicians can penetrate up to 1.0 mm below the skin surface with precise dosage control. Deeper penetration provides a greater catalyst for natural generation of new collagen to promote self-healing and remodeling.[18,54,55]

After 2 to 3 years of study, the fractional CO_2 was introduced to the market in December 2007. The Fraxel Re:pair (Solta Medical, Bothell WA) is a fractionally ablative microscopic CO_2 laser with a 10,600-nm wavelength. This laser approaches the efficacy of fully ablative lasers, but with markedly less downtime, less risk of adverse events and no reports of delayed hypopigmentation. A single treatment is carried out for most patients, although the treatment may be repeated 3 to 6 months later. There are 2 to 3 days of real downtime with severe erythema and oozing followed by marked redness fading to a lighter shade by day 6 or 7. Over the next month, the redness gradually fades. The primary clinical targets are wrinkle removal, skin tightening, severe photodamage, acne, and surgical scars. Whereas the Fraxel Re:store 1500 coagulates the epithelial and dermal tissue in the microthermal zone of injury, the Re:pair vaporizes the tissue centrally, leaving a rim of coagulation necrosis on the periphery of the injury and producing immediate skin tightening and wrinkle reduction. As pulse energy is increased, penetration depth also increases. As density is increased, more surface area is treated. With experience and carefully chosen parameters, varying both energy and density, one can safely treat virtually all skin types. The Re:pair delivers the deepest injury of any of the nonablative and ablative fractional lasers. Although the injury is pronounced, reepithelialization occurs within 48 hours.[18,54,55]

In 2009, the same manufacturer introduced the dual wavelength fractional laser (Fraxel Dual). This technology boasts two different wavelengths (1550 nm and 1927 nm). The additional wavelength enables the operator to better address pigmentation and dyschromia.

Recently, our group reported our experience with 716 patients who underwent fractional lasers in our center. Fractional lasers were carried out with three different laser wavelengths, depending on the condition(s) treated (wrinkling vs. pigmentation issues, etc.) and the patients' length of downtime. The fractional 1550/1927 dual wavelength laser was used in 222 patients; the fractional 1550 laser was used in 325; and the fractional CO_2 laser was used in 169 patients. Adverse events and complications occurred in 29 of 716 patients (4.05%). Complications were generally minor, and all resolved completely with treatment. Complications occurred in 1.12% of patients having the fractional 1550/1927, 4.05% having the fractional 1550, and 3.38% having the fractional CO_2 laser. Complications included minor burns/abrasions in 2 patients, acne outbreaks in 11, rash in 4, herpes outbreak in 3, and prolonged erythema in 2 patients.[57]

MULTIPLE OTHER ABLATIVE AND NONABLATIVE FRACTIONAL LASERS COMMERCIALLY AVAILABLE

The 1440-nm erbium: glass laser (Affirm, Cynosure, Westford, MA) is nonablative. It has some unique features that, in essence, deliver fractionated treatments to the skin surface. The unique aspect of this laser is the combined apex pulse (CAP) technology, which uses diffractive elements to bend the wavelength to treat larger surface areas. The laser also delivers both high- and low-energy light to the selected treatment areas, which "fractionates" the treatment. The CAP array in the 1440-nm Nd: YAG Affirm laser system was developed to combine both mechanisms in a single treatment, using high-fluence regions surrounded by low-level heating. This microthermal rejuvenation approach creates apices of high-fluence regions for collagen remodeling surrounded by a collagen-stimulating, low-fluence treatment zone. The CAP array is a special lens construction that consists of approximately 1000 diffractive elements affecting more surface area per single pulse. The high-fluence "apices" create a pattern of coagulated columns, while the background fluence gently heats the intervening uncoagulated tissue. Histologically, the high-fluence CAP columns are limited to approximately 300 μm in depth, constraining treatment to the zone of superficial photodamage. This combination of mechanisms is proposed to improve treatment efficacy, while maintaining the side effects profile of existing methods. The laser light is delivered via a stamping technology with a spot size of 300 μm, which is five times the spot size relative to repair. It is delivered with a pulsed technique. The handpiece must be replaced with each treatment and is the only consumable.[18,54,55]

The fractional 2940-nm wavelength Er : YAG laser (Harmony XL, Alma Lasers, Buffalo Grove, IL) is part of a platform system that offers multiple applications including 10 distinct technologies that treat a wide array of problems ranging from vascular lesions to photoaging. The 2940-nm Er : YAG, microoptic lens creates 49 (7×7) or 81 (9×9) pixel size ablation dots on the skin with an 11×11 mm treatment zone. The spot size is three times larger than the Fraxel Re:pair and has a fixed density of 20%. This laser delivers energy to a depth of 20 to 50 μm when using the fractional handpiece. The pulse duration is 1, 1.5, or 2 ms. Delivery of the laser is pulsed. Maximum coverage rate ranges from 98 mm^2/s to 121 mm^2/s. The handpiece must be replaced for each treatment. The laser is touted as providing the patient with the effectiveness of an ablative approach with the comfort level and convenience of a nonablative treatment. The laser can safely be used on the face, neck, chest, arms, and hands.[18,54,55]

Other available fractional lasers differ based on the spot sizes, depth of treatment, energy delivered, and mode of delivery (static vs. dynamic).

One system incorporates two fractional handpieces in the same device. The Icon (Cynosure, Chelmsford, MA) platform combines a 1540-nm and a 2940-nm fractional handpiece. Both handpieces use a diffractive optic to create a fixed pitch array of microthermal injuries. Multiple passes are made until the total density and depth of lesions are achieved for that particular application.

Another newer device (Halo, Sciton, Palo Alto, CA) applies a scanning technology that combines 1470-nm (nonablative) and 2940-nm ablative wavelengths simultaneously in the same pass and same handpiece. In this system, the provider can titrate the degree of ablative and nonablative fractional wounds to optimize outcomes in skin rejuvenation and scar treatments. The platform also incorporates a ratline surface temperature monitor to reduce the risk of bulk heating of the skin.

CLINICAL EXPERIENCE WITH FRACTIONAL RESURFACING PROCEDURES

Perioral wrinkles (Figs. 5.7 and 5.8) are most difficult to treat with all fractional lasers and require four to six

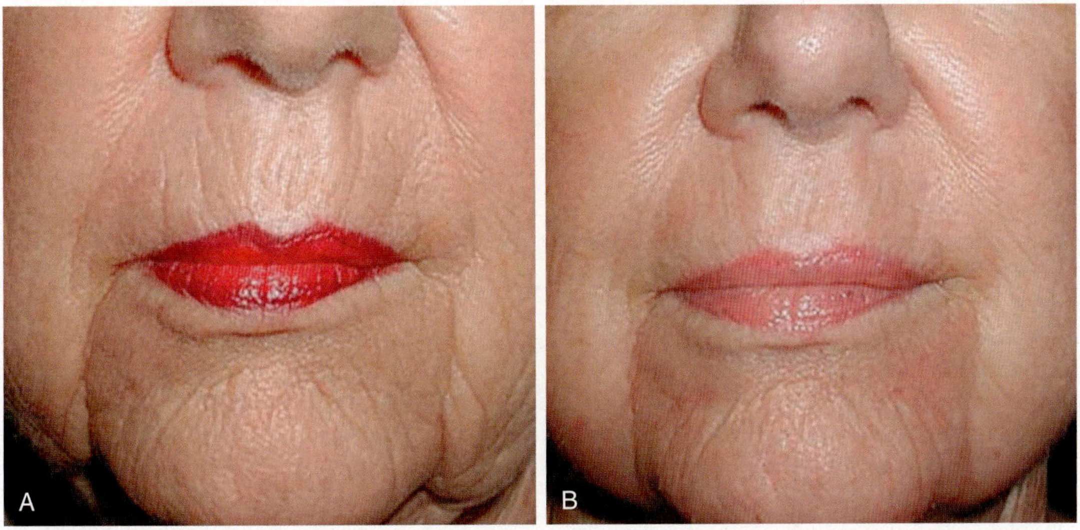

Fig. 5.7 1550-nm fractional erbium : glass laser for perioral wrinkles: (A) before and (B) 6 months after six treatments.

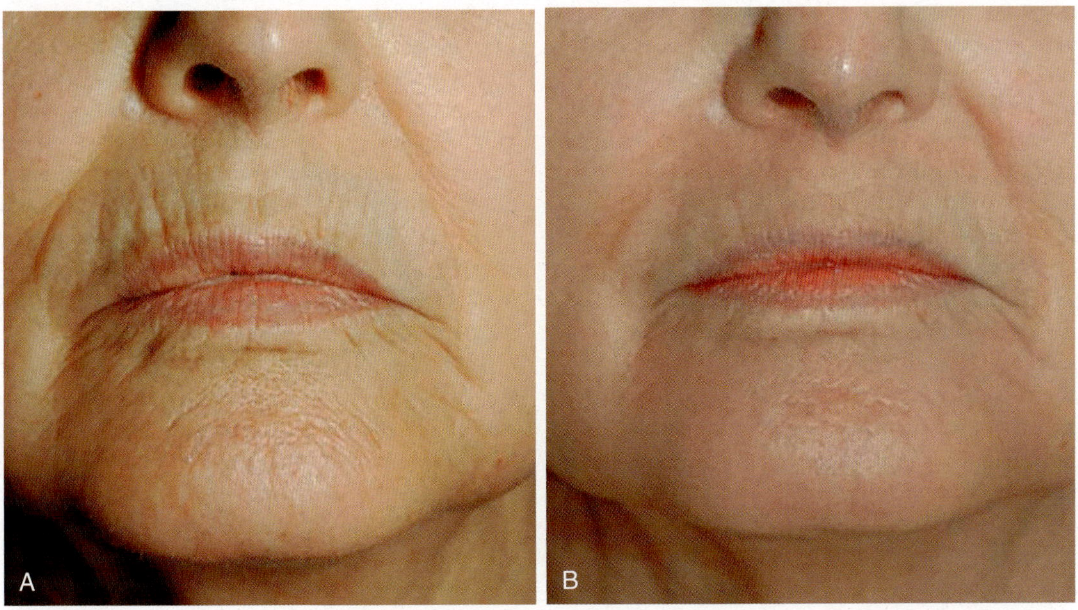

Fig. 5.8 Treatment of perioral wrinkles with fractional CO_2 laser: (A) before and (B) 6 months after a single treatment.

treatments, 2 to 4 weeks apart, depending on severity of the wrinkles. They are slow to respond and often require skin fillers. Higher energy is usually needed (three to four passes). That said, for deeper perioral wrinkles, we generally recommend a nonfractional CO_2 or Er : YAG laser (see Fig. 5.8). For acne scarring, one must be patient and allow time for collagen remodeling (see Fig. 5.4). With the 1550 erbium : glass fractional laser, four to six treatments, 3 to 4 weeks apart, are usually required. As aggressive as the skin type allows, higher energy is used.[1,18] Analgesic premedication may be needed. Hyperpigmentation is improved as well. Patients with melasma and dyschromia are pretreated with hydroquinone. In general, four to five treatments are used, spaced 10 to 14 days apart. Lower energy is used with more passes. Good results may be seen in Asian skin, although melasma may be very difficult to treat and eradicate. Treatment failures with melasma are not uncommon and may be disappointing. Realistic expectations must be set with the patient, and patient education is necessary to ensure they understand the limitations of treatment.[1,18,54,55]

Although infrequent, complications do occur. PIH can occur and can take 3 to 6 months to resolve. It is managed with hydroquinone and tretinoin (0.05% or 0.10%). We use the Obagi skin care system consisting of hydroquinone, tretinoin, vitamin C, and sunscreen. Patients with a history of herpes may experience an outbreak if not pretreated with Zovirax or a similar medication. If this history is known, we treat the patient for 48 h before fractional laser therapy.[1,18]

In our practice, prophylactic Valtrex (GlaxoSmithKline, Research Triangle Park, NC) 500 mg, 1 tablet PO bid, is started 48 h before treatment administration in all patients, regardless of a history of herpes simplex virus (HSV), at their pretreatment appointment. Administration of prophylactic antiviral and antibiotic (Keflex, unless allergy was noted, then clindamycin is given) medication is given to all CO_2 laser patients regardless of HSV history. Instructions are given to discontinue all irritating or abrasive products (Retina-A, glycolic, salicylic, lactic acids, benzol-peroxides, or any facial cleansing scrubs) 3 weeks before treatment and until 6 weeks posttreatment.

Over time, the patient can expect lessening of hyperpigmentation, then improvement of "crepey" skin tone, followed by lessening of fine lines and then deep lines. Changes in deep lines can be a delayed phenomenon and can take months to occur because of the collagen remodeling process. Significant tightening of the skin may result as a secondary response and appears to be cumulative. The tightening is particularly evident in the nasolabial folds and glabella. Results with the use of the 1550 erbium : glass fractional laser have been more consistent than those obtained with other nonablative systems. No comparative clinical outcome data for the other fractional lasers in this class are available, so it is difficult to assume equivalency, especially if lasers do not penetrate as deeply or if similar numbers of treatments are not delivered.[1,18,54,55]

Patients tolerate the 1550 erbium : glass fractional laser as well as the other Er : YAG or erbium : glass laser treatments when used with the Zimmer Cooler, Benadryl, and Tylenol (or similar medications). Men tolerate it less well than women and lower energy may need to be used. Women's skin may be more sensitive around their menstrual cycle.[1,18,54,55]

The best response is in solar-damaged skin, fine lines, and "crepey" skin. Very good outcomes may also be seen with periorbital lines. Using a lower setting and a higher density (6–8 mJ/cm^2; 250 MTZ/cm^2) results in a good response. Fractional photothermolysis can be used as an adjunct to surgery as well, but safety parameters have not been fully studied. Fractional laser of undermined skin flaps during facelift is unknown (Fig. 5.9).[1,18,54,55]

In patients undergoing fractional CO_2 therapy, our prelaser skin care regimen is similar to the less-invasive, 1550-nm erbium : glass fractional laser. Patients are prepped with topical anesthetic ointment for 1 h before the laser. Metal eye shields are routinely used. Many require an oral pain medication, and some require nerve blocks to divisions I–III of the trigeminal nerve for facial anesthesia. Full-face laser takes around 20 min. The energy and density are selected based on the patient's skin type and condition being treated. Lower energies and densities are used for darker Fitzpatrick skin types, and higher energies and densities are used for acne and deep wrinkles, depending on skin type. In general, lower energies and densities are used on the neck and chest as well.[1,18,54,55]

In the last few years, a multimodal approach for nonsurgical facial rejuvenation has become common practice. The use of ablative or nonablative lasers in conjunction with deeper heating long-pulse skin-tightening technologies (RF- or US-based) provides excellent aesthetic outcomes. In such treatment, lasers provide photothermolysis that results in the changes addressed previously in the chapter, while RF or US technologies deliver thermal energy to the deep layers and promote collagen regeneration, contraction, and skin tightening (Fig. 5.10).

POSTPROCEDURAL CONSIDERATIONS

Postprocedure Care

Postoperative care is aimed at providing an ideal environment for moist wound healing. Initially, a generous amount of bland ointment (white petrolatum, A&D

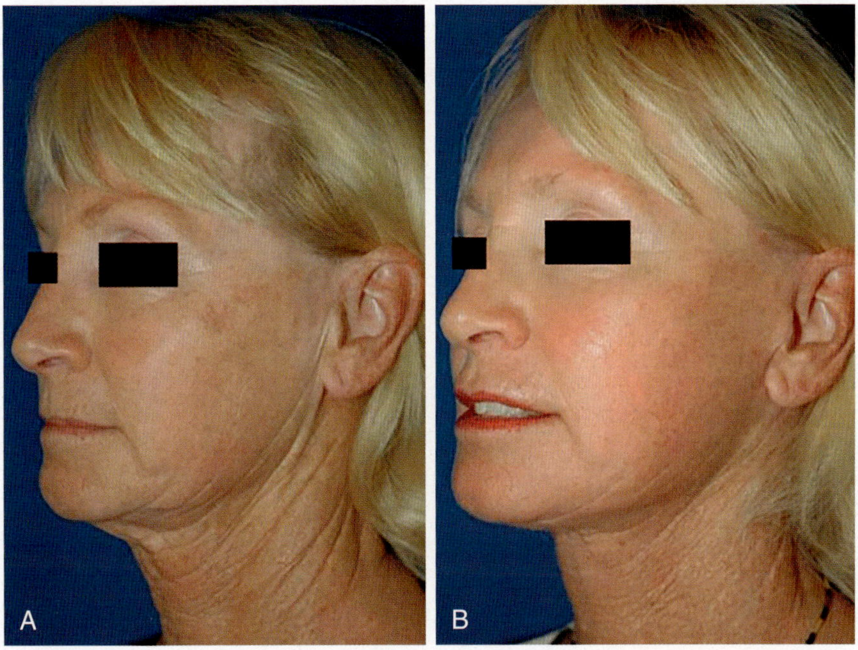

Fig. 5.9 Fractional CO_2 resurfacing done sequentially—superficial musculoaponeurotic system (SMAS) facelift followed by fractional CO_2 3 months later: (A) before and (B) 6 months after treatment.

ointment) is applied to the entire treated area. Crisco vegetable shortening historically had been used quite successfully but has been reformulated and now actually may be irritating to patients. Patients are instructed to reapply the ointment throughout the day, any time the face feels tight or dry. As the outer layers begin to shed, the patient is allowed to shower and gently wash the face with nonresidue soap using fingertips only. After showering, the face should be patted dry, and a new coating of ointment applied. Instruct patients not to pick at the face during the recovery period.[19,20] Following chemical peeling, some practitioners use topical agents that contain platelet products or growth factors. While these products have been reported to improve wound healing in other clinical situations, no randomized controlled clinical trials presently support their use in this setting. This is an area in which further research is ongoing. Understanding the process of reepithelialization and the importance of compliance with the prescribed posttreatment regimen is essential information for every patient. This includes awareness of likely facial edema that may contribute to symptoms such as diplopia. If antiviral therapy is instituted, continue therapy until reepithelialization is complete. In the early stages of wound healing, reexamine the patient within 48 h and again every several days. Instruct patients to refrain from trans-retinoic acid, sunscreen, or make-up until the face is healed to the satisfaction of the treating physician.[19,20]

Postlaser treatment generally consists of gauze and ice packs immediately after treatment, followed by vinegar and H_2O soaks every 3 to 4 h when awake for the first 2 to 3 days, depending on exudate and crusting. Benadryl capsule is recommended each evening for the first 3 days. Aquaphor ointment dressing is used for the first 3 days, then Cetaphil lotion for the duration of the healing process. Healing takes place over the first few days, with reepithelialization nearly complete by 48 h. Redness subsides over the next 3 to 4 days and gradually disappears over the next 3 to 4 weeks. Early results have been impressive.[19,20]

COMPLICATIONS AND OUTCOMES

Contraindications

Laser and chemical resurfacing have common contraindications. These include active bacterial, viral, fungal, or herpetic infection; open wounds; history of drugs with photosensitizing potential; preexisting inflammatory

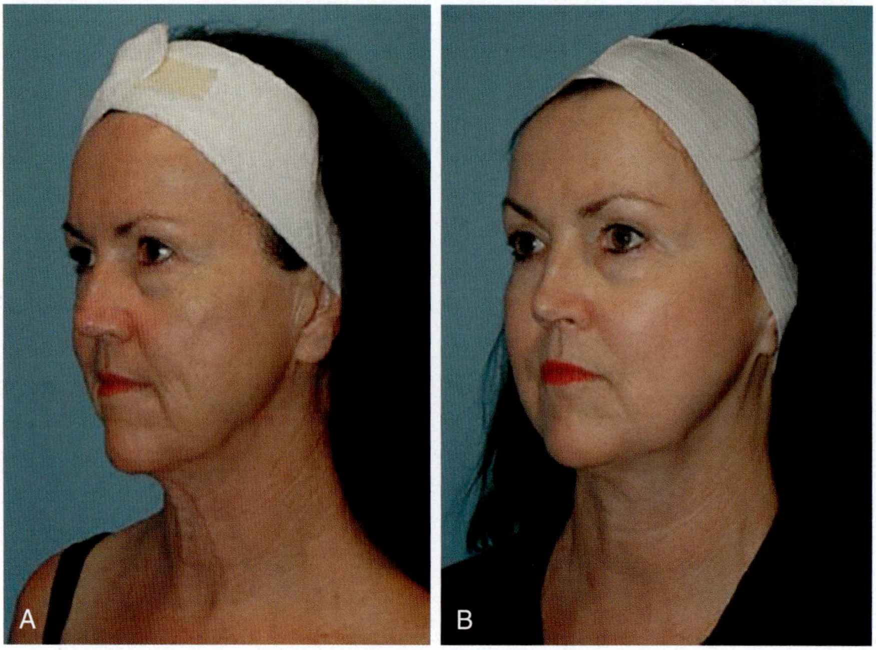

Fig. 5.10 Before and after ThermiRF (ThermiAesthetics, LLC, Southlake, TX) and Fraxel.

dermatoses; uncooperative patients; patients with unrealistic expectations; history of abnormal or keloid-type scarring.[19,20]

PIGMENTARY CHANGE

Pigmentary change is not an uncommon complication, especially with the deeper peeling agents, or deep penetration laser therapy. Taking proper precautions (as described earlier) can help prevent undesirable pigmentary changes. Usually, patients with lighter complexions have a lower risk of hyperpigmentation than darker skinned individuals. Skin priming using a combination of hydroquinone and tretinoin cream (Kligman formulation) before a superficial or medium-depth peel, and early introduction of this preparation after deep peels, might reduce the rate of this complication.[19,20]

SCARRING

Scarring remains the most feared complication of facial resurfacing. The contributing factors are still not well understood, but typically, outside of infection, the depth of the procedure is the primary risk factor in conventional resurfacing. In the case of fractional lasers, the depths and density of the microinjuries should be conservative enough to avoid bulk heating of the skin. By using the most appropriate resurfacing procedure for any given patient, the risk of scarring can be decreased. In addition, to further decrease the risk of scarring, the patient should be advised to refrain from touching or picking at the healing skin. Patients with a history of keloids should absolutely not undergo medium or deep treatments because of the risk of scarring. Weaker superficial treatments that only exfoliate the stratum corneum or superficial epidermis can be used for these high-risk patients.[19,20]

INFECTION

By using bacitracin for the medium and deep treatments and cleaning the face with a povidone wash, the risk of infection is decreased. However, some practitioners try to avoid using bacitracin because of the risk of contact dermatitis and use Aquaphor instead. Cold sores can be prevented with acyclovir (400 mg PO bid), beginning 2 days before the treatment and continuing 7 days after the treatment. Candidiasis also can develop, for which a short course of fluconazole can be used.

Cultures need to be taken, and appropriate antibiotics should be administered.[19,20] More recently, atypical mycobacterial infections have been reported after ablative fractional procedures.[58] Most likely, the penetrating nature of fractional approaches allows these opportunists to thrive. Measures to decrease the risk include thorough cleansing before treatment and avoidance of tap water at the wound site during and immediately after treatment. Physicians should note that the greatest association with infection is pain. If the skin is healing poorly and the patient reports marked pain, an infection is likely. The absence of pain does not remove the possibility of infection but markedly reduces its likelihood.

PROLONGED ERYTHEMA

Patients usually do not report erythema because it generally subsides in 30 to 90 days, but sometimes erythema continues. Prolonged erythema is usually not permanent, and topical hydrocortisone can be used to speed the healing process.[19,20]

ACNE

Some patients develop acne after a facial resurfacing procedure. This usually occurs between days 3 to 9. Cultures should be taken, and an antibiotic that covers gram-positive bacteria should be prescribed. If it is a true acne occurrence, then the appropriate topical treatment also should be started. If severe enough, isotretinoin may be initiated.[19,20]

MILIA

Small inclusion cysts, sometimes called *milia*, can appear in the healing process after a treatment. These usually appear about 2 to 3 weeks after reepithelialization and may be aggravated by ointments, owing to occlusion of the sebaceous glands.[19,20]

DISCLOSURES

Drs. Cohen, Saad, and Leong have no financial relationships with any commercial laser company discussed in this chapter. Dr. Ross receives honoraria from Palomar, Lumenis, Candela, and Cutera; Dr. Ross receives research support from Candela, Palomar, Sciton, Cutera, and Syneron.

REFERENCES

1. Alexander JT, Goldman MP, Roberts TL. Facial resurfacing. In: Mathes J, ed. *Plastic Surgery*. Vol. 2. 2nd ed. Philadelphia, PA: WB Saunders; 2006:339-384.
2. Smith L. Histopathologic characteristics and ultrastructure of aging skin. *Cutis*. 1989;43:414.
3. Brody HJ. *Chemical Peeling and Resurfacing*. 2nd ed. St. Louis, MO: Mosby-Yearbooks; 1997:29-38.
4. Anderson RR, Parrish JA. Selective photothermolysis: precise microsurgery by selective absorption of pulsed radiation. *Science*. 1983;220:524-527.
5. Ross EV, Swann M, Soon S, et al. Full-face treatments with the 2790-nm erbium:YSGG laser system. *J Drugs Dermatol*. 2009;8:248-252.
6. Gillitzer R, Goebeler M. Chemokines in cutaneous wound healing. *J Leukoc Biol*. 2001;69:513-521.
7. Glat PM, Longaker MT. Wound healing. In: Aston SJ, Beasley RW, Thorne CH, eds. *Grabb and Smith's Plastic Surgery*. Philadelphia, PA: Lippincott-Raven; 1997.
8. Anderson RR. Dermatologic history of the ruby laser: the long story of short pulses. *Arch Dermatol*. 2003;139:70-74.
9. Welch AJ, van Gemert MJ. Overview of optical and thermal interaction and nomenclature. In: Welch AJ, van Gemert MJ, eds. *Optical Thermal Response of Laser-Irradiated Tissue*. New York, NY: Plenum; 1995:1-14.
10. Anderson R, Ross E. Laser–tissue interactions. In: Fitzpatrick R, Goldman M, eds. *Cosmetic Laser Surgery*. St Louis, MO: Mosby; 2000:1-30.
11. Anderson R. Laser–tissue interactions. In: Goldman M, Fitzparick R, eds. *Cutaneous Laser Surgery – The Art and Science of Selective Photothermolysis*. St Louis, MO: Mosby; 1994:3-5.
12. Ross EV, Sajben FP, Hsia J, et al. Nonablative skin remodeling: selective dermal heating with a mid-infrared laser and contact cooling combination. *Lasers Surg Med*. 2000;26:186-195.
13. Ross E, Anderson R. Laser tissue interactions. In: Goldman M, ed. *Cutaneous and Cosmetic Laser Surgery*. Philadelphia, PA: Elsevier; 2006.
14. Alam M, White LE, Martin N, et al. Ultrasound tightening of facial and neck skin: a rater-blinded prospective cohort study. *J Am Acad Dermatol*. 2010;62:262-269.
15. Kelly KM, Nelson JS, Lask GP, et al. Cryogen spray cooling in combination with nonablative laser treatment of facial rhytides. *Arch Dermatol*. 1999;135:691-694.
16. Lask G, Lee PK, Seyfzadeh M, et al. Nonablative laser treatment of facial rhytides. In: Anderson RR, ed. *Lasers in Surgery: Advanced Characterization, Therapeutics, and Systems VII*. Vol. 2970. San Jose, CA: Society of Photo-Instrumentation Engineers; 1997:338-349.

17. Sadick NS. Update on non-ablative light therapy for rejuvenation: a review. *Lasers Surg Med.* 2003;32: 120-128. *A review of nonablative skin resurfacing modalities is presented.*
18. Cohen SR, Henssler C, Johnston J. Fractional photothermolysis for skin rejuvenation. *Plast Reconstr Surg.* 2009; 124:281-290.
19. Fabbrocini G. *Chemical Peels.* 2015. Available at: http://emedicine.medscape.com/article/1829120-overview.
20. Hilinski JM, Revis DR, Seagle MB. *Skin Resurfacing – Chemical Peels.* Available at: www.emedicine.com.
21. Fitzpatrick RE, Goldman MP, Satur NM, et al. Pulsed carbon dioxide laser resurfacing of photo-aged facial skin. *Arch Dermatol.* 1996;132:395-402.
22. Glogau RG, Matarasso SL. Chemical peels. Trichloroacetic acid and phenol. *Dermatol Clin.* 1995;13:263-276.
23. Ross EV, Zelickson BD. Biophysics of nonablative dermal remodeling. *Semin Cutan Med Surg.* 2002;21:251-265.
24. Saafan AM, Salah MM. Using pulsed dual-wavelength 595 and 1064 nm is more effective in the management of hemangiomas. *J Drugs Dermatol.* 2010;9:310-314.
25. Kauvar AN, Rosen N, Khrom T. A newly modified 595-nm pulsed dye laser with compression handpiece for the treatment of photodamaged skin. *Lasers Surg Med.* 2006;38:808-813.
26. Soon SL, Ross EV. Letter: use of a perforated plastic shield for precise application of intense pulsed light. *Dermatol Surg.* 2008;34:1149-1150.
27. Kono T, Manstein D, Chan HH, et al. Q-switched ruby versus long-pulsed dye laser delivered with compression for treatment of facial lentigines in Asians. *Lasers Surg Med.* 2006;38:94-97.
28. Taylor CR, Anderson RR. Ineffective treatment of refractory melasma and postinflammatory hyperpigmentation by Q-switched ruby laser. *J Dermatol Surg Oncol.* 1994;20:592-597.
29. Chan HH, Kono T. The use of lasers and intense pulsed light sources for the treatment of pigmentary lesions. *Skin Therapy Lett.* 2004;9:5-7.
30. Negishi K, Kushikata N, Tezuka Y, et al. Study of the incidence and nature of "very subtle epidermal melasma" in relation to intense pulsed light treatment. *Dermatol Surg.* 2004;30:881-886.
31. Wattanakrai P, Mornchan R, Eimpunth S. Low-fluence Q-switched neodymium-doped yttrium aluminum garnet (1,064 nm) laser for the treatment of facial melasma in Asians. *Dermatol Surg.* 2010;36:76-87.
32. Hwang CY, Lin CS, Tseng ML, et al. Spotted leucoderma after treatment of facial hyperpigmentation on hemodialysis patients employing 1064-nm Q-switched Nd:YAG laser. *J Cosmet Laser Ther.* 2010;12:47-50.
33. Taylor MB, Prokopenko I. Split-face comparison of radiofrequency versus long-pulse Nd:YAG treatment of facial laxity. *J Cosmet Laser Ther.* 2006;8:17-22.
34. Trelles MA, Alvarez X, Martin-Vazquez MJ, et al. Assessment of the efficacy of nonablative long-pulsed 1064-nm Nd:YAG laser treatment of wrinkles compared at 2, 4, and 6 months. *Facial Plast Surg.* 2005;21:145-153.
35. Prieto VG, Diwan AH, Shea CR, et al. Effects of intense pulsed light and the 1,064 nm Nd:YAG laser on sun-damaged human skin: histologic and immunohistochemical analysis. *Dermatol Surg.* 2005;31:522-525.
36. Lipper GM, Perez M. Nonablative acne scar reduction after a series of treatments with a short-pulsed 1,064-nm neodymium:YAG laser. *Dermatol Surg.* 2006;32:998-1006.
37. Jih MH, Friedman PM, Kimyai-Asadi A, et al. Successful treatment of a chronic atrophic dog-bite scar with the 1450-nm diode laser. *Dermatol Surg.* 2004;30:1161-1163.
38. Dahan S, Lagarde JM, Turlier V, et al. Treatment of neck lines and forehead rhytids with a nonablative 1540-nm Er:glass laser: a controlled clinical study combined with the measurement of the thickness and the mechanical properties of the skin. *Dermatol Surg.* 2004;30:872-880.
39. Paithankar DY, Clifford JM, Saleh BA, et al. Subsurface skin renewal by treatment with a 1450-nm laser in combination with dynamic cooling. *J Biomed Opt.* 2003;8:545-551.
40. Goldberg DJ. Nonablative dermal remodeling: does it really work? *Arch Dermatol.* 2002;138:1366-1368.
41. Jacob CI, Dover JS, Kaminer MS. Acne scarring: a classification system and review of treatment options. *J Am Acad Dermatol.* 2001;45:109-117.
42. Goodman G. Post acne scarring: a review. *J Cosmet Laser Ther.* 2003;5:77-95.
The acne scar is a historically difficult problem with pathology that varies considerably within and between patients. The authors emphasize the necessity of applying lesion-specific techniques in their review of evolving technologies to address acne scars.
43. Yaghmai D, Garden JM, Bakus AD, et al. Comparison of a 1,064 nm laser and a 1,320 nm laser for the nonablative treatment of acne scars. *Dermatol Surg.* 2005;31:903-909.
44. Alster TS, Tanzi EL, Welsh EC. Photorejuvenation of facial skin with topical 20% 5-aminolevulinic acid and intense pulsed light treatment: a split-face comparison study. *J Drugs Dermatol.* 2005;4:35-38.
45. Richey DF. Aminolevulinic acid photodynamic therapy for sebaceous gland hyperplasia. *Dermatol Clin.* 2007;25:59-65.
46. Dover JS, Zelickson B. Results of a survey of 5,700 patient monopolar radiofrequency facial skin tightening treatments: assessment of a low-energy multiple-pass

technique leading to a clinical endpoint algorithm. *Dermatol Surg*. 2007;33:900-907.

47. Gold MH, Eremia S, eds. *Skin Tightening with the Aluma Skin Tightening System in Office Based Cosmetic Procedures*. Cambridge, UK: Cambridge University Press; 2010:246-249.
48. Sadick NS, Shaoul J. Hair removal using a combination of conducted radiofrequency and optical energies – an 18-month follow up. *J Cosmet Laser Ther*. 2004;6:21-26.
49. Chess C. Prospective study on combination diode laser and bipolar radiofrequency energies for the treatment of leg veins. *J Cosmet Laser Ther*. 2004;6:27-31.
50. Hruza G, Taub AF, Collier SL, et al. Skin rejuvenation and wrinkle reduction using a fractional radiofrequency system. *J Drugs Dermatol*. 2009;8:259-265.
51. Gold MH, Foster A, Biron J. Clinical evaluation of a new fractionated bipolar radiofrequency device for the treatment of photoaging. *J Am Acad Dermatol*. 2011;64:AB171.
52. Kaplan H, Gat A. Clinical and histopathological results following TriPollar radiofrequency skin treatments. *J Cosmet Laser Ther*. 2009;11:78-84.
53. Boisnic S, Branchet MC. Ex vivo human skin evaluation of localized fat reduction and anti-aging effect of TriPollar radio frequency treatments. *J Cosmet Laser Ther*. 2010;12:25-31.
54. Bass LS. Rejuvenation of the aging face using Fraxel laser treatment. *Aesthet Surg J*. 2005;25:307.
55. Bernstein EF, Andersen D, Zelickson BD. Laser resurfacing for dermal photoaging. *Clin Plast Surg*. 2000;27:221.
56. Schenk P, Ehrenberger K. Effect of CO_2 laser on skin lymphatics. An ultrastructural study. *Langenbecks Arch Chir*. 1980;350:145-150.
57. Saad AN, Lim S, Goodacre A, et al. *Complications associated with fractional lasers: a review of 716 patients treated by medically supervised, nurse and physician assistant laser specialists*. Presented at the American Society of Aesthetic Plastic Surgery 2015 annual meeting, Montreal.
58. Palm MD, Butterwick KJ, Goldman MP. *Mycobacterium chelonae* infection after fractionated carbon dioxide facial resurfacing (presenting as an atypical acneiform eruption). Case report and literature review. *Dermatol Surg*. 2010;36:1473-1481.

6

Laser Hair Removal and Vein Ablation

Briana Paiewonsky, Gabriel J. Martinez-Diaz, Omer Ibrahim, and Carolyn I. Jacob

INTRODUCTION (PEARLS)

- Laser treatments are some of the most effective and minimally invasive options for removing unwanted hair and ablating veins.
- Lasers function based on the principle of selective photothermolysis, in which the pigment in the hair (melanin) or in oxyhemoglobin in the blood vessel is heated to destroy the chromophore without overheating the surrounding tissues to avoid epidermal damage.
- Lasers are selected based on wavelength, pulse duration, and depth of penetration to achieve the desired goal.
- Cooling during laser pulses is required to reduce epidermal injury and associated adverse events such as change in pigmentation, burns, blister, and scar formation.
- Laser hair removal and vein ablation are considered more effective than most other treatment options; however, they may still cause a rubber band snapping or pinprick-like sensation.
- Expectations and goals of treatment should be discussed with the patient before undergoing any form of laser treatment.
- Repeated sessions for clearance, and maintenance treatments for potential new veins, may be required to see and sustain the results of laser treatment.
- Common side effects of laser treatment include erythema and edema. Complications of scarring and permanent pigmentation changes may occur, but there is decreased risk with patient-centered laser selection, proper cooling, and laser settings.

BACKGROUND INFORMATION/ ANATOMIC PEARLS

Laser Hair Removal

Many postpubertal patients have unwanted hair and practice hair removal of some form. Common temporary methods of hair removal include waxing, plucking, shaving, and depilation. Temporary methods can last weeks to months, with waxing generally lasting the longest at 2 or 3 weeks longer than the others.[1] While these methods are typically temporary, they may incidentally damage the dermal papilla causing minimal permanent removal of hair.

Permanent hair reduction has been defined as a significant reduction in the number of terminal hairs after a given treatment, which is stable for a period of time longer than the complete growth cycle of hair follicles at the given body site.[2] Permanent methods of hair removal include electrolysis, laser therapy, or intense pulsed light (IPL) therapy. Electrolysis is labor intensive, and its efficacy largely depends on application of correct technique.[3] Laser hair removal may be a superior choice for long-term hair removal as it is more effective, faster, and less painful[4] (Fig. 6.1).

There are several wavelengths, measured in nanometers (nm), of lasers available for hair removal. They include the ruby laser (694 nm), alexandrite laser (755 nm), diode

Funding: There was no funding for this work
Disclosures: The authors have no relevant financial interests to disclose.

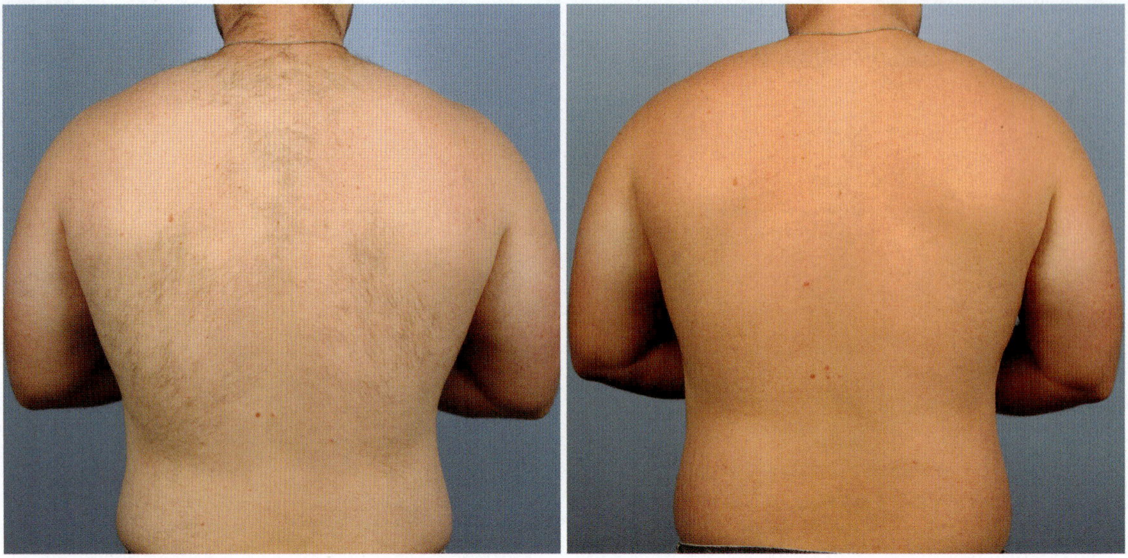

Fig. 6.1 Significant, long-term reduction in hair on the back of a male patient after a series of treatments using a long pulse 755-nm alexandrite laser.(Copyright retained by Melanie Palm, MD.)

laser (800 nm), and neodymium : yttrium-aluminum-garnet (Nd : YAG) laser (1064 nm). Separately, intense pulsed broadband light sources (590–1200 nm) can also be used for hair removal. Lasers are considered photo-epilation therapies that reduce hair through selective photothermolysis. Selective photothermolysis is a technique that asserts that applying a brief laser pulse to a pigmented target will generate and confine heat to that pigment as long as the laser penetrates deep enough, and the target has greater absorption than its surrounding tissue at a specific wavelength. The pulse should be brief and targeted such that the temperature exceeds that required to denature the pigmented target, in this case melanin in the hair bulb, without heating the surrounding tissue above its denaturing point.[5] Surrounding tissue often contains structures that may absorb the laser energy, such as skin pigment, which may lead to adverse effects or decrease the efficacy of the treatment.

The wavelength of the laser should be selected so that it is only absorbed by the melanin in the hair bulb and based on the desired depth of laser penetration. The main sources of interference for absorption in the hair are melanin in the skin and oxyhemoglobin present within blood vessels. However, it has been shown that a wavelength of 700 nm is selectively absorbed by melanin and, in turn, specifically destroys the hair follicle, leaving the blood vessels chiefly intact.[3] The longer the wavelength of the laser, the deeper penetration into the skin and the lower affinity for absorption by surface melanin. This allows for more selective absorption by the melanin in the hair bulb rather than epidermal melanin.

Adequate cooling between pulses is required to reduce epidermal injury and associated adverse events such as change in pigmentation and blister formation, especially individuals with darker phototypes. Cooling can be achieved through application of ice, application of a cooling gel, application of pulsed cryogen spray (dynamic cooling device [DCD]), or through addition of a contact cooling window attached to the handpiece of the laser. Cooling pieces include a sapphire handpiece or a cooled glass chamber.[2]

Laser hair removal, regardless of the laser used, creates pinprick or rubber band snapping against the skin sensation because of heat. That, in combination with the different pain thresholds throughout the body, results in areas of greater or lesser sensitivity to laser treatment.[6] The most sensitive areas include the bikini line and axilla, while the legs and arms are generally much less painful.

Laser Vein Ablation

Venous insufficiency can present with a variety of clinical symptoms ranging from superficial telangiectasia to chronic venous disease with severe skin ulceration. Treatment options include thermal or nonthermal vein ablation, sclerotherapy, or vein ligation and stripping, the latter of which are typically reserved for more severe disease and are associated with higher postoperative complications. When treating more superficial telangiectasias and varicose veins, sclerotherapy and thermal or laser vein removal are more appropriate treatments.

For the purpose of this text, we will discuss laser vein removal, as it is the most minimally invasive treatment option for cosmetic vein removal. It is most effective for telangiectasias, reticular veins, and small varicose veins. Specifically, laser or light vein therapy is optimal for use on vessels 1 to 2 mm in diameter, but it can be used for vessels as large as 4 to 5 mm.

Like laser hair removal, laser vein treatment applies selective photothermolysis. However, in the case of laser vein ablation, the target pigment is oxyhemoglobin rather than melanin. To target the oxyhemoglobin, a laser with the appropriate wavelength must be selected to avoid interference with competing melanin in the skin and hair. Specific lasers used for vein ablation target oxyhemoglobin using three broad absorption peaks at 418, 542, and 577 nm, or smaller peaks at 920 to 940 nm[7] and 1064 nm. The heat causes coagulation and collapse of the vein, resulting in decreased visualization of the vein and redirection of the blood flow through collateral vessels. Common lasers used on vascular lesions are long pulse lasers, including the potassium titanyl phosphate (KTP) (532 nm), pulsed dye laser (PDL) (585–595 nm), alexandrite laser (755 nm), diode laser (800 nm), Nd : YAG (1064 nm), and the IPL source (590–1200 nm). Similar cooling requirements, including use of cryogen spray, sapphire handpieces, chilled air or water, are needed for laser vein ablation as with laser hair removal. The pain associated with treatment is typically described as a pinching or stinging sensation.

PREPROCEDURAL CONSIDERATIONS

Laser Hair Removal

A proper history and physical examination should be performed on any patients undergoing laser hair removal. Special attention should be paid to discern any conditions causing the hypertrichosis, a history of herpes simplex, a history of keloids, previous laser treatment, and the results of that treatment.[2] If the patient has a previous history of herpes simplex, prophylaxis treatment with an antiviral should be considered before treatment. Pregnant patients should delay treatment until after delivery.

It is also important to set proper expectations for patients undergoing laser hair removal. Complete and permanent hair removal is uncommon. Patients should be counseled to expect less hair, thinner hair, and lighter hair after undergoing treatment. They should also be aware that repeated sessions and maintenance sessions are typically required to sustain these results.

Patients must prepare properly for the procedure. This includes avoiding any form of tanning or sunburning before the procedure, as increased skin pigmentation from baseline may lead to increased adverse effects because of absorption of the energy by the pigment in the epidermis. In addition, patients must avoid plucking, waxing, or any other methods of temporary hair removal for a couple of weeks before the procedure. For the lasers to be effective, there should be around 2 to 3 mm of hair present in the treatment area.[3] It is recommended that patients shave 2 to 3 days before the scheduled treatment.

Quite possibly the most important consideration for laser hair removal is selection of the appropriate laser. As previously mentioned, competitive structures with similar absorptive properties in the skin may interfere with the efficacy of selective photothermolysis. As a result, patients with darker hair and lighter skin tend to respond best to laser hair removal. However, certain lasers have been shown to be more effective for patients with darker phototypes. The ruby, alexandrite, diode, Nd : YAG lasers, and the IPL source will be discussed subsequently:

- The ruby 694-nm laser was the first laser studied. Typical of all lasers, this laser is most effective for use on dark hair on individuals with Fitzpatrick I–III phototypes.[2] Patients with darker skin tones or recent sun exposure may have increased risk of complications with the ruby laser.[8] This device is not commonly used now because of the better efficacy of the 755-nm laser.
- The 755-nm alexandrite laser penetrates deeper into the dermis than the 694-ruby laser. The deeper penetration means light is less likely to be absorbed by epidermal melanin, making alexandrite lasers safer than the ruby laser for use in patients with darker skin tones; however, other lasers may be better choices for indivuals with Fitzpatrick phototypes greater than III.

- The diode laser can operate at a range of wavelengths. At an 800 to 810 wavelength, the light can be absorbed by melanin, but less preferentially than with the ruby or alexandrite lasers, making it safer for use on indivuals with Fitzpatrick IV phototypes.[8]
- The 1064-nm long-pulsed Nd : YAG laser, however, appears to be the most appropriate laser for use in patients with darker skin tones, including Fitzpatrick IV–V phototypes. The 1064-nm wavelength is less avidly absorbed by endogenous melanin, making it less effective than the ruby or alexandrite laser. However, this also makes it less likely to cause adverse effects.[3,8] Patients with skin type Fitzpatrick VI phototypes typically do not have a great enough contrast between skin and hair color and therefore will not respond safely to laser therapy. They can, however, have treatment performed by microwave technology, which is color blind.
- IPL sources are different from the lasers discussed earlier. Lasers emit light at one wavelength, while IPL emits light at a range of wavelengths, specifically, between 550 to 1200 nm. By applying filters to the light source, specific wavelengths can be generated according to the patient's phototype, hair color, and coarseness. In addition, it has a relatively large exposure area, making this a good choice for large treatment areas and areas with coarse hair.[1]

Hair has three phases of growth, including the anagen phase, catagen phase, and telogen phase. The anagen phase is considered the actively growing phase, in which the hair matrix cells are rapidly dividing. It is during this anagenic phase that the hair is most sensitive to the thermal effects of laser hair removal, which may affect both the bulb and the bulge. Thus, treatments should ideally be conducted during the anagen phase of growth,[6] which is approximately every 3 to 5 weeks.

Laser Vein Ablation

As with laser hair removal, a full history and physical examination should be performed for every patient before undergoing treatment, noting for history of herpes simplex virus, history of keloid or hypertrophic scar formation, and previous laser treatment results. Pregnant patients should delay treatment until after delivery. If the patient displays signs or symptoms of venous reflux, this should also be managed before laser or light treatment. Furthermore, laser vein removal should not be considered in patients with a history of diabetes or peripheral vascular disease because of increased risk of delayed or inadequate wound healing. Laser vein removal may increase risk of deep vein thrombosis and should therefore be avoided in patients in a hypercoagulable state.

During the physical examination, the patient should be positioned upright to allow for proper examination of the vascular lesion. The physician should consider and investigate the cause of the varicose vein or telangiectasia. Whether or not there is an upstream vessel causing the target lesion may affect rates of recurrence after laser treatment and should be discussed with the patient.

Before treatment, patients should be briefed on the results to expect, as well as possible complications. The patient may observe immediate disappearance of the targeted vein after treatment; however, this may be caused by vasospasm rather than complete coagulation of the vein.[9] The patient should be advised that the target vein may persist or may simply appear less conspicuous despite the initial appearance of resolution. In addition, repeat sessions are generally required to achieve the desired results.

Patients must prepare properly for the procedure. This includes avoiding any form of tanning or sunburning before the procedure, just as with laser hair removal. Patients should also refrain from taking nonsteroidal antiinflammatory or anticoagulant agents before treatment, as this may increase risk of bruising.[9]

It is just as crucial to select the most appropriate laser for vein removal as it is for laser hair removal. To avoid targeting competing structures and adverse reactions, certain lasers are selected based on the size and location of the vein, as well as the Fitzpatrick phototype of the patient. In general, larger or deeper veins require the use of lasers with a longer wavelength, whereas shorter wavelengths can be used on smaller, more superficial lesions.[9] The KTP, pulse dye, alexandrite, diode, Nd : YAG lasers, and IPL sources used for vein treatment will be detailed subsequently:

- The KTP laser emits a green light with a wavelength of 532 nm to target oxyhemoglobin. This wavelength, however, overlaps with absorption by melanin, causing this laser to be best used in patients with Fitzpatrick phototypes I–III to avoid adverse complications from melanin interference. It works well on superficial leg veins less than 0.75 mm in diameter and may treat facial telangiectasias without causing purpura[10] (Fig. 6.2). In fact, this laser has proven to be more effective than the

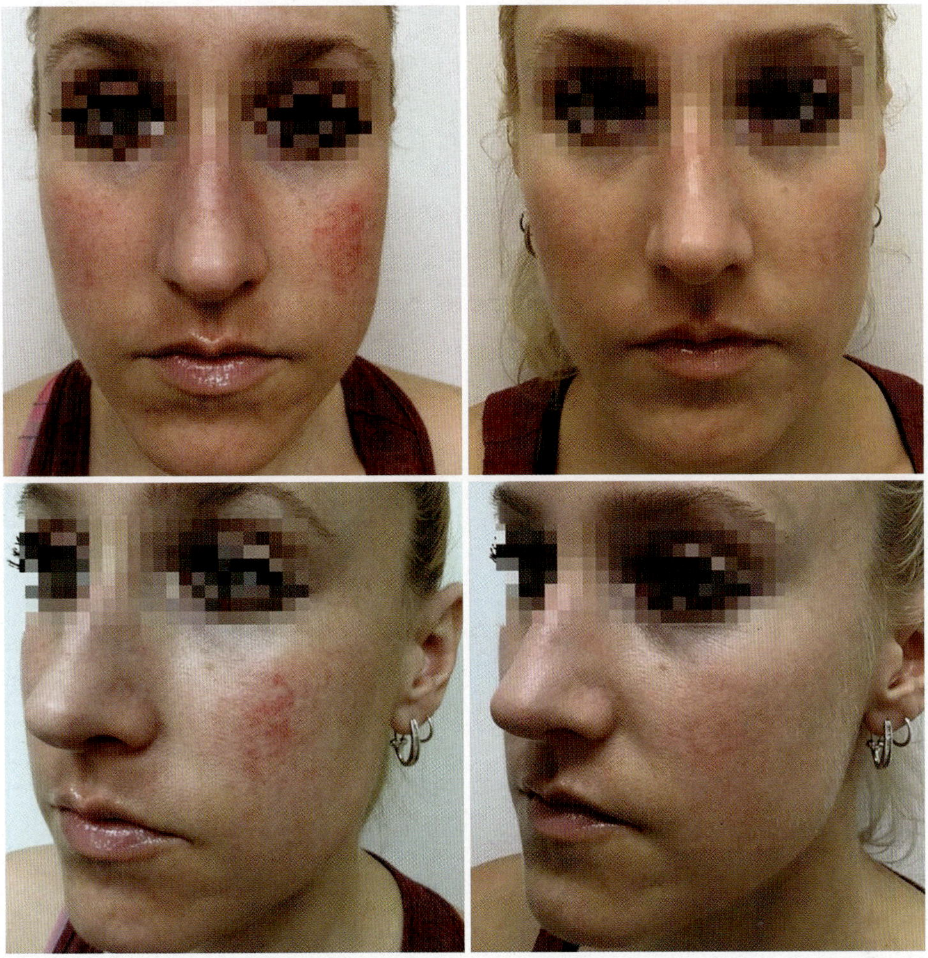

Fig. 6.2 Reduction in fine facial telangiectasias after a series treatments using a long pulse 532-nm potassium titanyl phosphate (KTP) laser. (Copyright retained by Carolyn Jacob, MD.)

Nd : YAG laser for smaller vessels.[9] Minimal pain and adverse effects are associated with this laser.[11]

- The long-PDL has a yellow wavelength of 585 to 595 nm. It is effective for treatment of deep vessels of up to 1.5 mm in diameter[10] but is most effective in vessels less than 1 mm.[9] It is also useful for treatment of facial telangiectasia. The pulse dye laser is superior to the KTP laser; however, it is more associated with persistent purpura and more pain.[12] Similar to the KTP, this laser is safer to use in patients with lighter phototypes.
- The alexandrite 755 nm laser has previously been discussed for laser hair removal. However, it is also effective for laser vein removal. Specifically, it is useful for veins around 2.5 to 3 mm deep and 0.4 to 3 mm wide.[13] Use of this laser for vascular purposes in darker skin tones has increased risk of adverse complications because of its absorption by melanin and should only be used in patients with Fitzpatrick phototypes I–III.
- The diode laser was also discussed for use for laser hair removal. This laser may operate at a range of wavelengths from 800 to 983 nm. The longer the wavelength, the more selective this laser is for oxyhemoglobin rather than melanin. The diode laser at 800 nm was shown to be most effective for vessels of 3 to 4 mm in diameter in patients with Fitzpatrick phototype III skin. This laser has less predictable results compared with the alexandrite laser, but it is

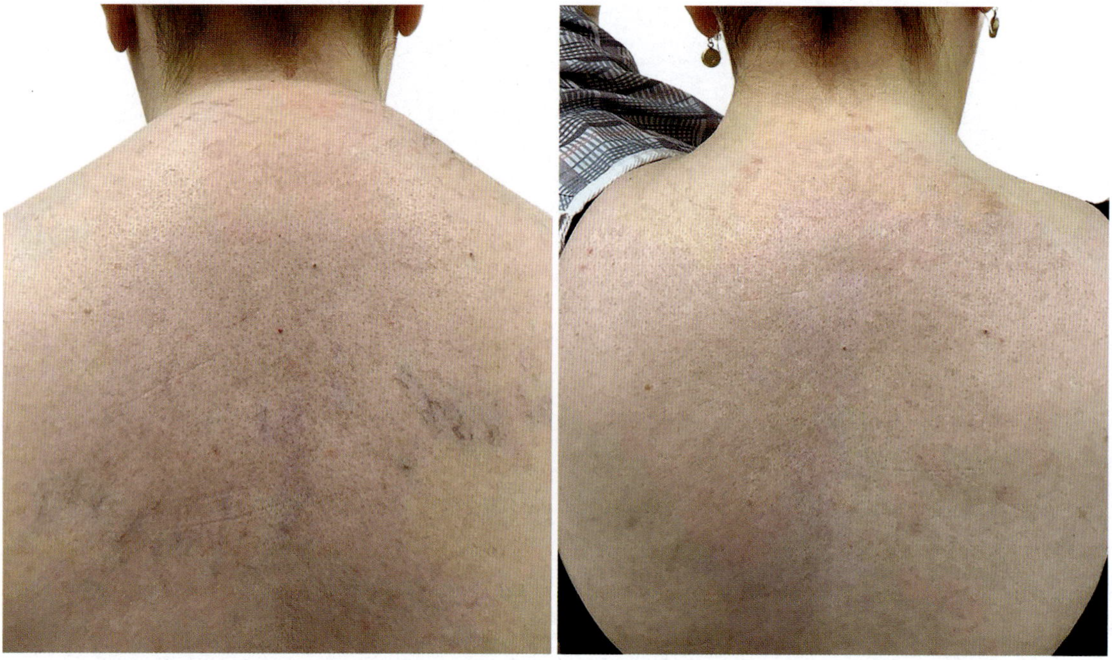

Fig. 6.3 Diminution of smaller and larger veins on the back after treatment using a combination of long-pulse 532-nm potassium titanyl phosphate (KTP) and 1064-nm neodymium-doped yttrium aluminum garnet (Nd : YAG) lasers. (Copyright retained by Carolyn Jacob, MD.)

safer than the alexandrite laser for patients with darker skin, including Fitzpatrick phototype IV.[14]

- The Nd : YAG laser emits a light with a wavelength of 1064 nm. Similar to its absorption by melanin, this longer wavelength is less avidly absorbed by oxyhemoglobin, making it less likely to cause adverse effects in patients with darker phototypes.[3,8] It is a versatile laser in that it effectively treats veins greater than 2 mm in diameter and has also been shown to be effective in smaller veins (Fig. 6.3). When compared to the alexandrite laser, diode laser, and IPL, the Nd : YAG is superior. The Nd : YAG laser can be used on facial telangiectasia if modified by the addition of a KTP crystal.[10]
- IPL sources, as previously mentioned, may be altered by the addition of filters to emit a specific wavelength. For laser vein removal, the 550 and 570 filters are typically used together. It can be used for treatment of small vessels, large vessels, and red facial telangiectasia but should only be operated by experienced physicians.[10]

PROCEDURE TECHNIQUES

Laser Hair Removal

First, the skin needs to be prepared, including removal of any make-up, creams, or other topicals. The laser treatment itself is associated with mild pain described as a pinprick or rubber band snapping sensation. To alleviate some of the patient's discomfort, topical anesthetic can be applied to more sensitive areas once the skin has been cleaned. EMLA or other compounded lidocaine cream of higher concentration is typically chosen and applied for 30 to 60 min before treatment. After sufficient numbing, the anesthetic is thoroughly removed. Although many lasers are equipped with a cooling handpiece, cooling gel may be applied at this time.

For the safety of the patient and the operator, protective eyewear should be worn during the treatment. Use of a smoke evacuator and adequate room ventilation are ideal to prevent respiratory irritation and unnecessary inhalation of the plume. Before conducting treatment throughout the entire target area, treatment may be conducted on a test spot, especially in patients with darker skin. The operator should use this spot to assess for combustion of the hair with mild erythema and swelling.[3] One should choose a test spot in the same area of intended treatment, especially if sun exposed. If excessive erythema, hypopigmentation, blistering, or lack of hair combustion is seen, laser fluence should be reconsidered. If adequate treatment results are seen (mild erythema and edema), the operator may continue treatment to the rest of the area.

During treatment, caution must be taken to avoid overlapping and treating an area twice while also ensuring to pulse the entire target area (Video 6.1). A treatment grid may be applied to the treatment area to ensure that no spots are missed and none are double-treated.

Laser Vein Ablation

Just as with laser hair removal, the skin needs to be prepared including removal of any make-up, creams, or other topicals. Capturing pretreatment photos is recommended to show progress from treatments. Laser vein ablation is associated with a mild pain, described as a pinching or burning sensation. For the comfort of the patient, topical anesthetic may be applied for 30 to 60 min before treatment. However, some clinicians believe that the topical anesthetic may lead to vasoconstriction, rendering the laser treatment less effective because of a smaller target. To ease movement of the laser handpiece across the skin, topical water-based gel or cooling gel may be applied to and around the target area, depending on the laser. In addition, it may be necessary to apply antifog drops to the laser window, if present, to prevent fogging during treatment.

Protective eyewear should be worn by both patient and physician for safety during the procedure. After the first pulse, it is important to evaluate for any excessive bruising or gray appearance to ensure the laser settings are correct and are not causing significant epidermal damage or skin necrosis. Mild purpura is common. If the first pulse appears successful, the physician can proceed with treating the rest of the lesion or area (Video 6.2).

After pulsing the laser, the vein should be coagulated and should no longer be visualized. With shorter wavelength lasers, a repeat pass or double-pulsing an area may be required to achieve occlusion or clearance of the vein. Some believe that double-pulsing is actually optimal as it allows for heating the vessel in a stepwise fashion, while allowing the adjacent skin adequate cooling time.[7] However, with lasers that emit longer wavelengths, such as the Nd : YAG (1064 nm), double pulses should be strictly avoided, particularly as it increases the risk of epidermal burn damage and subsequent scarring.

POSTPROCEDURE CONSIDERATIONS

Laser Hair Removal

After treatment, patients should expect erythema and swelling at the procedural site. They may also experience a sunburn-like sensation at the site for a few hours after the procedure. Application of ice packs may reduce the pain, swelling, and erythema if needed. If the erythema persists, topical application of steroids can be considered. Patients can expect some hair follicles to remain at the treatment site. These generally fall out within the first 2 weeks posttreatment. If any blistering or skin injury occurred, aggressive and appropriate wound care should be initiated. The patient should be advised against any abrasive treatment to the area, including shaving and picking. They should also avoid sun exposure for about 3 months after treatment.[3]

Laser Vein Ablation

Following treatment, patients may experience some bruising, erythema, or swelling. For any pain or swelling, ice packs may be applied. Some recommend avoidance of heavy lifting or strenuous cardio-intensive activity within the first 24 to 48 hours of treatment. All patients should avoid sun exposure or use proper sunscreen posttreatment to avoid hyperpigmentation. If any blistering or skin injury occurred, treatment with topical antibiotics should be prescribed. Some recommend the use of compression stockings for the first 3 to 5 days after the procedure, but their utility has yet to be confirmed by larger controlled studies.

COMPLICATIONS AND OUTCOMES

Laser Hair Removal

As previously mentioned, repeated sessions are required to achieve and maintain hair reduction. Repeat sessions can occur once hair regrowth has occurred, typically in about 6 to 8 weeks. Patients may need one to six sessions to achieve a significant reduction in hair. Once adequate hair reduction has been achieved, patients may require maintenance sessions occurring once every 6 to 12 months. Most patients respond favorably to treatment results.[2]

Perifollicular erythema and swelling are the most common side effects from laser hair removal. Infection is possible if skin injury or blistering occurs during treatment. Appropriate wound care to the affected sites should prevent further, more permanent complications.

Temporary pigmentary changes, such as hyperpigmentation or hypopigmentation, can occur and typically resolve on their own within the months following treatment. Permanent depigmentation, burns, and scarring are possible, but risk can be reduced by using the appropriate laser, fluence, and cooling techniques.

Laser Vein Ablation

Although the veins should appear to be resolved immediately after laser treatment, segments of the vessel may reappear within the next couple of weeks. Repeat treatments are often required and should be conducted at 4- to 8-week intervals. Clearance of the vessel should be seen within one to three sessions. As varicose veins tend to be a chronic problem, it is prudent to return for annual assessments to determine if maintenance treatments are necessary.

The most common adverse effects are pain, erythema, purpura, and itching. This typically resolves within hours to days of treatment and can be alleviated with use of ice packs as described earlier.

More serious complications include pigment changing, telangiectatic matting, scarring, thrombophlebitis, and skin necrosis. Pigment changes, including hyperpigmentation or hypopigmentation, are more common among patients with Fitzpatrick phototypes of IV–VI and may resolve within months to 1 year following treatment. During this time, it is important to avoid sun exposure to prevent permanent pigment changes. However, permanent pigment changes may occur regardless of sun exposure. Risk of any of these permanent complications can be reduced through selection of the most appropriate laser and through evaluation of a test spot before full treatment.

REFERENCES

1. Ramos-e-Silva M, de Castro MC, Carneiro Jr LV. Hair removal. *Clin Dermatol.* 2001;19(4):437-444.
2. Dierickx C. Laser-assisted hair removal: state of the art. *Dermatol Ther.* 2000;13:80-89.
3. Liew SH. Laser hair removal: guidelines for management. *Am J Clin Dermatol.* 2002;3(2):107-115.
4. Görgü M, Aslan G, Aköz T, Erdoğan B. Comparison of alexandrite laser and electrolysis for hair removal. *Dermatol Surg.* 2000;26(1):37-41.
5. Anderson RR, Parrish JA. Selective photothermolysis: precise microsurgery by selective absorption of pulsed radiation. *Science.* 1983;220(4596):524-527.
6. DiBernardo BE, Perez J, Usal H, et al. Laser hair removal: where are we now? *Plast Reconstruct Surg.* 1999;104(1): 247-258.
7. Ross EV, Domankevitz Y. Laser leg vein treatment: physical mechanisms and theoretical considerations. *Lasers Surg Med.* 2005;36(2):105-116.
8. Tanzi EL, Lupton JR, Alster TS. Lasers in dermatology: four decades of progress. *J Am Acad Dermatol.* 2003; 49(1):1-34.
9. Meesters AA, Pitassi LH, Campos V, Wolkerstorfer A, Dierickx CC. Transcutaneous laser treatment of leg veins. *Lasers Med Sci.* 2014;29(2):481-492.
10. Hercogova J, Brazzini B, Hautmann G, Ghersetich I, Lotti T. Laser treatment of cutaneous vascular lesions: face and leg telangiectases. *J Eur Acad Dermatol Venereol.* 2002;16:12-18.
11. Bernstein EF, Noyaner-Turley A, Renton B. Treatment of spider veins of the lower extremity with a novel 532 nm KTP laser. *Lasers Surg Med.* 2014;46:81-88.
12. West TB, Alster TS. Comparison of the long-pulse dye (590-595 nm) and KTP (532 nm) lasers in the treatment of facial and leg telangiectasias. *Dermatol Surg.* 1998; 24(2):221-226.
13. McDaniel DH, Ash K, Lord J, Newman J, Adrian RM, Zukowski M. Laser therapy of spider leg veins: clinical evaluation of a new long pulsed alexandrite laser. *Dermatol Surg.* 1999;25:52-58.
14. Trelles MA, Allones I, Alvarez J, et al. The 800-nm diode laser in the treatment of leg veins: assessment at 6 months. *J Am Acad Dermatol.* 2006;54(2):282-289.

7

Suture Lifts

Sachin M. Shridharani and Grace M. Tisch

INTRODUCTION

The pattern of facial aging is hallmarked by several facets, including the loss of volume in facial fat pads and diminished skin elasticity. In the midface, these processes lead to deepening of the nasolabial fold and diminished anterior cheek projection, while in the lower third of the face, the result of the maturation process can result in jowling, blunting of the cervicomental angle, and an indistinct inferior mandibular border. Skin laxity and descended features in the face and neck are common presenting complaints in aesthetic practice and are issues for which many patients seek both surgical and nonsurgical management.

Nonsurgical approaches to rejuvenation are increasing in popularity and allow for patients to avoid surgery and the associated risks and necessary downtime. However, nonsurgical modalities are often limited in their ability to provide full correction, particularly when used independently. Volume restoration with dermal fillers is unlikely to correct the consequences of laxity (e.g., deepening nasolabial or marionette folds) without overfilling, and treatment with energy-based devices alone such as microfocused ultrasound with visualization (MFU-V) or radiofrequency is often insufficient for repositioning descended tissues. Until recently, viable nonsurgical tools for tissue redraping have remained an unmet need.

Soft tissue redraping with suture and thread-based technologies has a complex history in aesthetic medicine beginning in the 1990s, and has included multiple "false-starts," including nonabsorbable sutures, which proved to be prone to migration or extrusion.[1] Sulamanidze and colleagues first reported the use of barbed threads (Aptos nonabsorbable polypropylene sutures) in 1998 in Moscow, Russia, although several reports noted high complication rates with this procedure.[1,2] Several similar techniques have since been developed, such as Woffles Lift (not commercially available), another nonabsorbable polypropylene thread with bidirectional barbs on either side of a central clear phone that allows the thread to be folded on itself in the temporal fascia as a self-fixating loop, and Isse Thread lift, which required surgical dissection of the scalp and fixation of the unidirectional barbed sutures to the temporal fascia.[3] Contour threads, polypropylene sutures with unidirectional barbs, lost U.S. Food and Drug Administration clearance for nonsurgical applications in 2007 because of patient complaints.[1] For these nonabsorbable sutures, complications included palpable thread ends with pain, thread migration, infection/granuloma, skin dimpling/irregularities, as well as more serious complications such as Stensen's duct rupture, nerve damage, chronic foreign body sensation, and scarring, which caused a decline in popularity and a growing need for alternative materials.[1] Today, the large majority of sutures and threads used in clinical practice for cosmetic purposes are entirely absorbable and do not require incisions or fixation to the fascia. Absorbable threads are made of polydioxanone, and absorbable

Disclosures: Dr. Shridharani is a consultant for Sinclair Pharma, Allergan, Endo Pharmaceuticals, Evolus, Galderma, Prollenium, and Sientra, and a clinical investigator for Allergan, Endo, Galderma, and Prollenium.

Statement of Funding: Funding for editorial support was provided though X-Medica, LLC (a CME provider) with funds from Sinclair Pharma, Inc.

sutures are made of poly-L-lactic acid and poly-L-glycolide (PLLA/PGLA). These nonsurgical devices are placed in the subcutaneous tissue where they mechanically support tissue and stimulate collagen. Because of their minimally invasive nature, biocompatibility, improved safety profile, and ability to address tissue descent, threads and sutures are increasing in popularity for facial and neck rejuvenation.

Manufacturer	Thread Material	Thread Type	Arrangement of Supportive Structure	Longevity
NovaThreads	Polydioxanone (PDO)	Smooth (monofilament or braided)	NA	Volume returns to baseline by 18 months
NovaThreads	PDO	Barbed	Bidirectional	Lift returns to baseline by 1 year
Mint	PDO	Barbed	Bidirectional, helical	Lift returns to baseline by 1 year
Silhouette InstaLift	PLLA/PGLA	Cones	Bidirectional	Retreatment generally required at 18 months in the mid- and lower face and at 9 months in the neck

BACKGROUND INFORMATION

Differentiating Thread and Suture Technologies

Absorbable threads and sutures may be categorized based on construction as smooth (monofilament or braided), barbed, or cone-based threads. Smooth threads are placed in the subcutaneous layer, often in a mesh pattern, for the primary purpose of stimulating collagen production. These threads are not intended to lift the tissue, but rather provide improved skin quality and texture over time via the induction of neocollagenesis. In contrast, both barbed and cone-based technologies are designed not only to stimulate collagen but also to engage ptotic tissue for the purpose of lifting. Within the United States, all commercially available threads are made of either polydioxanone (PDO; Nova Threads and Mint Threads) or PLLA/PLGA polymer (InstaLift, Suneva Medical, Inc, Irvine, CA). Both PDO threads and absorbable suspension sutures achieve their effect through the dual mechanism of lifting and collagen stimulation; however, the efficacy of the overall treatment can be shaped by their differing properties, described later.

Mechanical Lifting Capacity

The construction of barbed threads differs from that of PLLA/PLGA absorbable suspension sutures in a number of ways. In barbed threads, the barb is created either through molding or cutting into the suture. While molding is thought to be less likely to compromise the integrity of the thread, both give rise to a leaf-like structure, which is intended to support descended tissue. Barbs may be unidirectional, bidirectional, or multidirectional, depending on the product. In contrast, the mechanical capacity for lift in absorbable suspension sutures is provided by bidirectional cones, held in place by intercalated knots (Fig. 7.1). The cones of the absorbable suspension suture are unique in that they are designed to work in opposition to one another: on the superior side of the suture cones are placed in more fibrous tissue where they serve as anchors, while the cones on the inferior side are placed in more mobile tissue to provide lift and support to redraped tissue. From a mechanical

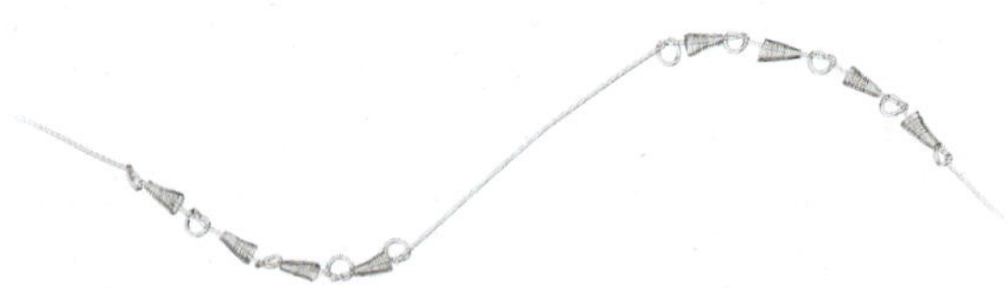

Fig. 7.1 The Silhouette InstaLift absorbable suspension suture is comprised of an 82% PLLA/18% PLGA polymer. Bidirectional cones along the length of the suture act together to support repositioned tissue in an elevated position. Two 23-gauge, 12-cm needles are appended to the suture ends to be used to place the suture and cones.(Image reprinted with permission from Sinclair Pharma Inc.)

perspective, cupped structures, such as those present in cones, provide significantly greater resistance to slippage than barbed structures,[3] an observation reflected in the clinical performance of available thread and suture technologies. In addition, the distribution of the supportive structures in absorbable suspension sutures make them a preferred modality when the primary aesthetic need is tissue redraping. For applications such as addressing facial asymmetry (or palsy), or maintaining postsurgical results, the mechanical capacity of the suture is of particular importance.

Collagen Stimulating Capacity and Biocompatibility

Both PDO and PLLA/PLGA have been shown to stimulate collagenesis; however, only the biocompatibility and biostimulatory activity of PLLA/PGLA has been established histologically in humans, both as a filler and when used as a suture.[4-6] The collagen stimulating potential of PDO has been reported in several animal models,[7,8] where it appears to be similar to that of PLLA. However, to our knowledge, no human histology studies have been done of PDO threads, either in isolation or as part of a comparison with absorbable suspension sutures.

Versatility

Absorbable suspension sutures are also a versatile modality that can be adapted to individual patient needs. Available in three suture configurations (8-, 12-, and 16-cone), the authors' experience is that the 8-cone suture is most often used to treat the face and upper neck. The 12-cone suture is typically used for treatment of larger surface areas in the lower neck or in larger faces to increase the purchase of recruited tissue.

Together, the long history of PLLA/PGLA use in both medicine and aesthetics confirmed biocompatibility and biostimulatory activity of PLLA/PGLA, and higher mechanical supportive capacity of absorbable suspension sutures make them one author's (SMS) preferred method of nonsurgical management of laxity in the face and neck. Notably, hyperdilute biostimulatory fillers have emerged as a way to improve skin quality and volume, providing an alternative approach to smooth threads for aesthetic improvement and biostimulaiton. The choice to lift ptotic tissue with either biostimulatory fillers or threads will likely be based on cost and patient/clinician preference.

Absorbable suspension sutures are approved for use in the midface,[7] but off-label use in the lower face and neck is both common in clinical practice and has been reported in smaller reports and literature studies.[9,10] In the midface, absorbable suspension sutures may be used to soften the nasolabial fold and can provide gradual revolumization because of stimulation of neocollagenesis by the suture's PLLA. In the lower face, absorbable suspension sutures may be used to efface the marionette lines, provide definition along the jawline, and correct jowling (Video 7.1). Finally, absorbable suspension sutures may be used in the neck to correct tissue laxity.

Though the use of absorbable sutures for facial tissue suspension has been described, there seems to be a paucity of literature on addressing the neck and lower third of the face. Importantly, patient selection, a critical aspect of optimal treatment outcome for this anatomic region, is not well described. Detailed procedural information on treatment of the midface can be found within the literature[11,12] and is not discussed in detail here. Comfort with use of absorbable suspension sutures in the midface is a prerequisite for the treatment of the lower face and neck, as vector planning and procedural considerations are more complex.

Here, the authors present videos of optimal treatment planning and technique for treatment of the lower face and neck and share valuable lessons learned surrounding patient selection, complementary treatments, and case studies illustrating the nature of treatment outcomes.

PREPROCEDURE CONSIDERATIONS

Patient Selection and Expectation Setting

The ideal patient for absorbable suspension sutures is not yet a surgical candidate but has ptotic skin or descent of facial fat pads that can be easily mobilized during physical examination. The skin must be of sufficient thickness to avoid palpability of the suture. Like most nonsurgical techniques, the procedure is not a surgical substitute and is unlikely to completely resolve issues that should be addressed with surgical interventions. However, patients who are better suited for surgery but who have comorbidities, limited downtime, or a fundamental lack of interest in surgery may be treated with absorbable suspension sutures as long as the patient has realistic expectations of treatment outcome.

A population particularly well suited to treatment with absorbable suspension sutures is patients with adequate volume who require redraping. For male patients in particular, the absence of surgical scars associated with treatment and the tendency for fillers to feminize the face when there is excessive fullness over the lateral zygoma or zygomaticomaxillary complex make absorbable suspension sutures an important tool in rejuvenation. Furthermore, patients who undergo nonsurgical management of jowl fat may have minor resultant skin laxity. A lower facelift in these patients is not warranted. While dermal fillers can camouflage mild age-related changes of the jawline, fillers have the potential to masculinize the normal female anatomy. As such, redraping the soft tissue with absorbable suspension sutures offers optimal correction in patients with early to moderate changes associated with aging.

As with all procedures, setting patient expectations is important for ensuring satisfaction. In the case of absorbable suspension sutures, it is essential for patients to understand that this medical device, along with all other minimally invasive/nonsurgical techniques, is not a substitute for traditional surgery. Accordingly, patients undergoing treatment should not expect a level of aesthetic improvement commensurate with a surgical face or neck lift. It is the authors' experience that before and after images do not generally capture the totality of treatment effect, and patients often find their own results to be more dramatic than those apparent in patient's images. In particular, improvements in skin quality, the degree of repositioning, and the effect of gradual revolumization on overall appearance are often difficult to appreciate in photographs. Furthermore, while the aesthetic effects of absorbable sutures can be visible for approximately 18 to 24 months, patients should understand that longevity and preservation of treatment outcomes will require interval maintenance treatments. Absorbable suspension sutures achieve optimal results when a long-term, multiple-treatment protocol is implemented. In addition, patients should be appropriately counseled regarding the social and physical downtime associated with suture placement. In contrast to other common nonsurgical techniques (e.g., dermal fillers, botulinum toxin injections), the social downtime that accompanies suture placement is of considerably greater duration (approximately 7–10 days) and requires additional limitations to physical activity postoperatively to maintain the strength and integrity of the sutures.

Poor candidates for the treatment include patients with significant skin laxity leading to pleats or facial folds when bimanually simulating a facial/neck lift. Patients who also have draping skin or facial folds when laid supine are noted to be poor candidates. Patients with prevalent platysma bands also are a trigger to proceed with caution, as the redraping laterally cannot overcome the midline muscle dehiscence/diastasis.

Planning for Complementary Treatment

In the clinical experience of one author (SMS), several co- and complementary treatments can further improve the outcome of treatment with absorbable suspension sutures. Between 2 and 4 weeks before suture placement in the neck, treatment of the platysma with botulinum toxin softens the appearance of the platysma bands and reduces the mechanical load placed on the sutures by mimetic forces. Because the sutures are placed in the subdermal layer over the platysma, reducing the appearance of platysmal bands can reduce the potential for suture visibility. In addition, treatment of submental fat and/or fat pads along the jowl with deoxycholic acid (ATX-101) injections at least 12 weeks before suture placement reduces bulk that may be difficult to reposition or may place additional downward pull on the sutures as well as improve mechanical load. However, additional lifting may be needed if the tissue is thinned or ptotic. Though the use of ATX-101 injection is beneficial for treating submental fullness and excess jowl fat, contouring of the jawline and neck can be further improved by redraping the skin and soft tissue envelope.[13-15]

Energy-based treatments such as MFU-V, helium plasma, or radiofrequency, particularly for the neck, strengthen and tighten skin and are ideally completed 2 to 3 weeks before treatment with sutures. It is best to avoid heating the skin after placing sutures because of a possible negative impact on longevity. If the patient insists on energy-based treatment following sutures, 3 to 5 months should pass to ensure that lifting has occurred to avoid disrupting the sutures. Resurfacing or fractionated laser could be done 6 to 8 weeks after suture placement.

For microneedling, sutures may be placed ~1 week following a microneedling procedure, or microneedling may be done between 2 and 4 weeks after suture placement. This period of time postsuture placement is to allow integration of the sutures before the mobility and manipulation required for an effective microneedling procedure take place, rather than any concern surrounding mechanical disruption of the suture.

For multimodal treatment using fillers and absorbable suspension sutures, volume should be corrected before placement of absorbable suspension sutures. Ordering the procedures in this way is analogous to performing fat grafting before surgery: the tissue is expanded first, then reset on the volume-restored face. Fillers may be injected on the same day, before suture placement, if they are in different anatomic areas. In the face, fillers typically are placed from top to bottom; so prior filler placement in the upper or midface will remove tension from the bottom of the face and may affect treatment plans. However, in cases where treatment of the jawline is needed, repositioning should be done first. An approach to rejuvenation that uses multiple treatment types can improve treatment outcome beyond what may be accomplished with nonsurgical redraping alone.

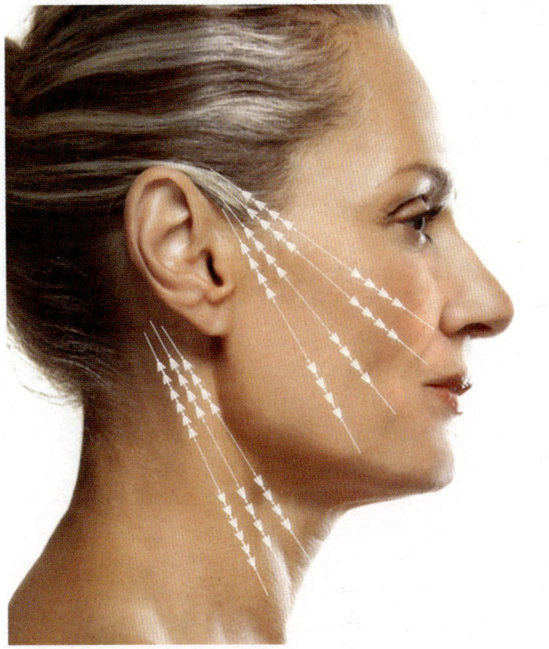

Fig. 7.2 Common vectors for treating the midface, marionette, jowl, jawline, and neck are shown. Absorbable suspension sutures are adaptable and various combinations of vectors are used to address specific patient needs.

PROCEDURAL TECHNIQUES

Pretreatment Vector Mapping

A full assessment of the patient should be performed before treatment (see Video 7.1). For all treatment areas, sutures should always be placed in a straight line. This principal of straight-line vector planning (SLVP)[10] maximizes lifting capacity of the cones and ensures that the forces acting on each set of cones within a single suture are in direct opposition to one another, keeping the suture in place, and maintaining support for redraped tissue. The neck and jawline are nearly always treated together, as laxity along the jawline diminishes the effect of neck treatment. Further, untreated laxity in the lower third of the face may lead to a disharmonious result. In general, more vertical vectors are used to address jowling and support jawline definition or tissue in the neck (Fig. 7.2). One author (SMS) prefers to use a star-shaped pattern, though other published reports show sutures placed parallel to the mandibular boarder and perpendicular to the nasolabial fold in the midface.[11] Regardless of treatment vector selected, the sutures should be placed in a straight line: curved or V-shaped suture placement should be avoided as these shapes diminish the lifting capabilities of the suture and increase risk of early loss of results and suture migration. A video detailing pretreatment SLVP for a case-study patient is presented in Video 7.1.

To obtain an optimal result, it is important to treat the patient with a sufficient number of sutures. Regardless of the anatomic area to be treated, using too few sutures results in excessive mechanical burden on the sutures that are used and may lead to shorter duration of treatment effect or inconsistent results. In clinical practice, the authors most often use a total of 14 sutures for complete treatment: two per side in the midface, two per side in the jowl, and three per side in the neck. The positioning and number of sutures may be varied to meet the needs of individual patients. For example, a patient's nasolabial fold may be especially pronounced and require the lift of three, rather than two, sutures. To achieve consistent results in the neck, a minimum of three sutures is used: two 8-cone sutures at the top of the neck and a 12-cone suture below. The use of the 12-cone suture allows treatment of a broader surface area and wider excursion across a larger anatomic area.

After the patient's face has been treated with a bactericidal skin prep (e.g., hypochlorous acid), vectors, entry points, and exit points are marked on the skin. Canonical treatment vectors are shown in Fig. 7.2. The exit point of the suture is marked 1.5 cm medial to the point of action, or the position of the inferior-most cone. The point of action is the lowest point of tissue support. Using the ruler provided with the absorbable suspension sutures, the central entry point for 8-cone sutures is marked 5.5 cm from the inferior-most exit point, and the superior-most exit point is marked 5.5 cm from the central entry point. For 12-cone sutures, the central entry point is marked 7.5 cm from the medial exit point and the lateral exit point is marked 7.5 cm from the central entry point.

To mark treatment vectors for the neck, reference the center portion of the lip, and mark the midline from the center of the lower lip to the sternal notch. The first entry point is marked 1.5 cm lateral to the midline and platysmal band at the level of the hyoid bone (see Video 7.1). In the neck, treatment vectors are tangential and oriented more vertically as one approaches the inferior aspect of the neck (see Fig. 7.2). The exit point should be behind the mastoid. As long as the sutures are placed in the correct plane, the external jugular vein and great auricular nerve are avoided. The suture vectors are approximately 1.5 cm apart, and the top two sutures are most often 8-cone sutures and the lower suture(s) is typically a 12-cone suture. While a minimum of three sutures are used to treat the neck, additional 12-cone sutures may be used to accommodate larger (most often male) patients.

Suture Placement

The primary objective of this chapter is to detail techniques for treatment of the lower face and neck. There are excellent, detailed descriptions of technique for midface treatment that may be found in the literature and are thus not repeated in detail here.[11] Placement for the lower face is similar to that for the midface, but the neck is a more challenging area because of complex anatomy and a thinner subcutaneous layer. Complete knowledge of the neck's anatomy and comfort with placement of absorbable suspension sutures in the midface are prerequisites for treatment of the neck.

A demonstration of the procedure for absorbable suspension suture placement in the lower face and neck is provided in Video 7.2. Following SLVP and marking of all entry and exit points, 0.5 cc of 2% lidocaine with epinephrine (1:100,000 dilution) is injected into the subdermal plane at each entry and exit site. Epinephrine causes local vasoconstriction, thereby reducing the risk of bruising.[16] Importantly, the suture paths are not injected with anesthetic, as this may interfere with proper placement. Placement of the sutures in the correct plane should be painless, and any pain experienced by the patient is an indication that the needle has passed into the incorrect plane.

Using a thumb and forefinger, present the entry site and penetrate the dermis in a perpendicular fashion with an 18-G needle. Gentle subcision around the entry site and rotation of the needle to dilate the entry point allows the cones to pass through more easily. In the neck, the platysma is close to the subcutaneous tissues, and care must be taken to ensure that the entry site is supraplatysmal. For the neck, the entry point for the lower 12-cone sutures may be over the sternocleidomastoid muscle, which must be avoided by placing the sutures in the correct (subdermal) plane.

Once the port site has been placed, the patient is ready to have the suture inserted (Video 7.3); however, before placement, the suture's knots must be tightened. The absorbable suspension suture knots are not tightened for packaging to ensure preservation of the integrity of the PLLA/PLGA monofilament in storage. To set the tension and secure the cones, hold the center of the suture and grasp the suture end on the side opposite to the last cone (rather than adjacent to the needle) and apply sufficient tension to tighten the knots. Repeat for the knots on the opposing side. To place the suture, insert the needle appended to the suture end into the entry site. There is a 5-mm depth gauge marked on the needle, and this may be used to ensure placement in the subdermal plane. Of note, the dermis of the neck is thinner than that of the midface, and the average depth of penetration is most often 3 mm rather than 5 mm. For male patients, the dermis may be slightly thicker. Once the needle is at the appropriate depth, the needle is turned tangentially and advanced through the subdermal plane. Either the superior or inferior side of the suture may be placed first, but in the neck, one author (SMS) has found that it is easiest to place the inferior side first.

The sutures must remain in the supraplatysmal space, and any exit from the subdermal plane into the musculoskeletal fascia will result in pain signals from musculoskeletal innervation. In addition, both bruising and bleeding will be more profound because of the vascularization of skeletal muscle. If the suture dips into the muscle, the mechanical forces in the muscle, which are much stronger than those in the subdermal plane, will diminish treatment efficacy and duration. Further, the mechanical capacity of the suture is inherently reduced because it is placed in a wave, passing through multiple planes, rather than acting in a single plane, thereby diluting the lifting force of the cones. For the neck in particular, it is helpful to use a thumb or forefinger to apply countertraction on the opposite side of the entry point during placement to prevent unnecessary pressure or pulling. The needle should glide easily, and there should be no resistance during placement or any sign of pain response. In some instances in which the patient has been previously treated with ATX-101 injections, there may be some resistance because of treatment-induced fibrosis. However, the needle should pass through with minimal additional pressure or rocking. Because the sutures are placed in the supraplatysmal space, it is possible to see the path of the needle though the dermis during advancement. If needed, tenting the tissue with the needle can provide a clear picture of the needle's path. For some patients, the cones may be slightly visible, but this visibility should diminish within a few days to a few weeks. The visibility of the cones in appropriately selected patients is largely driven by slight edema around the placed sutures and cones and lasts for a few days to a week. For patients with crepe-like skin who are less suited to treatment, the cones may be palpable and visible for months.

The needle then passes through the exit site, and the cones and knots are gently pulled though the entry site. It is important to pull the suture at a vector in the same plane as the intended treatment vector rather than pulling the suture at an upward or downward angle (see Video 7.3). Once the cones are in place, the central portion of the suture is held in place and, grasping the inferior portion of the suture PLLA/PGLA monofilament, the suture is pulled taut to check that no cones are caught on the dermis. If the suture was placed in the correct plane, there should be no dimpling when the suture is tensioned.

The superior portion of the suture is then placed in the same fashion using the same entry point. If the same entry point is not used to place both suture ends, the central portion of the suture will be too superficial, resulting in contour irregularities. For the first exit point on the neck, countertraction along the jawline can facilitate needle advancement, thereby ensuring the planned vector is captured. The exit point for the top-most suture is behind the mastoid; the actual exit point may be 1 to 2 mm from the planned exit point if needed. It is most important to avoid placing the suture too deep near the posterior exit point as the suture should not be anchored on the mastoid periosteum. After both ends of the suture are placed, the ends are pulled taut to ensure that the suture is properly placed and there is no dimpling in the dermis. The same procedure is repeated with the second 8-cone suture and the lower 12-cone suture(s). All sutures are placed before any attempts at redraping tissue or setting the sutures. The mechanical perturbations resulting from suture placement can disturb or unseat adjacent sutures or sutures placed on the contralateral side of the face or neck.

Suture Tensioning

Once all sutures are placed, the tissue may be redraped and sutures set. Video 7.3 shows the procedure for redraping and setting sutures. First, redraping is initiated by applying tension to the inferior end of the suture and advancing tissue over inferior cones, which will lock tissue into position. Tissue is advanced for each of the sutures in that anatomic area before engaging superior cones. The superior end of the suture is then tensioned and pulled so that the tissue engaged by the lower cones is further elevated. It is important to pull the superior end of the suture to set tension at maximum capacity, keeping in mind that it is incredibly difficult to overcorrect. Rippling and bunching are normal treatment sequelae, occurring in ~90% of patients. These effects will settle and dissipate within 3 to 4 days (Fig. 7.3). An

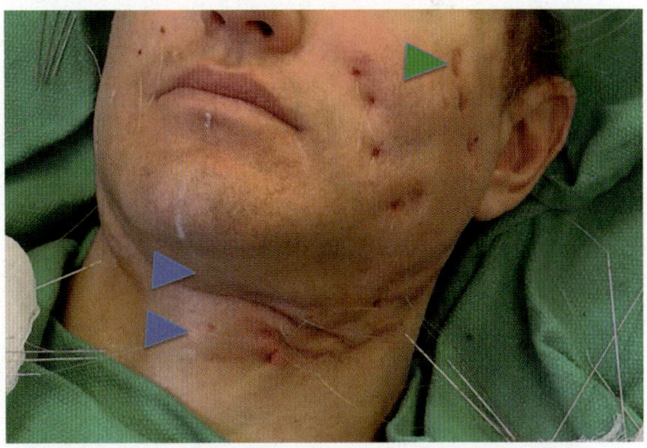

Fig. 7.3 A 42-year-old male patient treated with two sutures in the midface, one suture in the lower face, one suture along the jawline, and four sutures in the neck. The image shows the patient following setting of the sutures on one side. Note the divots near the entry site in the midface *(green arrow)*, the bunching and rippling following correction of the neck. The degree of tissue redraping is apparent when examining the center line *(blue arrows)*.

additional example showing the degree of correction necessary is shown in Fig. 7.4. The considerable pleating and bunching of facial and neck tissue immediately following suture placement is normal and resolved at 1 week. In the mid- and lower face, divots at the entry site may be apparent, and pleating or rippling may appear at the entry and exit sites or along the length of the suture. It is completely acceptable if one of the inferior or superior knots or cones is pulled through the exit points by redraping or elevation. The knot and associated cone can

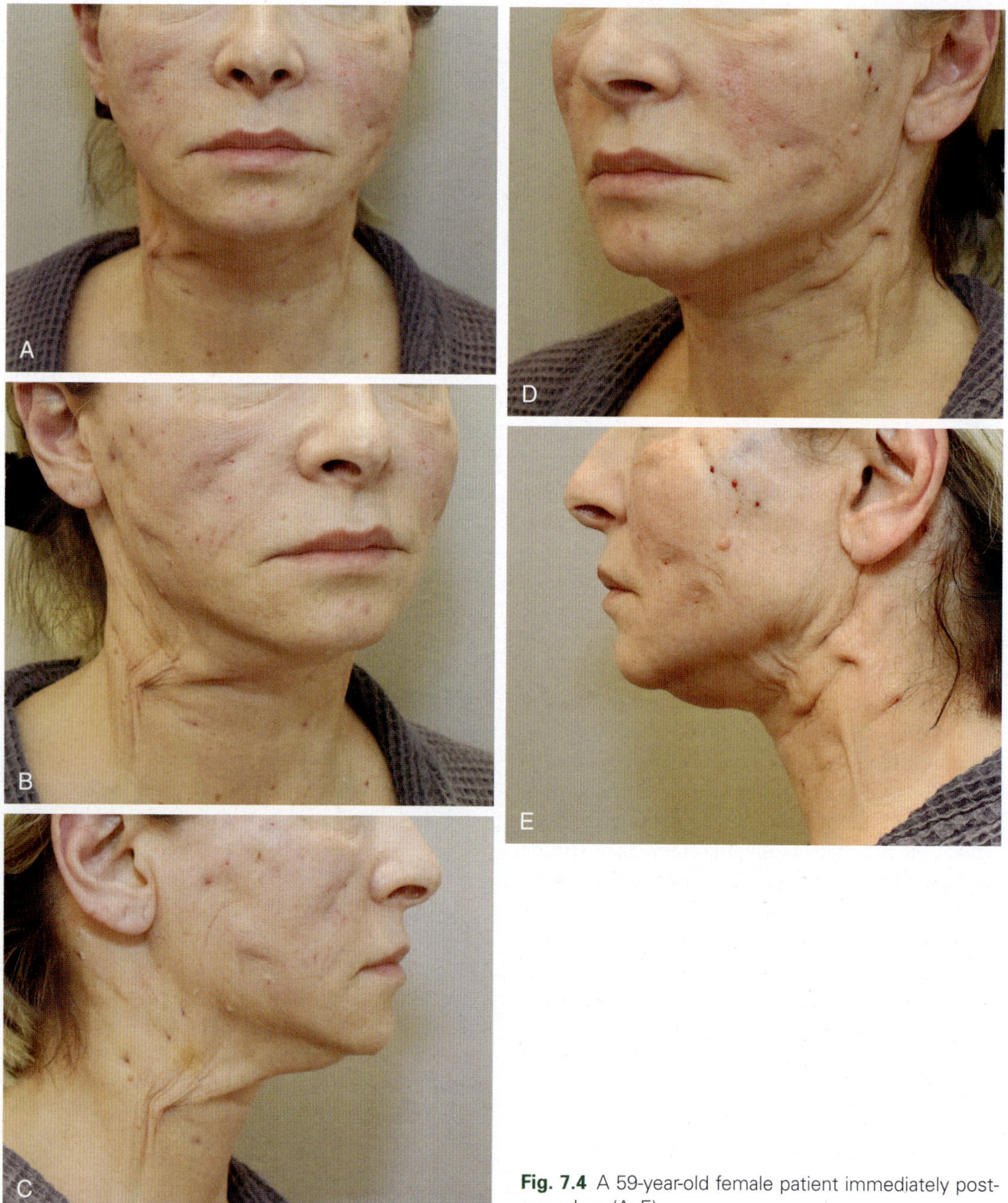

Fig. 7.4 A 59-year-old female patient immediately post-procedure (A–E)

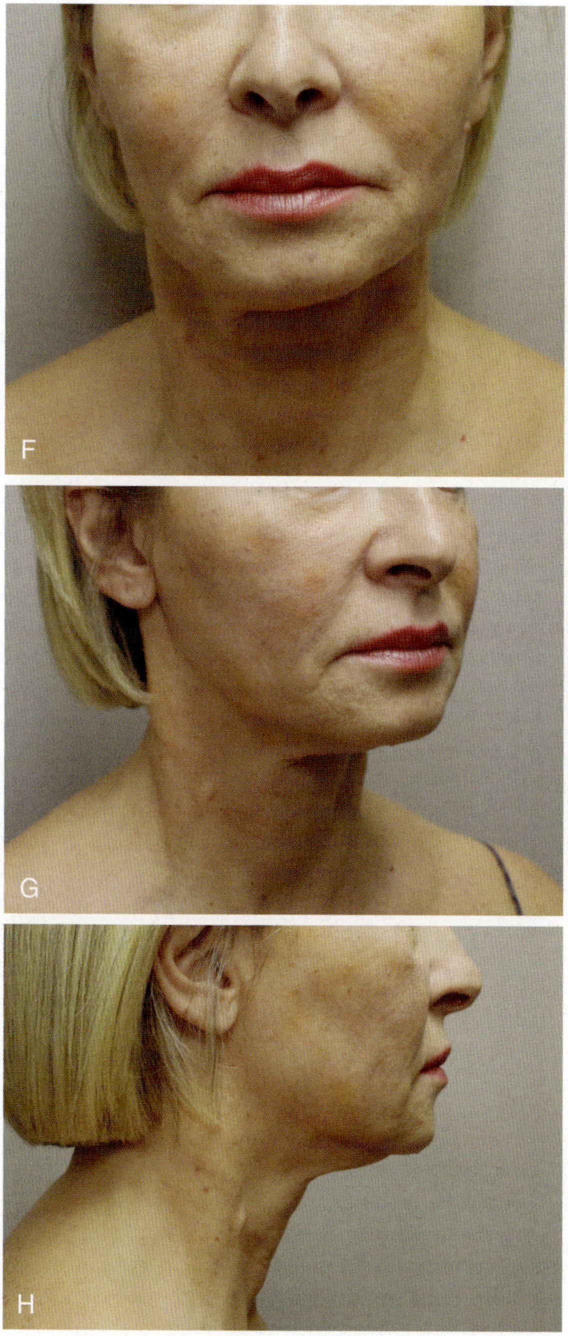

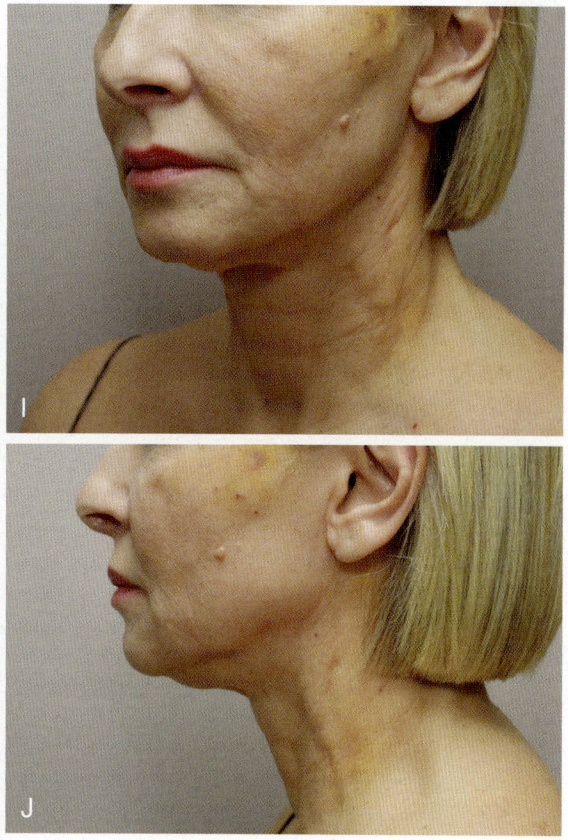

Fig. 7.4, cont'd. and 1 week postprocedure (F–J). Note the considerable pleating and bunching of facial and neck tissue immediately following suture placement and resolution of these effects at 1 week.

be trimmed at the end of the procedure. It is important to bring any knots or cones near the surface of the dermis though the exit point so that they are not left in the dermis, where they may stimulate prolonged inflammation. Fig. 7.3 shows the neck following correction of laxity on one side, illustrating the degree of correction required for optimal results. Note the position of the centerline.

The suture edges are then trimmed at the skin, and a finger is passed over the exit sites to ensure that the suture is entirely below the surface of the skin. Antiseptic ointment is then placed over the entry and exit points. The senior author favors placing Ocumend patches, as his anecdotal experience has been for patients to have reduced postprocedure edema and bruising.

POSTTREATMENT CARE

Following treatment of the mid- and lower face, patients are instructed to gently ice the area every 30 minutes for the first 48 hours. Patients are to wear their supportive neck garment continuously (other than when bathing) for the first 3 to 5 days. With treatment of the neck, patients are encouraged to wear the garment at night from day 5 to 7. Vigorous exercise is to be avoided for 1 week following treatment of the face and 2 weeks following treatment of the neck. The skin may be washed gently after 24 hours. Patients are also asked to adhere to a soft diet and avoid exaggerated facial expressions or otherwise straining the musculature of the face and/or neck for 1 week. Patients who have been treated in the lower face and neck may feel an urge to move their jaws and lift the chin, as treatment does result in initial feelings of tightness. Wrapping the neck snugly, while unnecessary for healing purposes, may serve as a physical reminder to remain less mobile until tissue integration has taken place and the sutures are stable. In the clinical experience of the senior author (SMS), this time period is approximately 2 weeks.

Outcomes for the neck in particular are impacted by patient adherence to postprocedure instructions. Patients should be advised that decreasing excess motion of the neck for 1 week is essential.

COMPLICATIONS AND OUTCOMES

Outcomes

Three case-study patients are presented in Figs. 9.5–9.8. Together, these case studies show the wide range of patients who can be successfully treated with absorbable suspension sutures. In each case, treatment results in better definition of the jawline, reduction of laxity, and improvements in skin quality.

Case Study 1

A 59-year-old female patient treated for midface descent and skin laxity of the face and neck with a total of 14 absorbable suspension sutures (four 8-cone sutures per each hemiface, two 8-cone sutures, and one 12-cone suture to each side of the neck; Fig. 7.5). The patient was also treated with 30 units of botulinum toxin to the platysma at 2 months. Note the improvement in skin quality, improved mandibular contour, and reduced appearance of laxity along the jawline and neck at 4 months postprocedure. At 7 months postprocedure, note the diminishing effects of treatment and the reoccurrence of laxity along the jawline and neck. The patient was pleased with the results and elected to undergo retreatment with a total of 10 absorbable suspension sutures to the midface, jawline, and neck at 7.5 months. The patient is shown at baseline 4 months and 7 months. The same patient is also shown immediately posttreatment in Fig. 7.4.

Of note, before treatment, both surgical and nonsurgical treatment options were discussed at length. The patient was advised that nonsurgical intervention would likely achieve suboptimal improvement because of the presence of severe skin laxity at baseline. However, because of a fundamental lack of interest in undergoing surgery, the patient elected for treatment with absorbable suspension sutures.

Case Study 2

A 36-year-old female patient treated for midface decent and skin laxity of the jawline and neck with a total of 14 absorbable suspension sutures (four 8-cone sutures per each hemiface, two 8-cone sutures, and one 12-cone suture to each side of the neck; Figs. 7.6 and 7.7). Note the improved definition along the inferior mandibular border, improved prominence of the gonial angle, and reduced appearance of jowling. The patient was very satisfied with her results. Patient is shown at baseline and 4 months.

Case Study 3

A 31-year-old female patient treated for mild skin laxity of the jawline and neck with a total of 12 absorbable

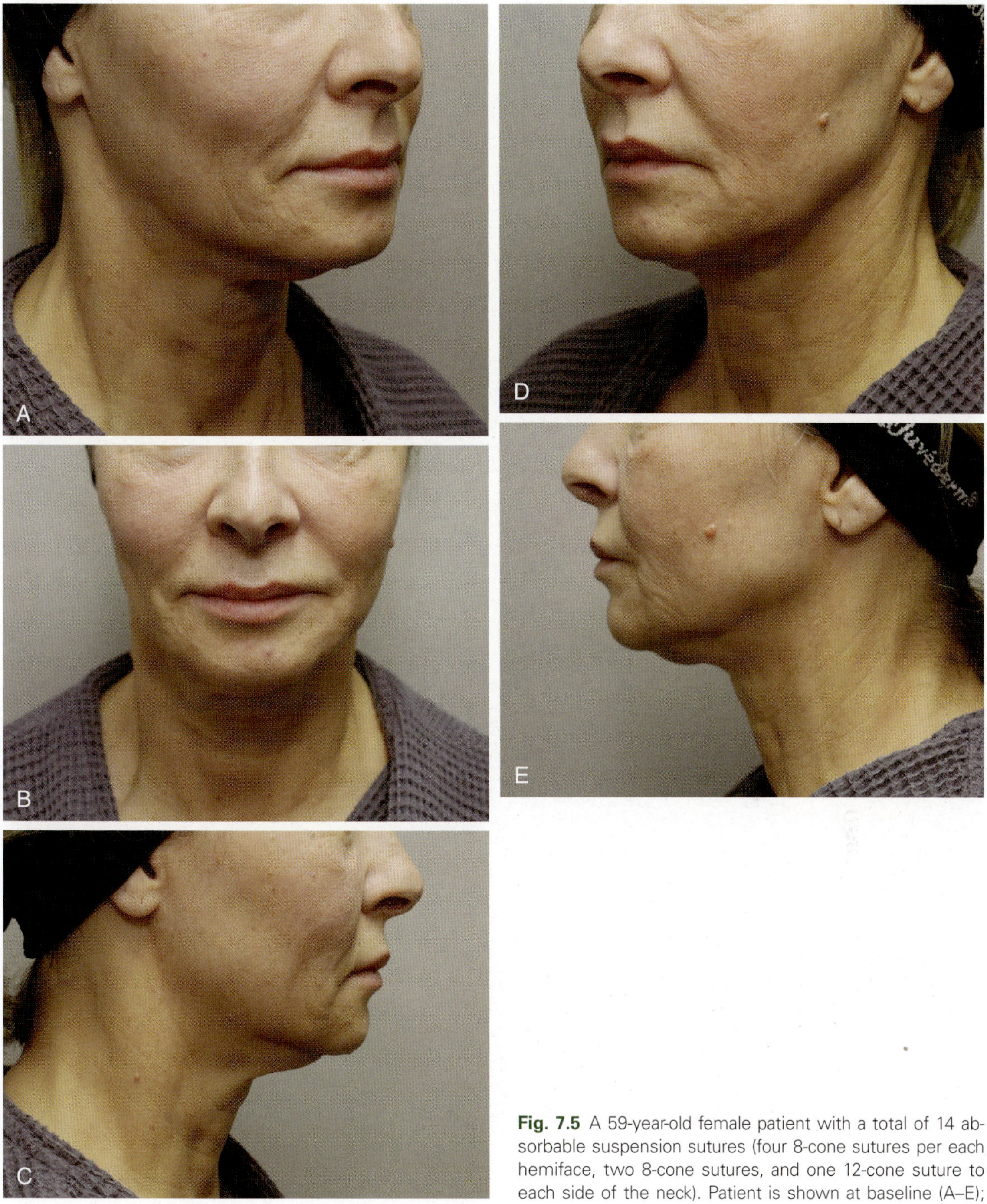

Fig. 7.5 A 59-year-old female patient with a total of 14 absorbable suspension sutures (four 8-cone sutures per each hemiface, two 8-cone sutures, and one 12-cone suture to each side of the neck). Patient is shown at baseline (A–E);

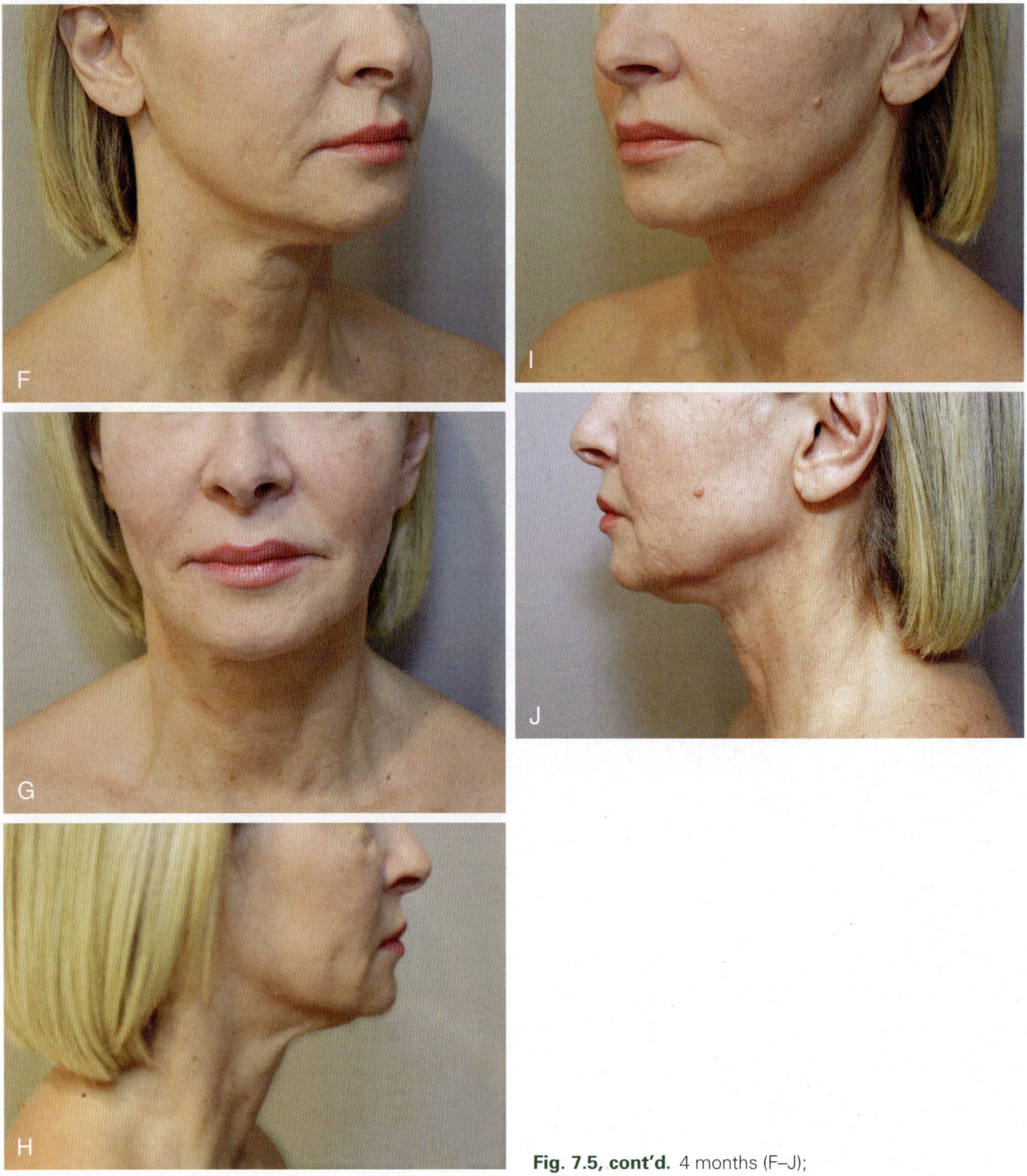

Fig. 7.5, cont'd. 4 months (F–J);

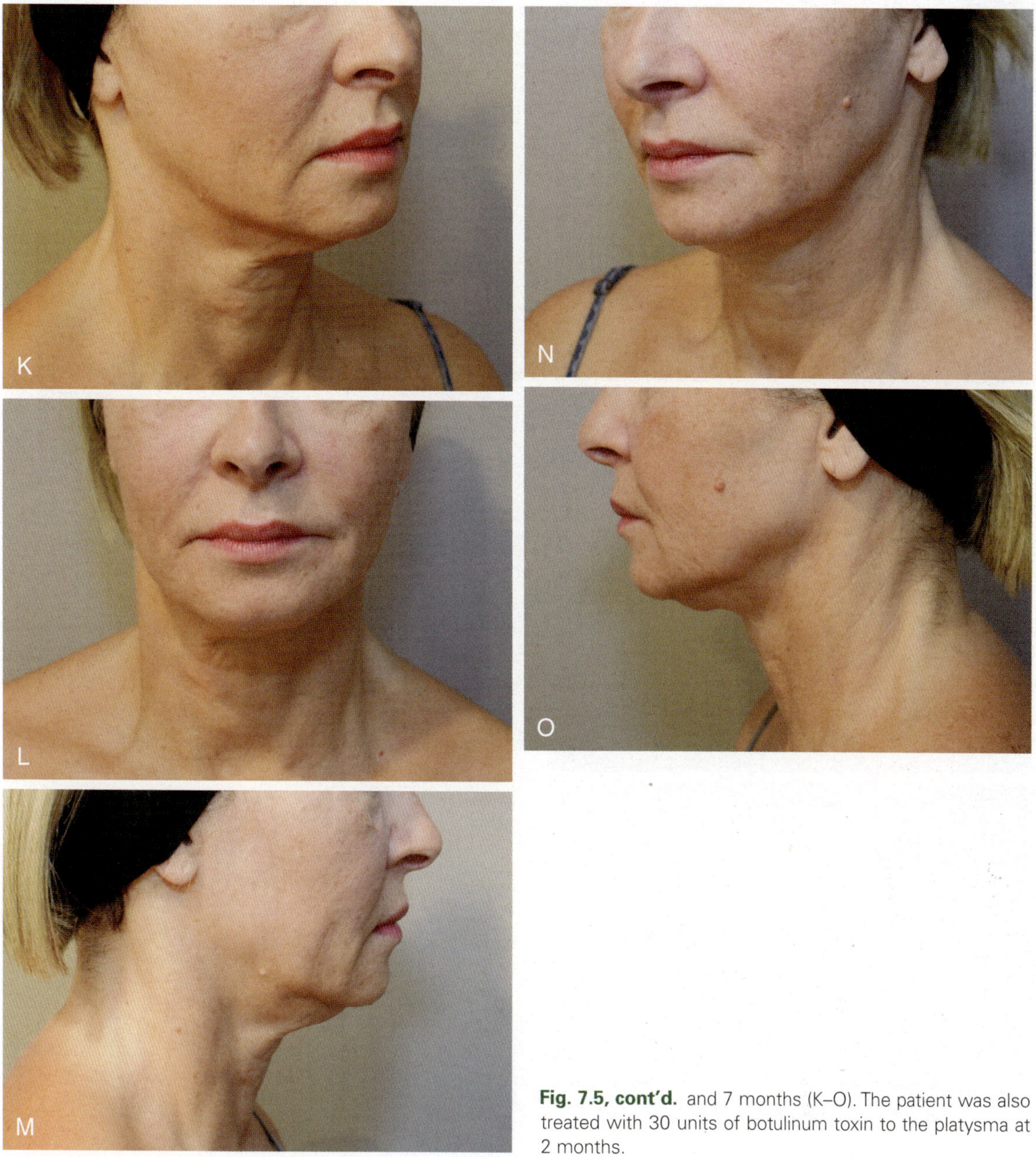

Fig. 7.5, cont'd. and 7 months (K–O). The patient was also treated with 30 units of botulinum toxin to the platysma at 2 months.

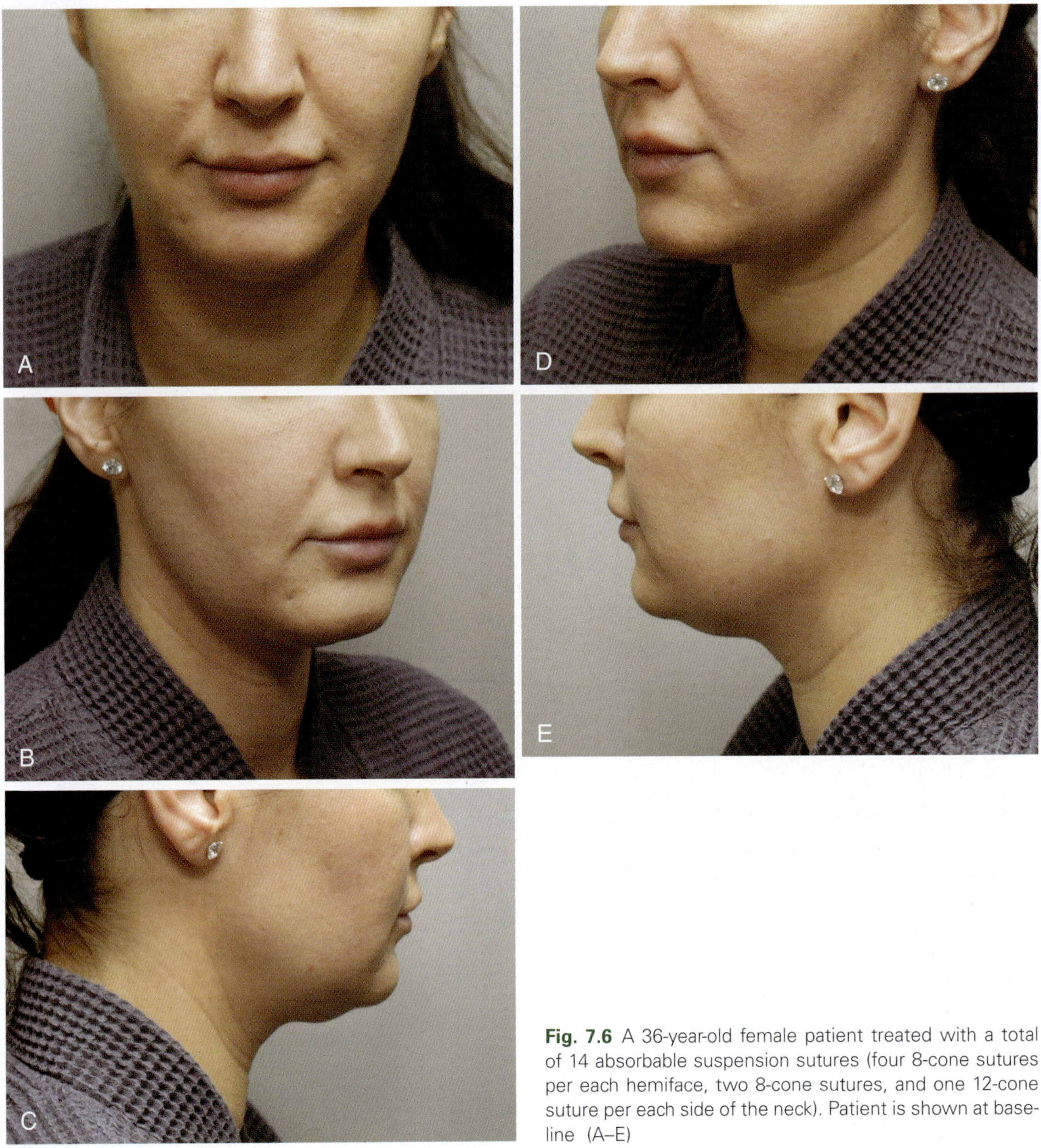

Fig. 7.6 A 36-year-old female patient treated with a total of 14 absorbable suspension sutures (four 8-cone sutures per each hemiface, two 8-cone sutures, and one 12-cone suture per each side of the neck). Patient is shown at baseline (A–E)

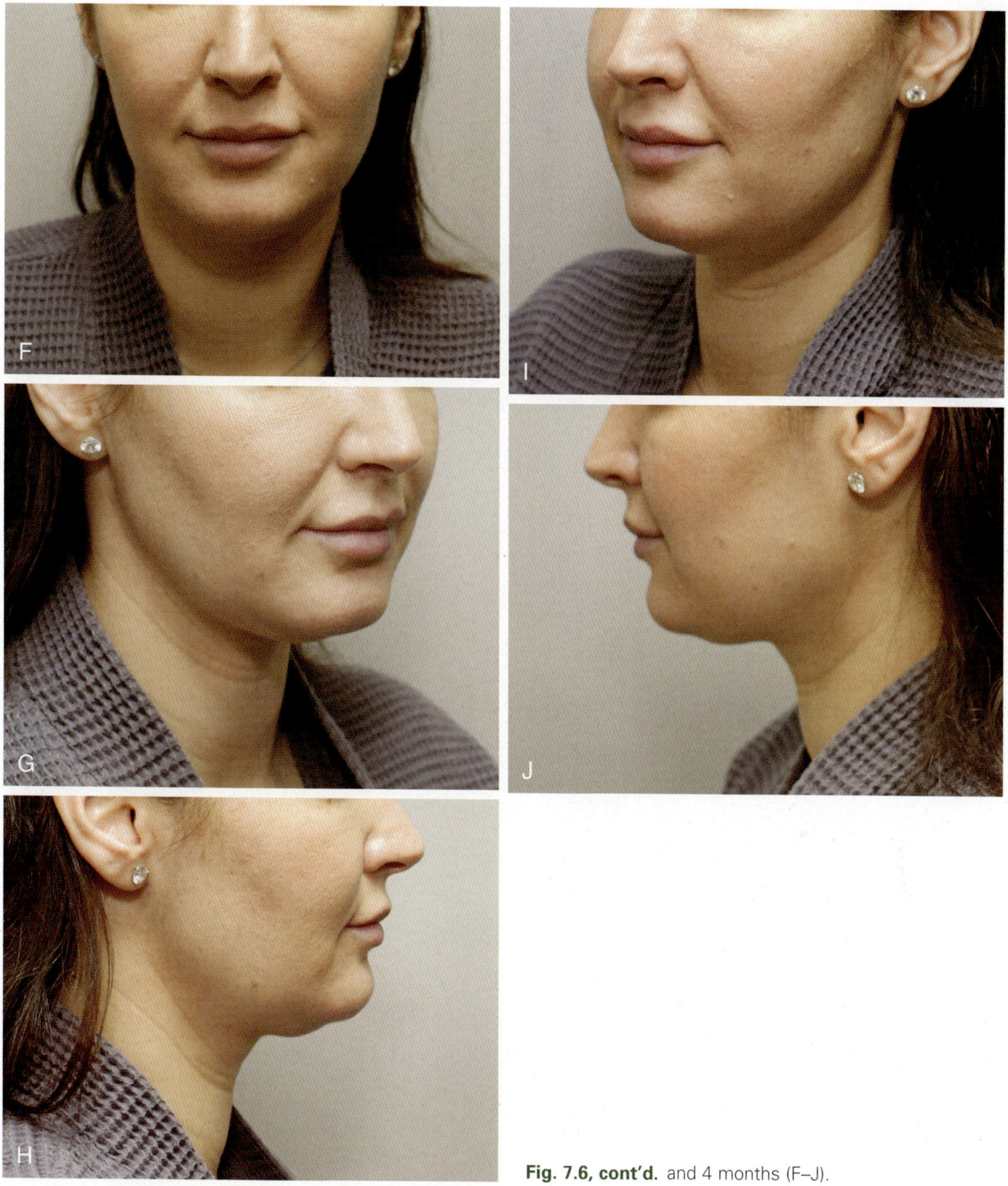

Fig. 7.6, cont'd. and 4 months (F–J).

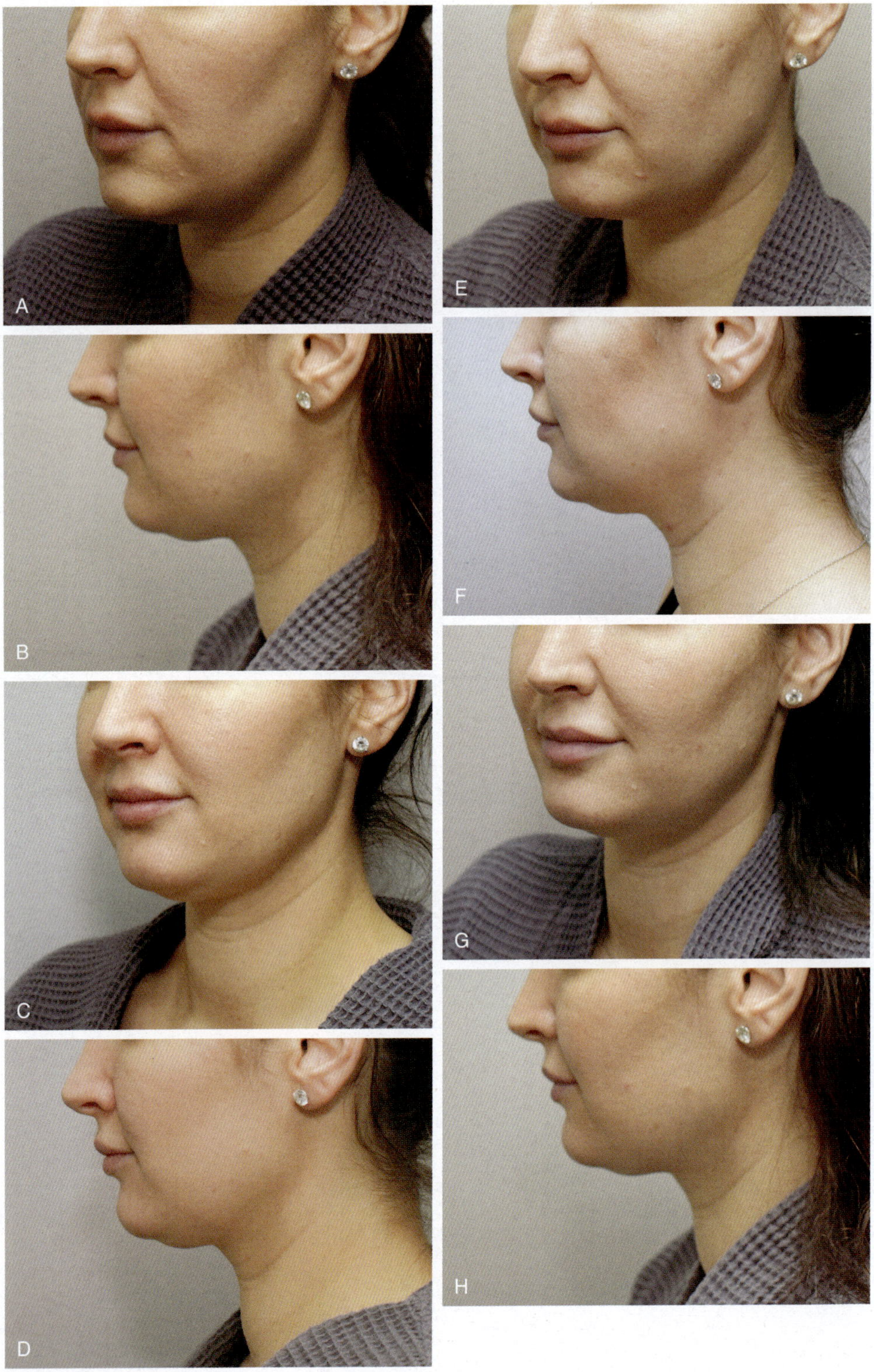

Fig. 7.7 Close-up view of case study patient presented in Fig. 7.6. The lower face and jawline are shown at baseline (A–B), 3 weeks (C–D), 6 weeks (E–F), and 4 months (G–H).

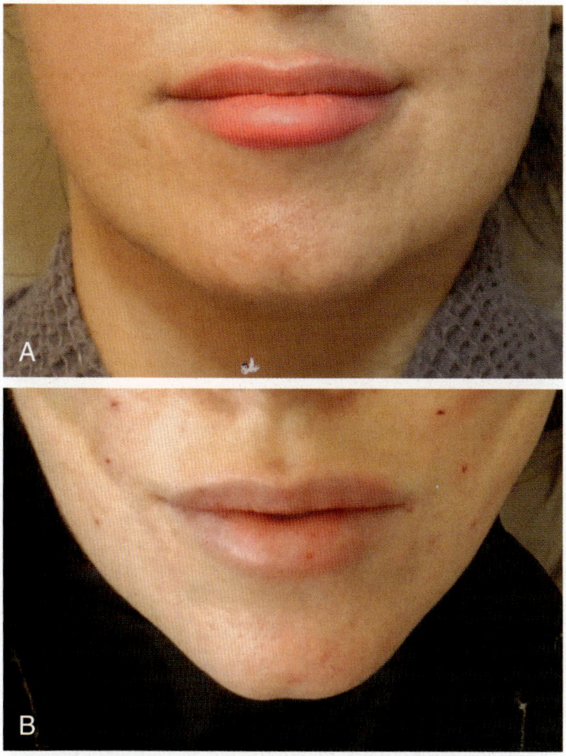

Fig. 7.8 A 31-year-old female patient treated with a total of 12 absorbable suspension sutures (four 8-cone sutures per each hemiface; two 8-cone sutures per each side of the neck) at baseline (A) and immediately posttreatment (B).

suspension sutures (four 8-cone sutures per each hemiface, two 8-cone sutures per each side of the neck; Fig. 7.8). Patient is shown at baseline and immediately posttreatment. Note the immediate lifting and repositioning of descended tissue along the jawline and the improved definition of the inferior mandibular border. The patient was very satisfied with her results.

Duration

In the clinical experience of the senior author (SMS), absorbable suspension sutures in the face have a duration of 18 to 24 months. For the neck, treatment duration is just over 1 year. It should be noted that patients rarely allow themselves to return to baseline, and the face is most often retreated at 18 months and the neck is most often retreated at 9 months. In patients who are better surgical candidates, durability of treatment is often reduced. For patients like those shown in Fig. 7.5, retreatment may be required sooner to prevent return to baseline.

Safety

Common treatment sequelae include bruising, which most often resolves within 7 to 10 days, and swelling, which most often resolves within 3 to 5 days. As mentioned in the description of optimal technique, skin bunching is expected with adequate redraping and occurs in 90% of patients. Most often, this is resolved within 7 to 10 days. In the 206 treatments performed by the senior author (SMS), no cases of hypersensitivity have been identified. Technique-driven adverse events include suture palpability or visibility resulting from placement that is too superficial. Patients with palpably thin skin can have visibility of cones for up to 3 months posttreatment. Additional potential side effects may include prolonged skin dimpling/skin irregularities, asymmetry, and sensory nerve injury.

DISCUSSION

Nonsurgical rejuvenation is of increasing importance in surgical practice. For the lower face and neck in particular, volume restoration and skin tightening are generally unable to completely manage tissue laxity and sagging, and nonsurgical tissue redraping has remained an unmet need. Absorbable suspension sutures are distinct from barbed threads in both their physiochemical and mechanical properties. Absorbable suspension sutures are comprised of PLLA/PLGA, molecules with a long history in surgical medicine and aesthetics and well-established collagen-stimulating properties.[5] The cone-shaped supports in absorbable suspension sutures offer a large surface area for support of redraped tissue, and the cup-like surface is more resistant to slippage than flat, barbed shapes.[3] Furthermore, the design of the device, when placed using the principles of SLVP, guards against migration or extrusion because the opposing cones hold it in place.[17] If used in the neck, barbed threads are better suited for improving tightness and reducing creping, while cones are better suited for redraping and repositioning sagging and ptotic tissues.[18] Rejuvenation achieved with threads in the face returns to baseline at 12 months,[19] while absorbable suspension sutures have been reported to maintain aesthetic effects for up to 24 months.[11,16] Patients who do not require lifting may prefer smooth PDO threads, which function solely to improve skin quality. Ultimately, the use of barbed PDO threads versus absorbable suspension sutures to lift ptotic tissue is based on clinician preference.

For patients seeking neck rejuvenation who are not yet candidates for surgery, absorbable suspension sutures are an effective treatment option. A full treatment with ~14 sutures takes about 1 hour in the office, and the procedure is associated with high patient satisfaction in published studies[11,17] and in the clinical experience of one author (SMS). More often than not, results are better appreciated in person than in before and after photographs. For treatment of the neck in particular, optimal outcomes are shaped by sufficient "overcorrection," use of a sufficient number of sutures, and patient adherence to postprocedure instructions. Complementary treatment with toxin in particular is advantageous because it reduces the mechanical burden on the suture while also giving the neck a younger appearance. For patients who are well suited to nonsurgical rejuvenation of the lower face and neck, absorbable suspension sutures are a valuable tool for treatment. The sutures are both biocompatible and have significant lifting capacity, making them attractive to both aesthetic surgeons and patients.

ACKNOWLEDGMENTS

The authors would like to thank Ginny Vachon, PhD of Principal Medvantage for her assistance in writing this manuscript. Funding for editorial support was provided by the CME provider X-Medica, LLC with funds from Sinclair Pharma, Inc.

REFERENCES

1. Tong LX, Rieder EA. Thread-lifts: a double-edged suture? A comprehensive review of the literature. *Dermatol Surg.* 2019;45(7):931-940.
2. Sulamanidze MA, Fournier PF, Paikidze TG, Sulamanidze GM. Removal of facial soft tissue ptosis with special threads. *Dermatol Surg.* 2002;28(5):367-371.
3. Wu WTL. Commentary on: effectiveness, longevity, and complications of facelift by barbed suture insertion. *Aesthet Surg J.* 2019;39(3):248-253.
4. Russo PR, Vercesi F, Migliorini L, Christen M. Histological findings after insertion of PLLA sutures with bi-directional cones in humans: two years follow-up. *J Plast Path Dermatol.* 2018;14(2):121-125.
5. Vleggaar D, Fitzgerald R, Lorenc ZP. Composition and mechanism of action of poly-L-lactic acid in soft tissue augmentation. *J Drugs Dermatol.* 2014;13(suppl 4):s29-s31.
6. Goldberg DJ. *Non-barbed suture lifting and neocollagenesis: why does the skin look healthier.* Oral presentation at: Vegas Cosmetic Surgery and Aesthetic Dermatology Annual Meeting; June 2018: Las Vegas, NV.
7. Kim J, Zheng Z, Kim H, Nam KA, Chung KY. Investigation on the cutaneous change induced by face-lifting monodirectional barbed polydioxanone thread. *Dermatol Surg.* 2017;43(1):74-80.
8. Kwon TR, Han SW, Yeo IK, et al. Biostimulatory effects of polydioxanone, poly-d, l lactic acid, and polycaprolactone fillers in mouse model. *J Cosmet Dermatol.* 2019; 18(4):1002-1008.
9. Archer KA, Garcia RE. Silhouette Instalift: benefits to a facial plastic surgery practice. *Facial Plast Surg Clin North Am.* 2019;27(3):341-353.
10. Ogilvie MP, Few Jr JW Jr, Tomur SS, et al. Rejuvenating the face: an analysis of 100 absorbable suture suspension patients. *Aesthet Surg J.* 2018;38(6):654-663.
11. Lorenc ZP, Ablon G, Few J, et al. Expert consensus on achieving optimal outcomes with absorbable suspension suture technology for tissue repositioning and facial recontouring. *J Drugs Dermatol.* 2018;17(6):647-655.
12. Few JW, Pintas S, Smith JR, Vachon G. Nonsurgical tissue repositioning: analysis of long-term results and patient satisfaction from 100 absorbale suture suspension cases. *Aesthet Surg J Open Forum.* 2020;2(1):ojz029.
13. Shridharani SM. Novel surface anatomic landmarks of the jowl to guide treatment with ATX-101. *Plast Reconstr Surg Glob Open.* 2019;7(10):e2459.
14. Shridharani SM. Improvement in jowl fat following ATX-101 treatment: results from a single-site study. *Plast Reconstr Surg.* 2020;145(4):929-935.
15. Shridharani SM, Chandawarkar AA. Novel expanded safe zone for reduction of submental fullness with ATX-101 injection. *Plast Reconstr Surg.* 2019;144(6):995e-1001e.
16. King M. The management of bruising following nonsurgical cosmetic treatment. *J Clin Aesthet Dermatol.* 2017;10(2):E1-E4.
17. de Benito J, Pizzamiglio R, Theodorou D, Arvas L. Facial rejuvenation and improvement of malar projection using sutures with absorbable cones: surgical technique and case series. *Aesthetic Plast Surg.* 2011;35(2):248-253.
18. Arora G, Arora S. Neck rejuvenation with thread lift. *J Cutan Aesthet Surg.* 2019;12(3):196-200.
19. Bertossi D, Botti G, Gualdi A, et al. Effectiveness, longevity, and complications of facelift by barbed suture insertion. *Aesthet Surg J.* 2019;39(3):241-247.

8

Noninvasive Liposculpting

Dennis J. Hurwitz and Armando Augusto Davila

INTRODUCTION

- Noninvasive advanced technology liposculpting treatments are increasingly supplanting, complimenting, and preliminary to excisional body contouring surgery.
- For optimal patient care and to maintain dominance in the body contouring market, a plastic surgeon needs to embrace reliable and safe technology, particularly for success in the office setting.
- Formidable barriers are a vast array of options, high capital purchase, costly disposables, maintenance fees, lack of experience, conflicting anecdotal reports, energy-related complications, marketing hyperbole, and rapid obsolescence.
- Competing marketed technologies have been rejected by plastic surgeons as being relatively ineffective, cost prohibitive, unsafe, or redundant compared to excisional surgery.
- Non–plastic surgeons are usurping patients through marketing of energy-based technologies. Their advanced technology offers scarless, rapid recovery and safer and less-expensive alternative to surgery. Having only machines, these clinics oversell their limited therapeutics beyond appropriate indications.

Disclosures: Dr. Dennis Hurwitz was a paid investigator for InMode from 2010 to 2011 and has stock options. He has accepted $5000 in fees for lectures. He has received no editing or direct financial support for this chapter.

BACKGROUND INFORMATION/ANATOMIC PEARLS

1. Overweight and obese patients are encouraged to lose weight and are offered an alternative diet of human choriogonadotropin (HCG)/500 calorie-a-day 6-week program. Goal body mass index (BMI) for patients for realistic results using noninvasives in the office setting are in the 25 to 30 kg/m^2 range. Patients in the 30 to 35 kg/m^2 range may see results when combined with more aggressive liposculpting and are better suited to the outpatient surgery center setting.
2. Energy-based technologies may supplant invasive surgery for mild to moderate skin laxity; often referred to as the gap deformity, that is, not bad enough for major surgery, but bad enough to do something about. They are also available to those who refuse excisional surgery.
3. Energy-based technologies have a reasonable return on investment by high patient satisfaction, increased variety of therapeutic alternatives, and can lead to traditional body contouring surgery.
4. Traditional vacuum and syringe with cannula liposuction are used for limited liposuction, and fat harvest for small lipoaugmentation.
5. VASERlipo (Solta Medical, Bothell, WA) is used for moderate to large volume liposuction, and adipose harvest for grafting to minimize residual tissue trauma and maximize connective tissue and dermal shrinkage.

6. Bipolar radiofrequency in the form of skin surface Morpheus8 microneedling and subcutaneous fat, vessel coagulation, and collagen fiber shrinkage through FaceTite, BodyTite, and AccuTite shrink tissues reliably and safely rejuvenates and shrinks skin.
7. Major body contouring operations are being modified to permit detailed sculpturing by ancillary procedures are the same time.
8. Topical electromagnetic, laser, and radiofrequency therapies such as EmSculpt, TruSculpt, and SculpSure reliably and safely rejuvenate skin, subcutaneous tissue, and muscle.

PREPROCEDURE CONSIDERATIONS (INDICATIONS FOR TREATMENT, IMPORTANT PREOPERATIVE PATIENT INFORMATION, PLANNING INFORMATION)

As experts in body contouring surgery, plastic surgeons are ideally positioned to provide and refine new technology as it emerges in the marketplace. This combination is clearly in the interest of our patients, particularly since many practitioners who cannot offer invasive body contouring may not present ideal and clear alternatives to patients who are not strong candidates for noninvasives. Based on a conscientious effort to sift through competing manufacturers' claims and our clinical cases, the authors present our chosen technologies and how we apply them to those concerned about their appearance.

Patients presenting for noninvasive or minimally invasive procedures vary widely, ranging anywhere from thin and wrinkled to obese with a hanging pannus. Naturally, these patients abhor their size, shape, bulges, unsightly scars, stria, and loose skin. In addition, larger patients are frequently concerned about oversized flanks and back, and sagging poorly shaped mons pubis, buttocks, and thighs. However, not all these patients will qualify for minimally invasive approaches. Overweight patients are encouraged to lose weight on their own or accept our preoperative 500-calorie-a-day diet/HCG injection 6-week program, but even after significant weight loss many will exceed the capacity of noninvasives. We discuss with the patient gender-specific contouring through artistic emphasis of shape to those both aware and ignorant of the differences.

As plastic surgeons, most patient discussion will involve invasive surgical options of removal of excess skin and fat, with patients' responses ranging from disapproval of invasive surgery to acceptance of whatever operation and resulting scars it takes to obtain optimal result. Nevertheless, most inquirers for torso contouring not only welcome but are intrigued by non- and minimally invasive technology to supplant or augment recommended surgery. Even when they elect complex excisional operations, patients appreciate our experience and explanation of the alternatives, but, for them, ultimately inadequate procedures.

Patients readily grasp that in the process of correcting their perceived localized contour deformity, their entire torso could be recontoured. A common example is request for correction of gynecomastia. Beyond addressing the residual chest skin laxity, further masculinization can be achieved through liposuction with etching of torso musculature and lipoaugmentation of the pectoralis and deltoid muscles (Fig. 8.1).

With or without excisional surgery, minimally invasive technology such as ultrasonic-assisted liposuction, bipolar radiofrequency skin tightening, and electromagnetic energy muscular enhancement remove adipose, damage collagenous support, and induce regeneration of connective tissue septi, dermis, and muscle. These patients may present primarily to the office requesting these technologies, particularly during effective office advertising campaigns, but this is often the exception and not the rule. Know when to integrate these technologies with precision to enhance or supplant other techniques.

PROCEDURAL TECHNIQUES (STEP-BY-STEP GUIDE ON PERFORMING TECHNIQUES)

Looking at the big picture, comprehensive contouring of the torso involves eight interactive tools. Complex and lengthy excisions may be complimented by preoperative weight reduction and intraoperative energy-based technologies. Items pertinent to non- or minimally invasive approaches are discussed in detail.

1. HCG/500-calorie-a-day diet to reduce excessively high BMI.[1,2]
2. VASER ultrasound-assisted lipoplasty to debulk fat, undermine flaps or excision sites, and harvest adipose tissue.[3,4]

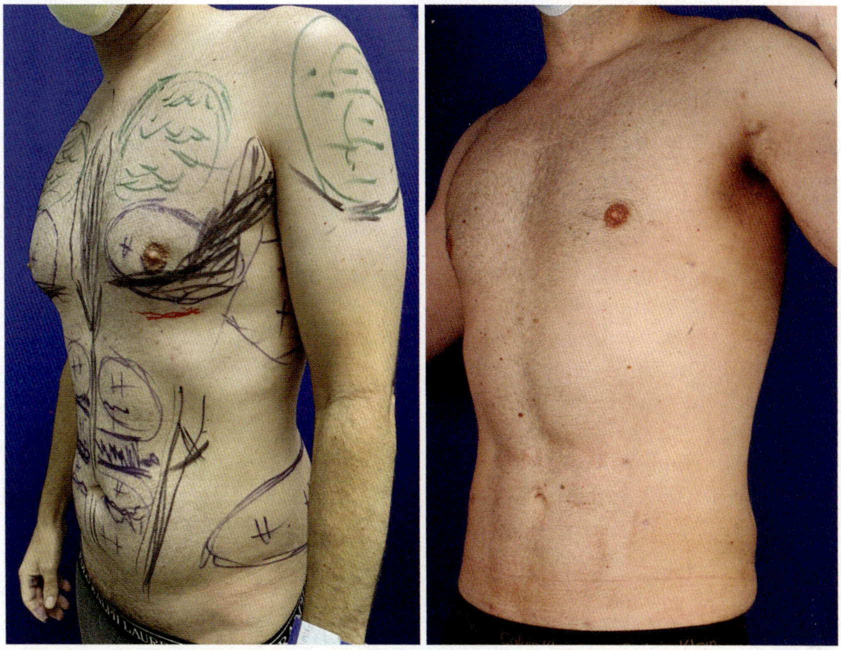

Fig. 8.1 A 44-year-old with body mass index of 25.1 kg/m^2 requests correction of his gynecomastia. COVID-19 restrictions have reduced his workouts and for the 7 pounds he has gained, he also requests body liposuction, improved muscular definition, and reluctantly accepts recommendation of pectoralis and deltoid muscle lipoaugmentation. Left anterior oblique views show before with surgical markings *(left)* and 3 months after *(right)*. VASERlipo, and syringe injection lipoaugmentation of filtered extract with 60 cc into each pectoralis and 35 cc into each deltoid muscle. After 2800 cc infusion of saline with 3 mg of epinephrine, 500 mg xylocaine into the abdomen (1000 cc), 10 min pulsed VASER followed with 5 ring probe at 80%, and then 600 cc aspiration through 3.7 mm. VentX cannula; into the flanks (600 cc), 6 min VASER followed and then 600 cc total aspiration; and into the chest (1200 cc), 12 min VASER followed with 1 ring at 80% and then 500 cc aspiration. From the aspirated 1700 cc, 190 cc of filtered fat was available for injection. An anticipated glandular pull through direct excision was not needed. Three months after *(right)*, the VASERlipo correction of the gynecomastia is complete with pleasing mid-pectoralis bulge and presternal vertical depression. The deltoid augmentation is not well seen. The rectus muscle is etched with a smooth transition to the pubis and no skin laxity. Subtle hip prominence appears in the wake of reduced flanks.

3. BodyTite, FaceTite, bipolar radiofrequency to subcutaneous tissue for mild to intermediate surgical tissue laxity.[5,6]
4. Morpheus8 Body with Burst bipolar radiofrequency microneedling to dermis and subdermis to tighten and rejuvenate skin.[7]
5. Lipoabdominoplasty with or without lower body lift when flank/transverse laxity is absent.[8]
6. Oblique flankplasty with lipoabdominoplasty (OFLA) to narrow a sagging waist, tighten the torso, and lift the buttocks and lateral thighs in cases of greater laxity, particularly in the female torso.[9]
7. Oblique flankplasty with TULUA abdominoplasty allows for VASERlipo abdominal etching and lipoaugmentation, especially in the male.[10,11]
8. J Torsoplasty with breast/chest reshaping to compliment OFLA or lower body lift.[12]
9. High-frequency ultrasound (HFUS) for intraoperative tomographic guidance: autologous augmentation of positive contours and targeted peripheral nerve nonnarcotic pain control.
10. EmSculpt high-frequency electromagnetic energy (HIFEM) for natural muscular development and toning.[13]

11. Topical but limited therapies for those who refuse minimally invasive procedures and invasive surgery such as TruSculpt, SculpSure.

PREOPERATIVE RAPID WEIGHT LOSS HCG 500-CALORIE-A-DAY 6-WEEK DIET

Overweight individuals, especially those with prominent intraabdominal girth, requesting body contouring are at increased risk for delayed healing and poor aesthetics. Rather than rejecting them, for the past 14 years Hurwitz center has offered a 500-calorie-a-day diet with daily injections of HCG that the senior author learned directly from plastic surgeon Hassan Tazia in Casablanca, Morocco. This high-protein, HCG-injection 6-week program was originated by Internist Alfred Simeon in Italy.[1,2] The HCG hormone induces visceral fat metabolism and reduces hunger for a weight loss of nearly a pound a day. Preoperatively treated, about 80% of the last 300 patients have lost enough weight to successfully proceed with extensive body contouring operations. Our demonstrative patient is a 32-year-old woman who lost 30 pounds on the HGC program to lower her BMI from 32 to 27 kg/m^2 (Fig. 8.2). Her lipoabdominoplasty included imbrication of her diastasis recti and umbilical herniorrhaphy, plus VASERlipo of the flanks and lipoaugmentation of her breasts. Two years later, she has gained only 5 pounds, maintained her new figure with no recurrence of the hernia or diastasis recti. While significant rapid weight loss can precipitate significant tissue laxity that may transition a patient from minimally invasive to more invasive procedure, HCG is an important tool that can assist a patient to meet their final goal before a procedure.

POSTPROCEDURE CONSIDERATIONS (POSTOPERATIVE CARE RECOMMENDATIONS, RESTRICTIONS)

Because of poor compliance, approximately 20% of users are unable to lose to goal weight. We have avoided

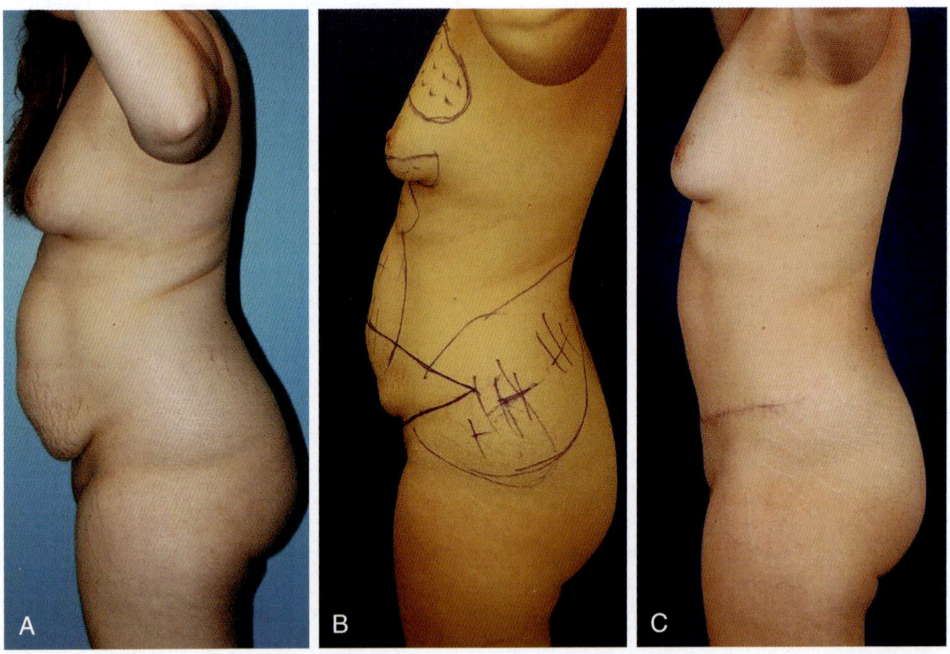

Fig. 8.2 Reduction of obesity with human choriogonadotropin (HCG)/500-calorie-a-day diet before lipoabdominoplasty and VASERlipo of the flanks as seen left lateral views. (A) Presentation of a 32-year-old with body mass index 31 kg/m^2 for abdominoplasty and repair of diastasis recti. (B) After 30-pound loss because of the diet, patient is marked for lipoabdominoplasty and VASERlipo of the flanks. Notable is the reduction of abdominal protuberance and absence of back rolls. (C) Two years after her lipoabdominoplasty, VASERlipo of the flanks and 150 cc lipoaugmentation of the breasts, her abdomen is flat and the flanks are hollowed.

patients with unstable endocrine disorders but have often treated patients with stable diabetes and patients on hypertensives without adverse sequalae. About 10% of successfully treated patients request a repeat 6-week diet to treat their postsurgical weight gain.

Complications and Outcomes (General Complications and Outcomes Information)

Limiting to no more than two consecutive 6-week treatments, there have been no metabolic or medical adverse events. The visceral fat target has led to loss of intraabdominal fat, which explains no recurrence of repaired diastasis recti. While patients on HCG/500-calories-a-day diet have increased energy and libido, they are being starved and should not undergo surgery until 1 week after completing the program to avoid delays in wound healing.

BODYTITE, FACETITE, ACCUTITE BIPOLAR RADIOFREQUENCY ENERGY APPLIED TO SUBCUTANEOUS TISSUE

Advanced bipolar radiofrequency technology, whereby, the energy flows from a small, deeply situated electrode to a larger skin paddle, was originated and continues to be upgraded by InMode (Yokum, Israel) in the form of progressively smaller handles with decreasing total wattage and maximum temperature allowances known as BodyTite, FaceTite, and AccuTite. After entry through a stab wound, a blunt 1.2-to-3-millimeter probe on a scissor-like bipolar handpiece emits a steady stream of energy directed to the disc receiving electrode in contact with the skin surface (Video 8.1). The probe is positioned in the proper plane during the forward stroke and the energy is applied on the slow back stroke for multiple passes until predetermined external and internal temperature limits are achieved, delivering a measurable amount of kilojoule energy to the tissues. Preset temperature high-limit cutoffs prevent overheating and excess thermal damage. Care in proper tissue level placement and stroke pattern prevents superficial and deep burns. The end points are observable skin shrinkage, achieving designated high-temperature settings, and predetermine levels of kilojoules per area. Any liquified fat can then be evacuated by gentle liposuction. Incompletely damaged collagenous supporting connective tissue heals shortened and rejuvenated. When properly performed, minimal scar tissue develops, which allows for repeat BodyTite treatments to incrementally tighten tissues.

These minimally invasive radiofrequency devices can treat generalized skin laxity with and without excess adipose. While AccuTite and FaceTite are focused for small, localized tightening, BodyTite expands treatment options by treating laxity on those with mild to moderate deformity, or who refuse excisional surgery. Since the late 2016 reintroduction of BodyTite to the senior author's practice (DJH), bipolar radiofrequency minimally invasive procedures to the face, neck, arms, torso, and thighs have been applied to 368 patients. From an unknown skin tightening technique, new patients now request it by name, and with our extensive experience, they accept their role as we assign to them. To avoid overpromising results, I emphasize that BodyTite does not replace the gold standard of excisional surgery and should be more considered "body-not-loose" rather than "body tight," and results even in mild deformity are likely to not exceed more than a 50% to 70% maximum expected result of an equivalent excisional procedure. A secondary radiofrequency procedure 6 months later can have an additive effect and is easily executed because of limited scarring from the initial procedure. Simply informing patients of the possible need for a secondary BodyTite application emphasizes the uncertainty of results. In our practice, secondary BodyTite has been performed in approximately 25% of patients.

As an isolated procedure, BodyTite of one or two regions is performed in our office operating room under super wet local anesthesia and mild oral sedation. When BodyTite compliments major excisional body contouring, it is performed in the operating room in conjunction with the invasive operation. When adipose bulk needs to be removed, we prefer preaspiration application of VASER ultrasonic energy to dislodge the fat, followed by BodyTite, and then traditional liposuction. Since BodyTite functions best when the connective tissue is naturally stretched to length by the fat cells and hydrated, we do not perform thorough aspiration of fat before application. When there is little to no adipose excess or VASER is unavailable, preliminary liposuction is not performed.

In the following case presentations, photographs validate clinical descriptions of contour deformity but are unable to document skin laxity. Furthermore, liposuction of bulging tissues usually leaves additional laxity. The assessment of the contribution of supplemental bipolar energy radiofrequency needs to be left up to the treating surgeon. The ideal candidate for bipolar radiofrequency therapy exhibits sagging fullness with youthful elastic skin, such as our 39-year-old woman with excess adiposity and sagging skin of the neck. Pleased with her lasting result from BodyTite reshaping of her arms performed by the senior author (DJH) in 2009 for an InMode sponsored clinical trial for U.S. Food and Drug Administration (FDA) approval, she wondered if the same technology could be used for her oversized neck. Since FDA approval, the obvious improvement in instrumentation was the addition of an accurate immediate temperature sensor with energy cutoff on the deep probe. Without complication and within 3 weeks of applying 14 kJ of energy with internal limits of 40 °C and external skin 68 °C and liposuction of 20 cc of fatty emulsion, her neck took on the proper shape and skin tightness that has lasted 4 years (Fig. 8.3).

VASERlipo and BodyTite are an ideal combination for a minimally invasive contouring of a mild sagging adipose deformity. After super wet infusion of saline with xylocaine and epinephrine, the VASER probe cavitates the adipose, allowing for easy access of the BodyTite probe to injure the supporting connective tissue in a radiofrequency conductive wet environment, followed by gentle VentX aspiration of fatty emulsion. An abdominal example is a 54-year-old woman with a "gap" deformity that has annoying adipose with skin laxity, but not enough to warrant an abdominoplasty (Fig. 8.4). After application of pulsatile VASER, then 24 kJ of

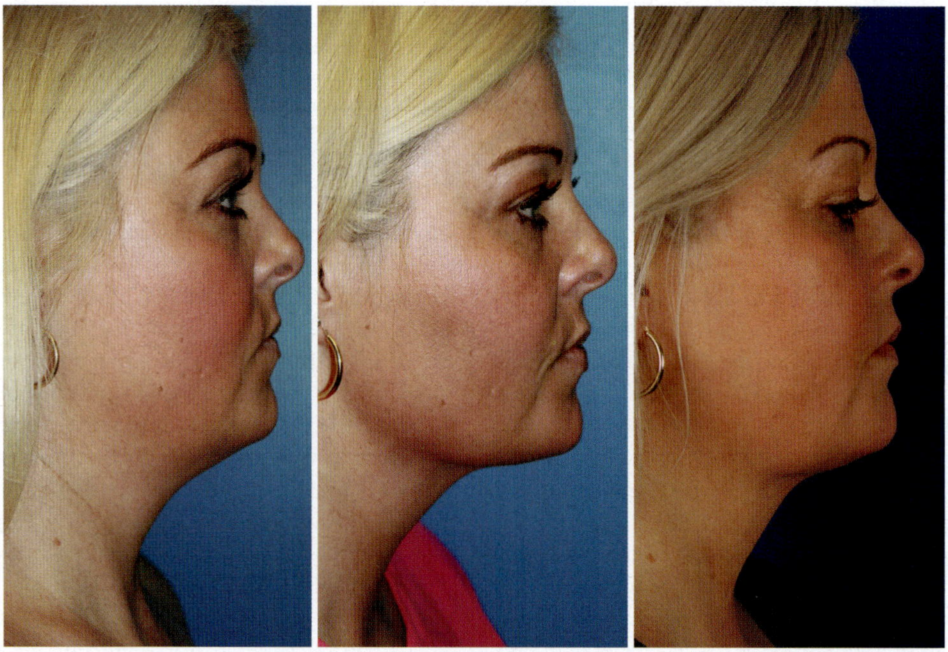

Fig. 8.3 *(Left)* Before right lateral face/neck views show hanging adipose, and the result 6 months *(middle)* and *(right)* 4 years after neck FaceTite with 20 cc of syringe liposuction of the neck and 20-pound weight gain. This 39-year-old woman requested FaceTite of her neck with liposuction, because of her long-lasting improvement for a similar problem in her arms. Upper row shows sagging adipose neck deformity. After infiltration of 100 cc of saline with xylocaine and epinephrine. Ten cc of fatty emulsion was aspirated through a 2-mm diameter cannula and 20-cc luer lock syringe. FaceTite was inserted through stab wound incisions in the lateral neck and submental region for application of 7 kJ of energy in each location. After pushing the probe through superficial subcutaneous fat, the energy is released during multiple backward pulls with the temperature cutoffs set at 40 degrees external and 70 degrees internal. Then the last 10 cc of fatty emulsion including some denatured fat was aspirated from the superficial adipose of the neck. In the submental area, subplatysma fat is also aspirated. At 6 months, the submental and jawline is nicely contoured, and is nearly as defined 3.5 years later and 20 pounds heavier.

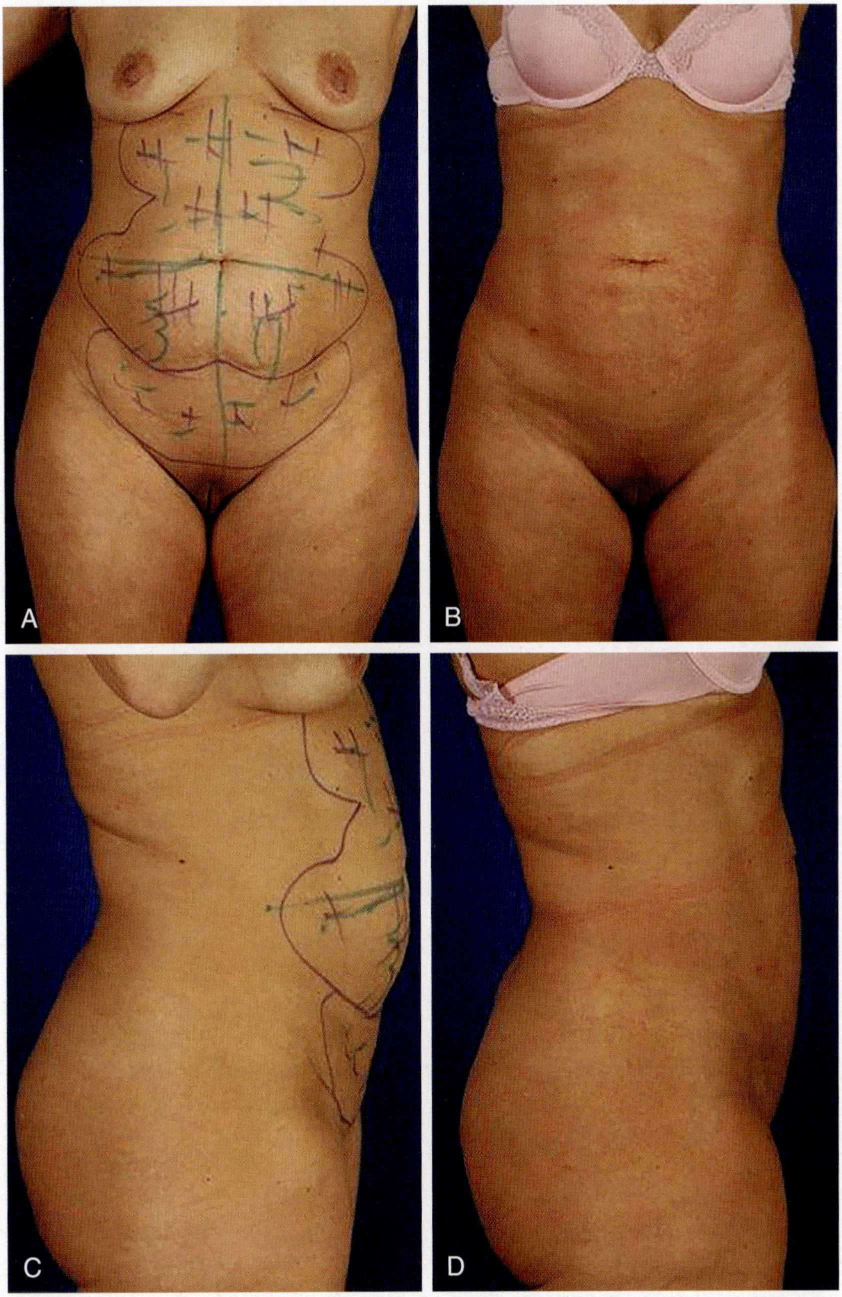

Fig. 8.4 Combining VASERlipo with BodyTite for a minimally invasive abdominal contouring in a 54-year-old woman. She has a "gap" deformity that has annoying adipose with skin laxity, but not enough to warrant an abdominoplasty. (A) Before, frontal view condition with presurgical markings for VASERlipo and BodyTite of anterior abdominal wall, and (B) 4 months after, frontal images. (C) Before, right lateral condition with presurgical markings, and (D) 4 months after, right lateral images. She has a flat, smooth abdomen with naturally appearing muscular etching.

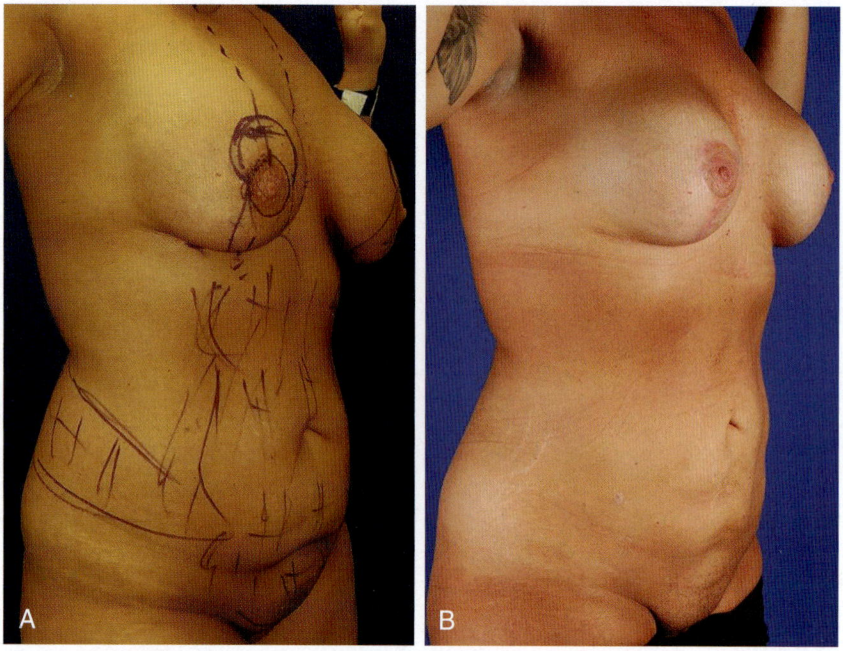

Fig. 8.5 Combining VASERlipo with BodyTite for a noninvasive abdominal contouring in a 32-year-old and VASERlipo of her flanks. Dr. Hurwitz performed implant exchange and Wise pattern mastopexies, while the physician assistant performed the minimally invasive surgery. (A) Before, presenting condition with presurgical markings for the mastopexies and VASERlipo and BodyTite of anterior abdominal wall and VASERlipo of her flanks. Note the depression superior to her ptotic mons pubis. (B) Six months after, right anterior oblique images. She has a "gap" deformity that has annoying adipose laden skin laxity, but not enough to warrant an abdominoplasty. She obtained a flat, smooth abdomen with elevation of the mons pubis. Her smaller breasts with raised nipples are no longer ptotic.

BodyTite, 100 cc of slurry fat was aspirated. Her before and 4-months postoperative result reveals a flat, nonsagging, and well-defined abdomen.

Another combination of VASERlipo with BodyTite for abdominal contouring for a "gap" deformity is a 32-year-old that also had VASERlipo of her flanks. The senior author (DJH) performed implant exchange and Wise pattern mastopexies, while his physician assistant performed the minimally invasive surgery (Fig. 8.5). She obtained a flat, smooth abdomen with elevation of the mons pubis and effacement of the suprapubic depression. Her breasts are smaller and without ptosis.

A third young patient with sagging adipose laden abdominal skin and ptotic mons pubis declined a lipoabdominoplasty at the time of her implant exchange with mastopexy. Instead, she had VASERlipo of the abdomen followed by BodyTite that extended across the mons pubis (see Fig. 8.5). Four months after the procedure, she has a reduced and well-contoured abdomen and suspended mons pubis (Fig. 8.6). A fourth young patient added EMSculpt enhancement of her rectus muscles to the previously described combination of VASERlipo with BodyTite for a minimally invasive abdominal contouring. In addition, this 27-year-old overweight woman underwent VASERlipo of her flanks and saddlebags and lipoaugmentation of her lateral gluteal areas. Three months lateral, she has a series of four EmSculpt HIFEM treatments. She now has a smoothly proportioned and natural feminine muscular appearance.

BodyTite may also limit the extent of excisional surgery of the abdomen, arms, and thighs to reduce the trauma of surgery and scar burden. Frequently, our limited abdominoplasty is combined VASERlipo with BodyTite of the midtorso, as in a 36-year-old mother with a depressed C-section scar and small hanging pannus (Fig. 8.7). She also had VASERlipo of her flanks and fat grafting of her lateral buttocks and superior poles of the breasts. Her epigastrium is not loose enough to

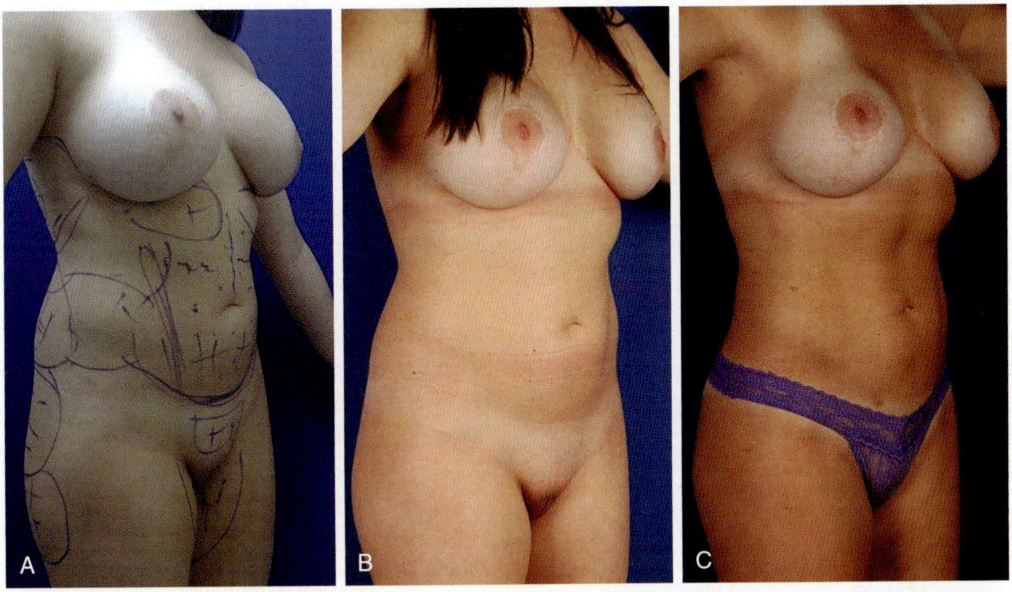

Fig. 8.6 Right anterior oblique views showing combining VASERlipo with BodyTite for a minimally invasive abdominal contouring in a 27-year-old overweight woman, along with VASERlipo of her flanks and saddlebags and lipoaugmentation of her lateral gluteal areas. Three months later, she undergoes four EmSculpt HIFEM treatments. (A) Before, presenting condition with presurgical markings for VASERlipo and BodyTite. (B) Before, without markings. (C) Four months after, right anterior oblique images. She has a smoothly proportioned, tight skinned muscular appearance.

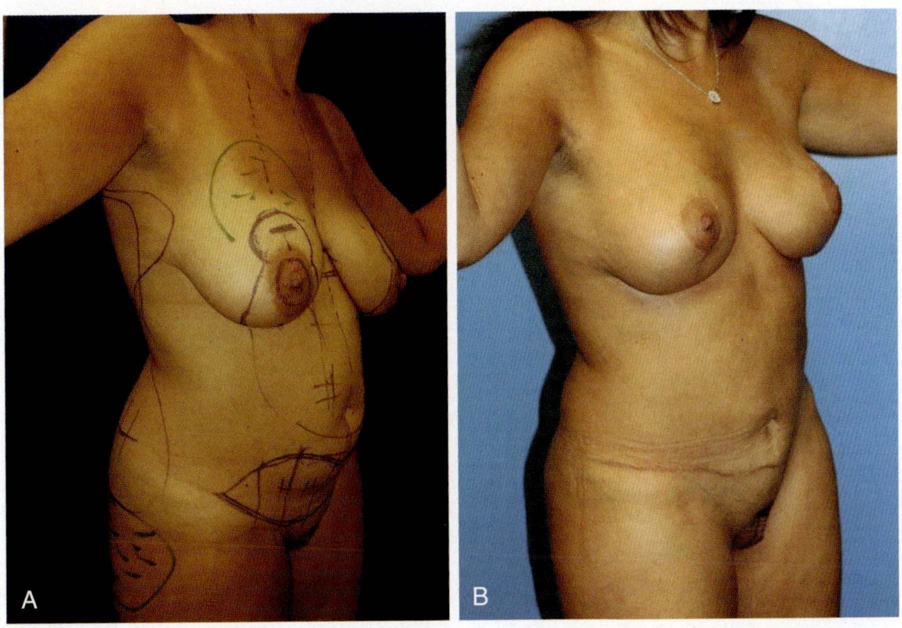

Fig. 8.7 A limited abdominoplasty is combined VASERlipo with BodyTite of the epigastrium and lateral torso in a 36-year-old mother with a depressed C-section scar. She also had VASERlipo of her flanks and fat grafting of her lateral buttocks and superior poles of the breasts. (A) Before, presenting condition with presurgical markings for the mastopexies, limited abdominoplasty, and VASERlipo and BodyTite of anterior abdominal wall and VASERlipo of her flanks, and (B) 6 months after, right anterior oblique images. Her epigastrium is not loose enough to complete a full abdominoplasty with a low-lying scar, but loose enough to need BodyTite. She receives a flat, smooth abdomen to her mons pubis. Her smaller breasts with raised nipples are no longer ptotic. Her lateral breast roll was removed.

complete a full abdominoplasty with a low-lying scar, but loose enough to benefit from by BodyTite. She obtained a flat, smooth abdomen to her mons pubis. Her smaller breasts with raised nipples are no longer ptotic. Her lateral breast roll was removed.

Patients with heavy and loose-skinned upper arms and thighs are understandably weary of the long brachioplasty and medial thighplasty scars. When there is minimal skin laxity, BodyTite is added to VASERlipo fat reduction for essentially scarless improvement that is usual pleasing. When their skin laxity requires surgical reduction, most patients more readily accept reductions that leave a scar that only goes halfway down the extremity, with the distal arm treated by bipolar radiofrequency tightening. A thin 68-year-old woman underwent a limited L brachioplasty that equally reduced considerable skin laxity of the lateral chest and proximal arm as it crossed the axilla and BodyTite of the distal half of the upper arms. The distal third of the arm was circumferentially treated with BodyTite (Fig. 8.8). Fourteen months later, there is an artistic reduction of the lateral chest, axilla, and entire upper arm. Since this treatment was performed before the availability of Morpheus8 bipolar radiofrequency skin microneedling, the dermis was not also treated, so wrinkling of the distal upper arm skin, much to her dismay, was accentuated.

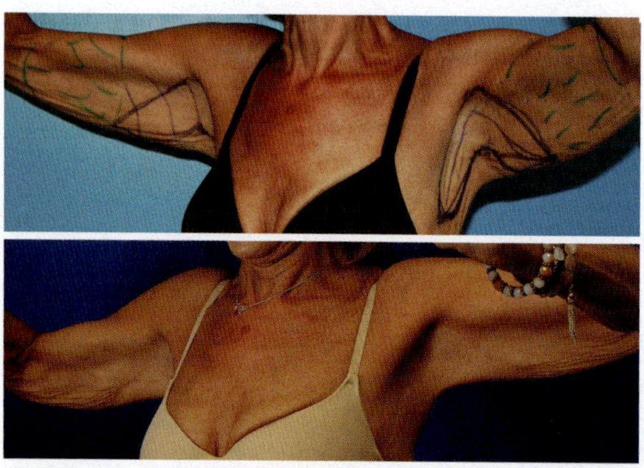

Fig. 8.8 Left anterior oblique arm views of a thin 68-year-old woman desiring limited-scar arm reduction. *Upper.* Presurgical markings for a limited L brachioplasty and BodyTite (green) of the distal half of the upper arms. *Lower.* Fourteen months later, artistic reduction of her lateral chest, axilla, and entire upper arm is accompanied by distal wrinkling of the untreated skin.

POSTPROCEDURE CONSIDERATIONS (POSTOPERATIVE CARE RECOMMENDATIONS, RESTRICTIONS)

As with liposuction, postoperative continuous uniform elastic compression is essential for the first 4 days, and then extended for up to 6 weeks. Swelling obscures results. With the regeneration of supportive collagen, the final result may not be fully appreciated for 3 to 6 months.

Complications and Outcomes (General Complications and Outcomes Information)

The entry stab wound area may sustain thermal injury because of excessive overlap of energy, leaving a thicken scar that would benefit from a later excision. Undulating depressions, because of under- and/or overtreated spots, are difficult to avoid and may need to be touched up. Patients need to be warned, and many are accepting of minor contour irregularities instead of a long scar. Sun damaged, severely aged, and wrinkled skin may become more wrinkled after BodyTite as subcutaneous tightening is not indicated for treating wrinkles or stretch marks. However, frequently encountered stretch marks are indicators of poor native contractility of the skin postliposuction, and the patient may benefit from BodyTite.

MORPHEUS8 BODY WITH BURST BIPOLAR RADIOFREQUENCY TO TIGHTEN AND REJUVENATE SKIN[6]

Morpheus8 Body with Burst supplies radiofrequency via gold-coated tip radiofrequency enhanced percutaneous microneedling, which provides dermal and subdermal level skin tightening and smooths out the skin. Morpheus8 has a comfortable pistol grip handpiece with interchangeable disposables, which provide 12, 24, and 40 retractable electrode pins that penetrate 2 to 7 mm (Video 8.2). Upon stretch of the skin and firm pressure on the skin, the distinct pattern of microperforations is made. The handle is rapidly lifted and placed down again with about 50% overlap. The device can be set to a variety of energy levels and depths, limited via the electronic software depending on the disposable tip placed on the device. The 12-pin Prime tip is focused on small, delicate areas such as the undereye, while the 40-pin Body tip provides deep radiofrequency energy to

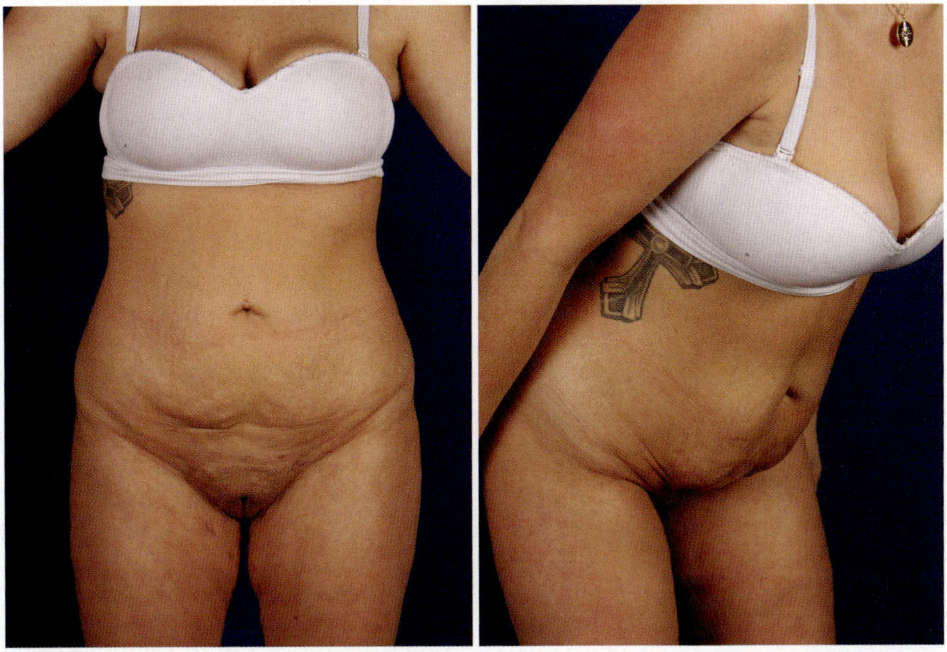

Fig. 8.9 A 28-year-old mother desires a flat abdomen without an abdominoplasty. Before shows lower abdominal fullness with small hanging pannus *(left)*. A four-quadrant abdominal application of 10 kJ each of BodyTite followed by lipoaspiration of 400 cc of fat and then application of Morpheus8 Body Burst of 35 kJ at 2, 4, and 7 millimeters. *(Right)* The result 6 weeks later.

8 mm and can apply three-level energy using burst mode in a single cycle. Finally, the resurfacing 24 pin is locked at the 1-mm depth to provide aggressive resurfacing of the epidermis in patients with higher Fitzpatrick levels who are poor candidates for laser resurfacing. Deeper levels of treatment often require tumescent infiltration, as topical solutions are not sufficient to penetrate subdermally. Over the next several months of healing, the retracted skin wrinkles smooth out. This is in contrast with the BodyTite subcutaneous tightening, which can worsen these superficial skin wrinkles. When more skin tightening is desired, InMode labels the combination of BodyTite and Morpheus8 Embrace. They tout a synergistic effect, which seems to be related to the multilevel radiofrequency energy applied. The next patient is a 49-year-old female, with a history of two pregnancies, who desired correction of her oversized and sagging abdomen. She refused abdominoplasty and elected to undergo VASERlipo with BodyTite and Morpheus8 Body. After 500 mL of tumescent (saline, xylocaine, and epinephrine) was infused into the subcutaneous tissue of her abdomen, a three-ring VASER probe was applied at 90% for 4 min and 30 s. Then BodyTite was applied for a total of 24 kJ with subsequent evacuation of 300 mL of emulsion through liposuction. Finally, two passes of Morpheus8 Body with a Burst at 2-, 4-, and 7-mL penetration was performed to reduce dermal laxity and stria. Her own platelet rich plasma was immediately wiped over the needle punctures. Her improved shape is seen at 2 months with additional contraction expected with time (Fig. 8.9).

POSTPROCEDURE CONSIDERATIONS (POSTOPERATIVE CARE RECOMMENDATIONS, RESTRICTIONS)

Regenerative creams are applied daily for 5 days. Platelet rich plasma can be used as a topical serum after the procedure to reduce the patient's recovery and downtime. The system cannot be used without administering radiofrequency energy and so a wet interface is not acceptable. Early postoperative swelling was reduced by twice weekly Hyvamat electrophysiologic lymphatic massage for six treatments.

Complications and Outcomes (General Complications and Outcomes Information)

When meticulously applied, the Morpheus8 and Morpheus8 Body Burst may cause temporary urticaria-like swelling but otherwise is remarkably free of complications at all Fitzpatrick skin types. For maximal skin contraction, Morpheus8 radiofrequency energy may need to be applied over three treatments at least 1 month apart.

OBLIQUE FLANKPLASTY WITH TULUA ALLOWS FOR SAFE VASERLIPO ETCHING OF THE ABDOMEN

Major body contouring operations are being redesigned to allow for safe and effective defining of torso contours during the same stage. For some years now with the limited central undermining of the epigastrium of lipoabdominoplasty, we like Saldana have cautiously liposuctioned the epigastric flap, with primarily flank and lateral flap liposuction to create the negative spaces of the lateral oblique muscle depressions.[8] Especially adapted for the male, the TULUA substitutes the limited epigastric undermining for only VASERlipo and demands wide transverse imbrication of the muscular fascia between the pubis and umbilicus. Upon closure of the lower abdominal wound and creation of a neoumbilicus, aggressive thinning and etching of the anterior abdomen is safely performed.[10,11] The lack of undermining allows this aggressive approach to be possible, and while the technique can be applied to the muscular female with mild to moderate adiposity and lower skin laxity, it is uniquely suitable for the male torso. Since Oblique flankplasty transversely tightens the epigastric region through the posterior rotation advancement of the superior flap, closure of the flank and abdomen wounds provides circumferential skin tightening for optimal midbody narrowing. Previously described radiofrequency devices such as BodyTite can also safely be applied to the abdominal flap to deepen etching or Morpheus8 for stretch marks. A 28-year-old transgender man with prior mastectomies desires a masculinizing single-stage torso transformation (Fig. 8.10). For his barrel-like torso, TULUA and Oblique flankplasty was combined with VASERlipo etching of the abdomen, lateral chest, and lipoaugmentation of the pectoralis and deltoid muscles. Rid of bulges and loose skin, his superficial torso muscles are distinct with a narrow lower body topped by a broader upper.

POSTPROCEDURE CONSIDERATIONS (POSTOPERATIVE CARE RECOMMENDATIONS, RESTRICTIONS)

The customary postoperative care for major body contouring procedures applies. We favor narrow foam rubber strip compression of etching. Lymphatic massage is started about the fourth day. Interi continuous high-negative pressure manifold drain system (IC Surgical, Grand Rapids, Michigan) appears to better prevent seromas and dehydrate swollen tissues through a multi-tailed fluted drain exiting single drain site.

Complications and Outcomes (General Complications and Outcomes Information)

Proper selection of a patient with excess epigastric subcutaneous adipose is essential for the TULUA. Combining with an oblique flankplasty removes otherwise persistent transverse abdominal skin excess. Our personal experience is too limited to appreciate its complications or to fully endorse this procedure, but aggressive liposuction and lack of undermining in four challenging patients demonstrates promise.

HIGH-FREQUENCY ULTRASOUND FOR INTRAOPERATIVE TOMOGRAPHIC GUIDANCE: AUTOLOGOUS AUGMENTATION OF POSITIVE CONTOURS AND TARGETED PERIPHERAL NONNARCOTIC PAIN CONTROL

While defining negative spaces is often the focus in body contouring, the complementary positive spaces are critical in defining the male and female anatomy. These procedures can be performed through the same minimally invasive approach as the negative defining techniques. The use of ultrasonic VASERlipo easily facilitates fat harvest, with the emulsification of the fluid substrate surrounding the adipose cells allowing for gentle fat extraction and excellent fat graft quality. Further processing

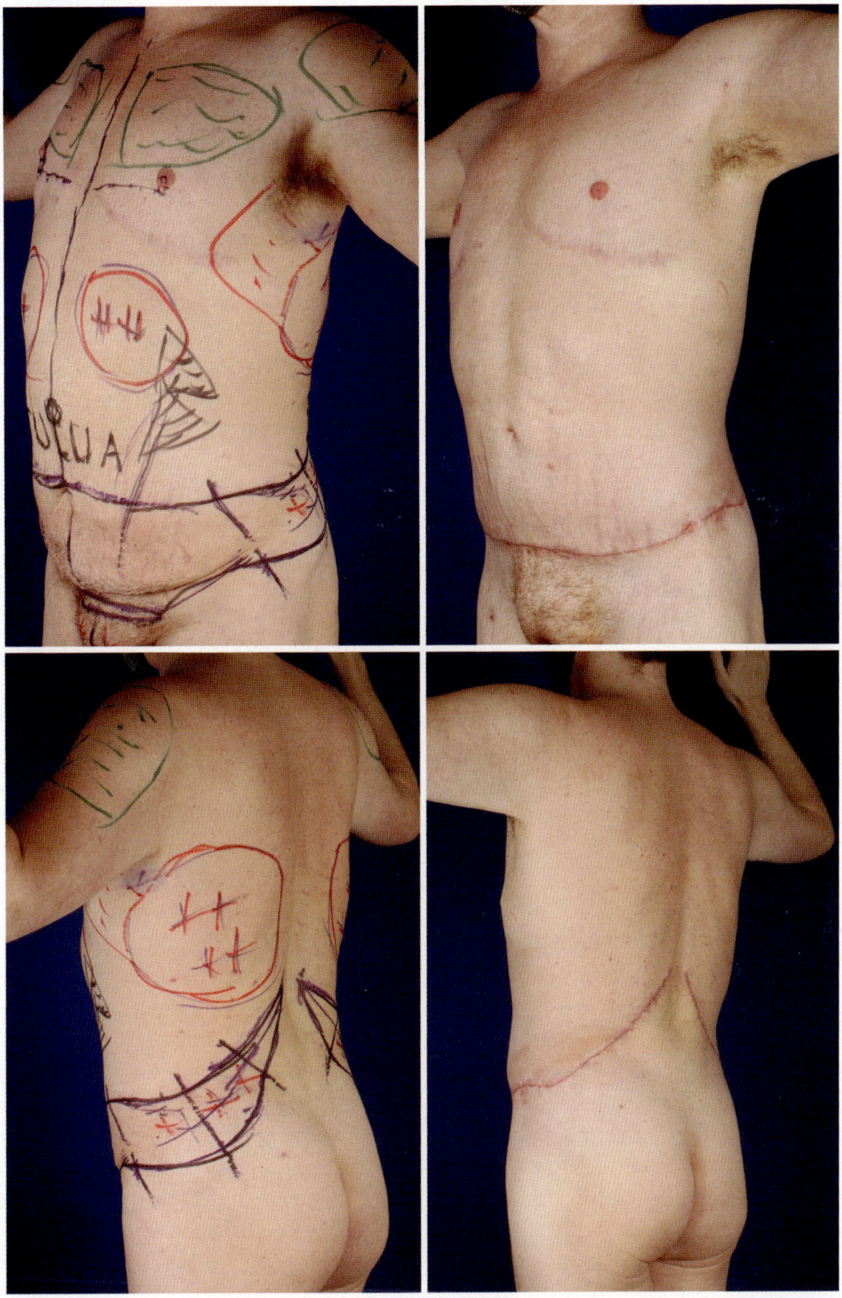

Fig. 8.10 Left oblique body views of combining TULUA and oblique flankplasty with etching VASERlipo of the abdomen, lateral chest, and lipoaugmentation of the pectoralis and deltoid muscles for a male transexual who desired as masculine transformation in a single stage. *Upper*. Before presenting condition with surgical markings for TULUA and VASERlipo and lipoaugmentation. He exhibited a barrel-shaped loose skin torso. *Lower*. Six weeks after show absence of unwanted bulges and loose skin with narrowing of the lower body and accentuation and widening of the now masculinized upper body.

using self-contained devices such as the Revolve or Puregraft systems eases transfer and time-consuming decantation or centrifugation. Regardless of method, subtle volumes of autologous fat can accentuate the muscular definition of deltoids, triceps, pectoralis, calves, in the male physique, or soften the curves of the female figure in the subcutaneous plane of the cleavage lines, trochanteric depressions or buttocks (see Fig. 8.10). The plane of injection can be fully visualized for safety, accuracy, and volume assessment using high-frequency, high-resolution, handheld ultrasound. The authors use the Clarius L7 HD Linear probe, with 4 to 13 MHz frequency and depths up to 11 cm. Portability is key during intraoperative assessment with the ultrasound operator guiding the cannula under direct guidance. An assistant injects on command using short IV tubing for small volume, and larger suction tubing for large volume injections. A similar technique is used for targeted peripheral blocks such as the quadratus lumborum, transversus abdominus plane, serratus, and PEC 1 & 2 blocks. Difficult to provide long-acting local/regional anesthetic in liposuction procedures, these blocks can be used in combination with Exparel liposomal bupivacaine mixtures to provide unparalleled pain control both during a wide-awake, office-based, lipocontouring and during the postoperative recovery. PAJUNK sononeedles assist with visualization during these blocks because of the reflective gradations along the needle path and ideal tip inclination angles.

POSTPROCEDURE CONSIDERATIONS (POSTOPERATIVE CARE RECOMMENDATIONS, RESTRICTIONS)

Liposomal bupivacaine blocks can reduce narcotic requirements and ease wide-awake procedures, but the wide dermatomal distributions encountered during lipocontouring do not allow for a completely pain-free experience. Patients are frequently counseled on the possibility of poor graft take and need for multiple grafting sessions, making it essential that these touch-up procedures can be streamlined to be performed easily in the office operating room setting.

Complications and Outcomes (General Complications and Outcomes Information)

Fat embolism, while rare with thoughtful and precise injections, are a possibility that should be discussed with the patient. Reports of fat embolism in the upper torso musculature is poorly elucidated compared with gluteal muscle augmentation, which is not recommended.

EXTERNAL APPLICATION OF ENERGY (SCULPSURE, TRUSCULPT, EMSCULPT)

The most popular topical application of energy is the external freezing of adipose. Aware of CoolSculpt saturation in the Pittsburgh market, and its occasional paradoxical adipose hypertrophy, we have purchased both the laser SculpSure and its monopolar radiofrequency alternative, TruSculpt. The market for these completely noninvasive devices can be competitive, with many nonsurgical physicians offering these services. As such, the integration of these technologies as adjuncts to minimally invasive or invasive procedures, creates a unique niche for the plastic surgeon. Administered by our certified aestheticians, Hurwitz Center has about a 70% patient satisfaction in over 100 patients with using SculpSure. The set of three 20-min applications of the penetrating CO_2 laser with immediate skin cooling requires mild sedation to overcome the pain to obtain subtle reduction of bulges. This need for mild sedation can be a limiting factor for treatment, as well as several treatments over 6-week intervals may be necessary. TruSculpt distributed by Cutera is a monopolar radiofrequency treatment just as effective as SculpSure, but with less pain. Several treatments spaced months apart are the best administration. In over 100 patients, we have had 80 satisfactory outcomes, with the other 20 often electing excisional surgery. There have been no complications, thermal or otherwise. It is our go-to technology to reduce post–invasive surgery adipose bulges with a high degree of patient satisfaction. While patients may seek these technologies in isolation, it will be the rare patient who has significant correction of a moderate to severe deformity, and mild cases without multiple treatment. The devices can have a “disposable” component, and so cost to the persistent patient who seeks completely noninvasive, low-recovery contouring can rise rapidly and so it is critical to set appropriate expectations to the patient. These devices are much more utilitarian in soothing a disgruntled postoperative patient who is very focused on small asymmetries or contour deformities.

On the contrary, the use of EmSculpt can be a strong preoperative motivator and adjunct to the lean or slightly overweight patient. Especially in those under 50 years, muscle bulking of rectus abdominus, pectoralis, gluteus, and upper arms and thigh is routinely achieved after six sessions. Quarterly maintenance treatments are encouraged. We are applying EmSculpt preoperatively and to early postoperative abdominoplasty and VASERlipo patients and have seen improvement in core strength and shape (see Fig. 8.6). Abdominal etching is complemented through muscular hypertrophy.

The device functions through using electromagnetic external pulses of 30 min per treatment over 3 weeks duration. The electromagnetic external pulsation has resulted in stronger and more toned abdominal and gluteal muscularity in both young patients and postabdominoplasty patients with roughly 85% satisfaction. The results are variable, particularly with regards to the advertised adipose reduction, which can be minimal. As such, patients with more significant adiposity should be adjunctly treated with either monopolar topical radiofrequency or VASERlipo. The second generation EmSculptNEO integrates synchronized radiofrequency treatments, with the electromagnetic pulses eliminating the need for multiple devices.

SUMMARY/DISCUSSION

Candidates for body contouring present a wide variety of complaints and deformities. Through searches of the Internet and experience of friends, most are aware of many non- and minimally invasive alternatives to open surgery. Moreover, increasing numbers are presenting with minimal deformity amenable to the limited capabilities of energy-delivered alteration of tissues. However, even larger patients or those with more laxity can benefit from these technologies as adjuncts. Our presentation selects a wide range of clinical scenarios for independent and complimentary use of ultrasonic-assisted lipoplasty and multilayer use of bipolar radiofrequency tissue remodeling and tightening.

We emphasize that tissue response to properly applied radiofrequency energy is not entirely predictable. Plastic surgeons used to precise excisions and measurements may feel initial discomfort with this uncertainty. Furthermore, patients may have unrealistic expectations of result. An appropriate balance needs to be struck, contrasting radiofrequency tightening with the effect of more invasive traditional excisional surgery.

Cost also plays a significant role, with many patients believing that the lack of invasiveness of these procedures justifies significantly reduced surgical fees. However, the majority of these noninvasives are laborious, time-consuming endeavors with high-cost disposables and need for multiple treatments. Many patients can expect to spend an equivalent amount in surgical fees, perhaps only reduced because of the savings provided by lack of general anesthetic. As a busy surgeon, one must allocate significant time for these adjuncts and not be fooled by their lackluster nature intraoperative. Oft monotonous, lack of focus can lead to serious thermal injuries, hematomas, and prolonged tissue edema.

Patient discomfort and tolerability during wide-awake anesthetic procedures can also be deceptive. Surgeons accustomed to local only, small volume lipocontouring may find that bipolar radiofrequency may be overly painful because of the levels of heat generated, particularly in the thin patient, or when the bipolar energy is closer to the muscular fascia or close to larger sensory nerves. The devices are not selective; excessive application of energy can damage nerves, of particular importance when performing NeckTite or AccuTite of the face.

An excellent safety profile of these devices predicates their synergistic nature, each with a target focus, from deep muscle stimulation to whole-body epidermal resurfacing. The addition of noninvasive or minimally invasives into the armamentarium provides a broad menu of options for the consumer, savvy patient, and the artistic plastic surgeon. Despite the high cost of acquisition, this expanded offering is a definite practice enhancement.

REFERENCES

1. Hurwitz DJ, Wooten A. Plastic surgery for the obese. *Int J Adipose Tis*. 2007;1:5-11.
2. Hurwitz DJ. *Comprehensive Body Contouring: Theory and Practice*. New York: Springer Verlag; 2016:3-4.
3. Hurwitz DJ. Ultrasonic-assisted liposuction in the massive weight loss patient. In: Garcia Jr O Jr, ed. *Ultrasonic Lipoplasty Current Concepts and Techniques*. New York: Springer Nature; 2020.
4. Hurwitz DJ. *Comprehensive Body Contouring: Theory and Practice*. New York: Springer Verlag; 2016:12.
5. Hurwitz D, Smith D. Treatment of overweight patients by radiofrequency-assisted liposuction (RFAL) for aesthetic reshaping and skin tightening. *Aesthet Plast Surg*. 2012;36:62-71.
6. Theodorou SJ, Del Vecchio D, Chia CT. Soft tissue contraction in body contouring with radiofrequency-assisted liposuction: a treatment gap solution. *Aesthet Surg J*. 2018;38(suppl 2):S74-S78.

7. *Morhpeus8 Body Clinical Experience*. Available at: http// www.Inmoderesources.com. Accessed February 6, 2021.
8. Saldanha O, Ordenes AI, Goyeneche C, et al. Lipoabdominoplasty with anatomical definition. *Plast Reconstr Surg*. 2020;146(4):766-777.
9. Hurwitz DJ, Beidas O, Wright L. Reshaping the oversized waist through oblique flankplasty with lipoabdominoplasty (OFLA). *Plast Reconstr Surg*. 2019;5:960-972.
10. Villegas FJ. A novel approach to abdominoplasty: TULUA modifications (transverse plication, no undermining, full liposuction, neoumbilicoplasty, and low transverse abdominal scar). *Aesthet Plast Surg*. 2014; 38(3):511-520.
11. Hoyos A. TULUA male high-definition abdominoplasty. *Plast Recontr Surg*. 2022;149(1):96-104.
12. Clavijo-Alvarez JA, Hurwitz DJ. J torsoplasty: a novel approach to avoid circumferential scars of the upper body lift. *Plast Reconstr Surg*. 2012;130:382e-383e.
13. Kinney, BM, Lozanova P. High intensity electromagnetic therapy (HIFEM) evaluated by magnetic resonance imaging (MRI): safety and efficacy of a dual tissue effect based on noninvasive abdominal wall shaping. *Lasers Surg Med*. 2019;51(1):40-46.

9

Hair Transplantation

Adeeb Derakhshan, Lisa E. Ishii, and Linda N. Lee

INTRODUCTION

- Androgenetic alopecia (AGA) is the most common cause of hair loss in both men and women, and is significantly mediated by dihydrotestosterone (DHT).
- The two primary methods of hair transplantation are follicular unit transplantation (FUT) and follicular unit extraction (FUE).
- FUT is a highly reliable procedure involving removal of occipital scalp tissue, microscopic dissection of follicular units, and subsequent reimplantation into desired areas.
- FUE is a more recent technique for harvesting grafts, whereby follicular units from the donor site are individually extracted using a punch device and implanted into recipient areas.

BACKGROUND AND PHYSIOLOGY OF HAIR LOSS

The human hair consists of a shaft and a root. The shaft is the visible part of the hair, while the root extends down into the deeper layers of the skin, surrounded by the hair follicle (a sheath of skin and connective tissue), and connected to a sebaceous gland. The hair follicle is attached to a small muscle (arrector pili muscle) that can make the hair stand up. It also contains many nerve endings which sense hair movement. The hair root widens at its base to form the hair bulb. At the base of the hair bulb is the papilla, which supplies the hair root wiht blood. New hair cells are produced near the papilla within the hair bulb. (see Figure 9.1).

Alopecia is a common physical disorder that can significantly impact patients' quality of life.[1,2] AGA is the most common cause of hair loss in both men and women, affecting around 50% of men and 25% of women by the age of 50 years.[3,4] Prevalence increases with age and is higher in white populations compared with Asian and black cohorts.[5]

The life cycle of a hair follicle consists of three primary phases. Anagen is the active growth stage, lasting between 3 and 5 years and comprising approximately 90% of hair follicles at any one time. Catagen is characterized by apoptosis and loss of a hair follicle's dermal attachments, resulting in its migration to the skin surface as a club hair over 1 to 2 weeks. Telogen describes a 2- to 3- month resting phase, during which the dormant club hair remains temporarily anchored in place while a new hair bulb forms within the papilla[6,7] (see Figure 9.2).

The primary hormones driving the effects seen in AGA are testosterone and its downstream analogue, DHT. Stimulation of dermal papilla cells' androgen receptors (ARs) by these molecules results in site-specific effects, ultimately contributing to male and female pattern hair loss (MPHL and FPHL). In androgen-dependent areas such as the beard and axilla, hair follicles increase in size upon androgen stimulation. Conversely, follicles in the frontal and vertex scalp miniaturize with androgen exposure, resulting in the classical presentation of MPHL.[8] The temporal and occipital scalp contains largely androgen-insensitive hair follicles. These differing hormonal responses are thought to be secondary to differences in embryologic origins of scalp dermis.[9]

Androgens progressively reduce the anagen phase of the hair cycle, resulting in shorter follicles, which ultimately may not breach the epidermis.[10] Notably, DHT has a fivefold increase in AR affinity compared to its precursor testosterone and is therefore considered the dominant

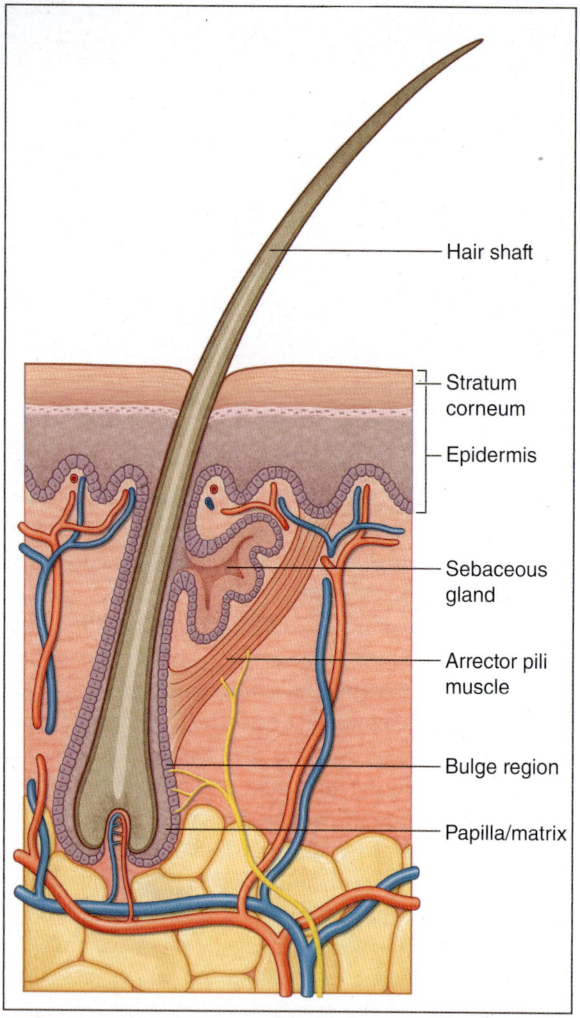

Fig. 9.1 Hair follicle anatomy. (From Procedures in Cosmetic Dermatology: Lasers, Lights, and Energy Devices. Ibrahimi, Omar A.; Kilmer, Suzanne L.; Moustafa, Farah. Published December 31, 2022. © 2023.)

androgen responsible for follicular changes seen in AGA.[11] As such, a mainstay medical therapy for MPHL seeks to block the conversion of testosterone to DHT by inhibiting the responsible enzyme, 5-alpha reductase.

The phenotypic appearance of MPHL and FPHL are most commonly described by the Norwood and Ludwig classifications, respectively.[12] The Norwood classification system groups men's hairlines into seven stages based on severity. Increasing progression of hair loss from anterior to posterior results in higher staging (see Figure 9.3). The Ludwig system stratifies women into three groups based on generalized thinning and central hair loss. The frontal hairline is typically spared, but thinning at the vertex often results in a characteristic "Christmas tree" pattern of alopecia (see Figure 9.4).

PREPROCEDURE CONSIDERATIONS

While the effects of alopecia on physical health are limited, its psychosocial impact results in lower self-esteem, diminished quality of life, and reduction in patient identity.[13-15] Patients can exhibit body dysmorphia, and often have feelings of social disadvantage compared to their peers.[16] A recent health utility study performed by Abt et al. found that patients were willing to trade in 7% to 9% of their remaining life to permanently cure their hair loss.[17] These data collectively demonstrate the profound negative effect of alopecia on patients' mental health. Studies examining the psychosocial state of the post–hair transplant patient are more limited. However, Bater et al. found that men were perceived more attractive, successful, and approachable following hair transplant than their pretransplant counterparts.[15] Abt et al. further demonstrated that individuals who had undergone hair transplant were perceived as healthier than those with hair loss.[17] These encouraging findings can help guide preoperative counseling for select individuals.

Patient Selection

Appropriate selection of a hair restoration candidate is dependent on patient expectations and their understanding of what surgery can achieve.[18] In-depth interview and consultation allows for the patient to communicate their goals, expectations, and desires for hair transplant. The dynamic nature of balding, variable progression of the disease, and finite number of suitable follicles for transplantation must be emphasized to patients as treatment limitations. Individuals aiming to have a return to a "full head of hair" for the remainder of their lifetime will undoubtedly be disappointed by their surgical outcome. The procedure should be deferred for patients unable or unwilling to accept the surgical limitations.

Good candidates for hair restoration express realistic goals, have stable donor hair, and possess a recipient area that will support growth of transplanted follicles.[18] Patients undergoing a rapidly evolving hairline should consider delaying treatment until a new baseline is achieved. The effects of facial aging will also alter the perception of patient's hairlines; transplanted hairlines

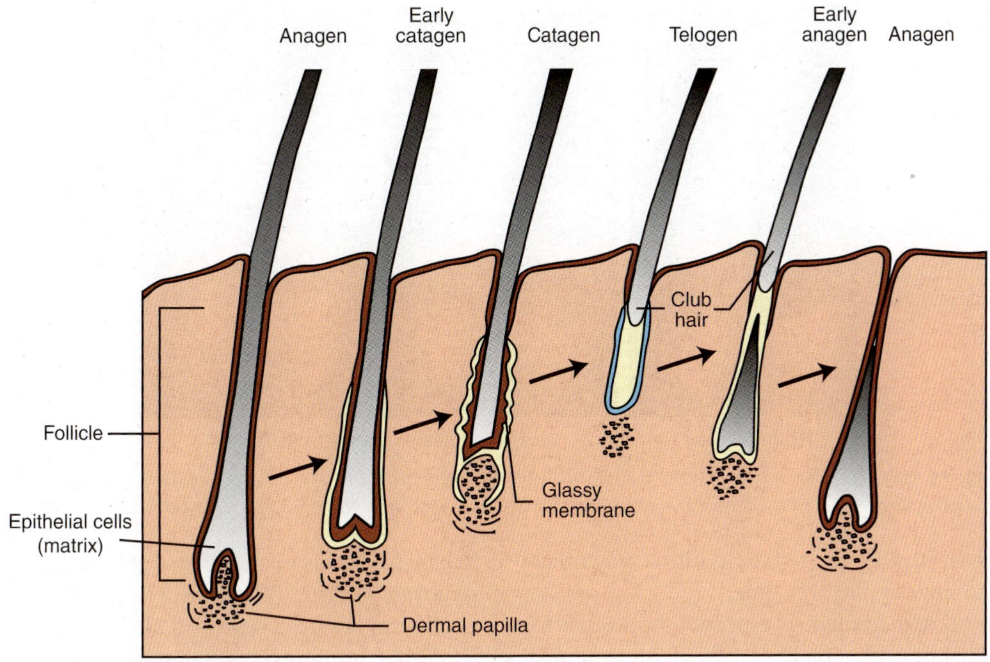

Fig. 9.2 Hair Growth Cycle (From Thomas Colville, Joanna M. Bassert; Clinical Anatomy and Physiology for Veterinary Technicians, Fourth Edition, Copyright Elsevier Inc.)

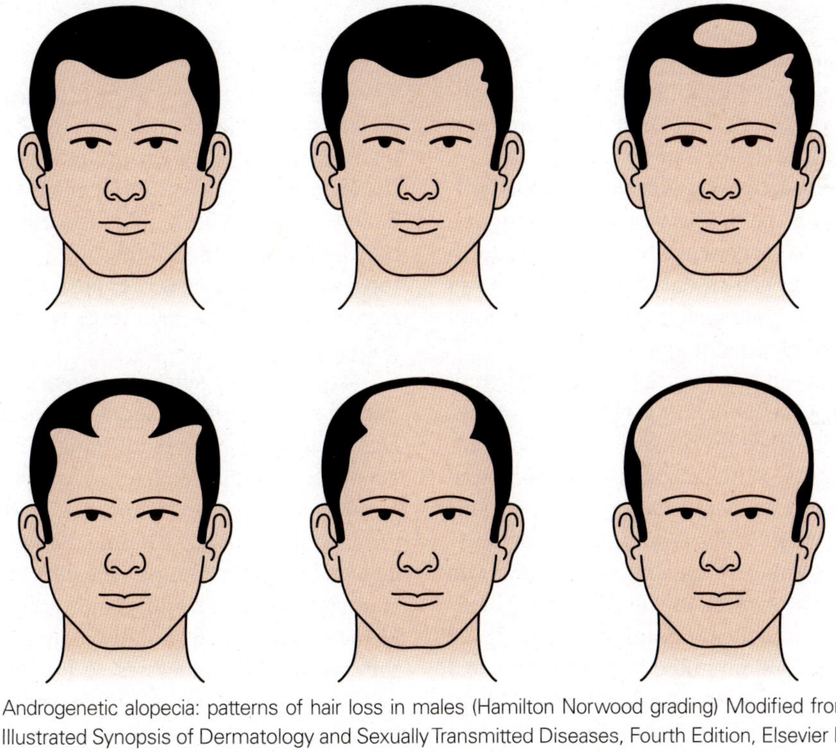

Fig. 9.3 Androgenetic alopecia: patterns of hair loss in males (Hamilton Norwood grading) Modified from Neena Khanna, Illustrated Synopsis of Dermatology and Sexually Transmitted Diseases, Fourth Edition, Elsevier Inc., 2012

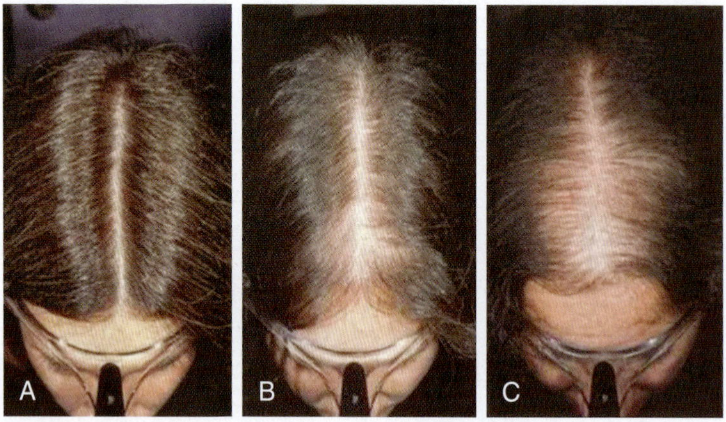

Fig. 9.4 Hair loss pattern showing the Ludwig classification for female alopecia (From Yen & Jaffe's Reproductive Endocrinology: Physiology, Pathophysiology, and Clinical Management, Ninth Edition; Copyright Elsevier Inc.)

do not recede, making their static position potentially artificial and undesirable over time.

Expectation management is especially important for younger patients, with emphasis placed on continual maturation of the patient's hair line. Young candidates should be counseled on the higher risk of extensive hair loss, given additional years and faster rate of loss they face.

Contraindications

Relative contraindications exist to performing hair restorative surgery, given the high likelihood of suboptimal outcomes. These conditions commonly stem from intrinsic issues with the donor hair or recipient site.

Diffuse unpatterned alopecia is an uncommon variant of AGA, in which the donor areas of the temporal and occipital scalp also experience balding. These locations are typically androgen-insensitive; transplantation of androgen-sensitive donor hairs can therefore result in poor growth and subsequent loss of grafts.[18]

Telogen effluvium can also induce a diffuse pattern of hair loss. Triggered by physiologic or psychosocial distress, the condition is hallmarked by excessive hair follicles entering the telogen phase simultaneously and resulting in significant hair loss.[19] Causes are numerous and include childbirth, chronic systemic illness, and thyroid dysfunction.[20,21] Careful screening of patients should occur to identify such potential sources, as the condition is self-limiting and resolves once the root cause is addressed.

Inflammatory and autoimmune causes of hair loss present a suboptimal environment for graft take. Conditions that result in cicatricial or scarring alopecia, such as lichen planopilaris, result in degenerative changes and hypovascularity of the recipient bed. Although hair transplantation has been described in such cohorts,[22] patients should be cautioned that their underlying pathology reduces their likelihood of success. Similarly, patients with autoimmune diseases such as alopecia areata are at higher risk of graft failure given the possible attack of transplanted follicles by the immune system.

Preparing for Transplantation

The underpinning foundation of hair restorative surgery is donor site dominance, the concept that transplanted hairs retain their original characteristics rather than adopting those of the recipient region.[23,24] Concordantly, donor follicles should be androgen-insensitive, thereby avoiding the balding effect of DHT on the frontoparietal counterparts they are replacing. The occipital region contains the area most commonly selected for donor grafts.

Adherence to general reconstructive techniques is critical to maximizing success of transplanted grafts.[25] Harvested grafts take 48 to 72 hours to begin developing a new blood supply courtesy of capillary inosculation.[25] Many perioperative factors can reduce likelihood of graft survival during this time. Tissues must be handled delicately under loupe magnification, minimizing trauma from crush injury and transection. Vascularity of the recipient bed should be carefully considered; although the scalp possesses an inherently rich vascular supply, it can be reduced in comorbid patients as discussed previously. The use of vasculogenic factors, such as platelet-rich plasma, has been described to help optimize the recipient area.[26,27] Finally, follicles must be stored in an appropriate medium once harvested to avoid dehydration. The ideal storage parameters are a subject of debate; considerations include ionic concentrations, pH, osmolality, and additive substances.[25]

PROCEDURAL TECHNIQUES

While reports of hair transplantation date back to the late 19th century,[28] the modern era of hair restorative surgery began in the 1950s with the work of Orentreich.[24] Orentreich conceptualized donor site dominance and successfully performed free donor occipital grafts to areas of hair loss. This provided the basis for the two primary harvesting techniques used today, FUT and FUE.

Hair grafts were initially harvested using 4-mm punch biopsies, creating a patchwork appearance of the recipient site with clusters of 15 to 20 hairs. In the 1980s, the "follicular unit" was identified as a natural grouping of one to four hairs with associated sebaceous glands, neurovascular bundle, erector pili muscle, and fine villous hair.[29] This allowed for refinements of harvest techniques, creating minigrafts (5–10 hairs) and micrografts (1–4 hairs). Strip excision was subsequently popularized over punch biopsies, and in 1994 microscopic dissection of a single donor strip into small micrografts was described.[30] Thereafter, the modern era of FUT was created. In addition, increasing sophistication of punch biopsy techniques concurrent with the advent of specialized motorized devices led to the popularization of FUE over the past 15 years.

Follicular Unit Transplantation

Patient and surgeon comfort are of utmost importance to help maintain stamina and maximize efficiency. The procedure is typically performed with the patient awake and alert in an outpatient setting, making administration of local anesthetics paramount. Oral anxiolytics can help ease certain patients.

The occipital scalp serves as the harvest area for FUT. For most men, this donor bank provides 6000 to 10,000 hairs, which can be transplanted.[31] On average, the area contains 80 to 100 follicular units per cm^2; given each follicular unit contains an average of 2.3 hairs, there are approximately 230 hairs per cm^2 of occipital scalp. Sufficient aesthetic coverage of the recipient area is typically achieved with a density of 25 follicular units per cm^2, although high-density transplants of 40 to 45 follicular units per cm^2 are sometimes used in the frontal hairline in select patients.[32]

The patient can either be seated upright or lying prone during the harvest. The donor site is prepared by clipping hairs down to about 5 mm. The hair is trimmed just to the edge of what is to be harvested based on the approximate number of grafts needed. The inferior limit of the donor strip is the fringe scalp below the occipital protuberance extending toward the ears bilaterally.[31] The width of the strip is typically 10 to 15 mm, but can extend up to 2 cm if a higher number of graft harvests is needed. The length should not exceed the posterior aspect of the helical rim.[32]

Analgesia is provided using 1% lidocaine with epinephrine diluted 1:100,000 for a vasoconstrictive effect. Small amounts of 0.25% bupivacaine can also be administered for a longer anesthetic effect. After the onset of anesthesia, tumescent should be infiltrated into the subcutaneous plane to aid with hemostasis and achieve hydrodissection away from the galea aponeurosis. Incision is carried out along the direction of the hair follicles to ensure those on the border of the strip are not transected. The dissection is performed down through the subcutaneous tissue and the strip is removed en bloc. Immediately thereafter, the strip is passed to the processing team. The tissue is sectioned into follicular unit grafts consisting of one to four hairs apiece. The grafts are kept on saline-soaked Telfa to prevent desiccation.

Closure of the donor site is then performed. The majority of hemostasis is achieved with skin closure, as this stops most skin edge bleeding. Suture ligation may be needed for a more significant bleed; bipolar cautery should be used cautiously, with care taken to avoid use near remaining follicles. The laxity of the virgin scalp typically allows for primary closure without need for extensive undermining. A trichophytic closure of the donor site can be achieved by trimming a 1-mm strip of skin from the edge of either flap. Piercing towel clamps can be placed to reapproximate the wound edges and facilitate closure. A single running layer of 4-0 polyprolene suture is typically sufficient for a tension-free closure.

The recipient site is then prepared for grant implantation. Additional local anesthesia is provided via a supraorbital nerve block and injection along the hairline. Tumescence is again used. Scalp puncture is performed using 19-gauge needles or specialized blades that can be customized to the width and depth of the patient's grafts. Sites should be oriented in line with natural hairs. At the same time as site creation by the surgeon, the follicular unit grafts are created by the processing technicians. Site creation determines the position, angulation, and depth the follicular units will be seated in; thereafter, the grafts are individually placed into the microincisions. Platelets and fibrin initially secure the grafts, while tissue ingrowth occurs over the course of the first week. Although the transplanted hair shafts usually shed over the first few weeks, the transplanted follicular unit will regrow a new hair thereafter.

Follicular Unit Extraction

FUE differs from FUT in the method used for graft harvest. In lieu of strip excision, FUE extracts individual follicular units from the donor site using a punch device 0.7 to 1 mm in diameter. The first article on FUE was published in 2002,[33] at which time the technique was well defined but not regularly practiced. Over the ensuing 15+ years, advancements in technology have increased its popularity among both patients and surgeons.[34] Motorized devices were the first replacement for the manual punch, allowing the idea of FUE to come to fruition. Rotating, oscillating, and vibrating motorized systems exist for harvest. Most devices require manual extraction of the graft following punch excision, unless the device has an associated suction. Punch devices can be characterized as sharp, blunt, or hybrid.[34] Sharp punches are the most traditional and are present on conventional systems; they are powerful dissectors and thus require more superficial skin incisions (around 2 mm) to avoid hair transection. Blunt punches avoid the risk of hair transection but must be introduced deeper into the skin (around 4 mm). Hybrid systems contain a sharp outer edge to incise the skin and a dull inner surface to separate the follicular unit from adherent tissue without transecting the hair.

Donor site preparation typically involves trimming the entire occipital and temporal hairs down to 2 mm. While "no shave FUE" is possible, it is significantly more time consuming and technically challenging.[35] The optimal donor site is marked out, as are surrounding transition areas going from dense to sparse hair. The safe donor zone is evenly divided and marked into boxes based on number of estimated grafts needed, with each box intended to provide the same number of grafts. Local anesthesia is provided in a ring block, and tumescence is injected into the subcutaneous plane. The patient is then laid prone. Harvest is begun systemically, with the surgeon extracting each follicular unit and assistants collecting the graft and immediately placing it in storage solution.

Care must be taken to ensure correct direction of the punch, correct depth, and proper pressure are applied. The visible hair shafts provide the correct trajectory and angle in which the punch should be performed to avoid transection of the follicular unit. The depth of punch must be modulated based on the type of device used. Pressure is provided both by the punch itself as well as the counter-tension from the surgeon's nondominant hand. The counter-tension from the off-hand can be applied to orient the skin in a near-perpendicular fashion to the punch, reducing the diameter of the hole created.

Graft implantation for FUE does not differ from that of FUT.

POSTPROCEDURE CONSIDERATIONS

The donor site for FUT typically leaves a well camouflaged scar in the occipital region, with surrounding hair ultimately making it difficult to discern. No dressings are required. Gentle shampoo of the hair is recommended starting around 48 hours following surgery. Patients should sleep relatively upright to avoid rolling onto the recipient area for the first 3 to 5 days after transplant. Donor site sutures for FUT are typically removed 1 to 2 weeks following the procedure. Hair dying or cutting can be resumed after 2 to 3 weeks. Patients should be instructed about the possibility of telogen effluvium developing in the postoperative period, resulting in a thinner hairline than before for the first 3 to 4 months. The condition is temporary, and patients should be reassured as such should it occur. Early transplant results can be expected in 6 to 8 months, with full results achieved in approximately 1 year (see Figure 9.5 and 9.6).

COMPLICATIONS AND OUTCOMES

Significant complications following hair transplantation are rare. The majority of suboptimal outcomes from the surgery results from poor surgical planning. Poor donor site choice, inappropriate patient selection, and graft mishandling can each lead to unsatisfactory results for both the patient and the surgeon.

As with any surgical procedure, there is a risk of bleeding and infection. Injection of lidocaine may induce

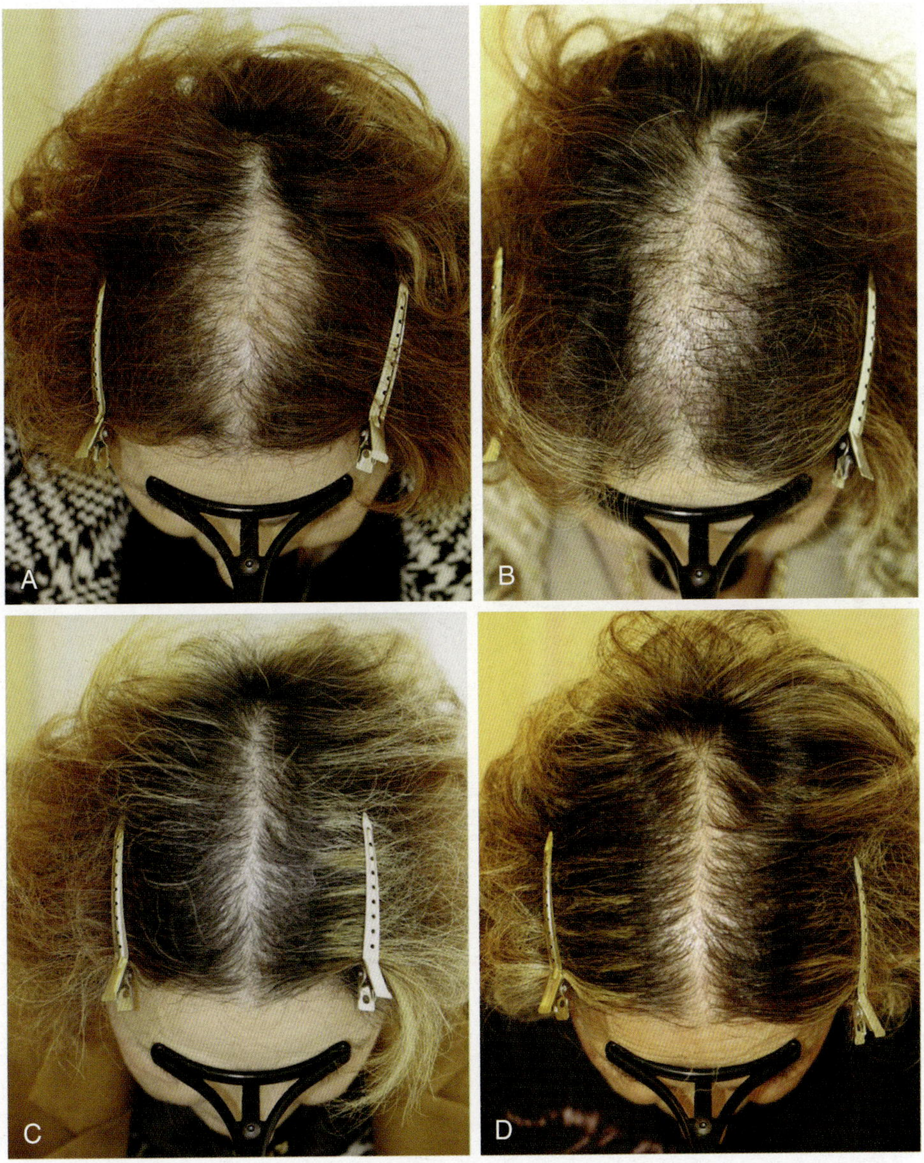

Fig. 9.5 Hair transplantation (From Mariya Miteva; Alopecia; Copyright Elsevier Inc.)

vasovagal reactions or lidocaine toxicity. Periorbital swelling may develop following inflammation and use of tumescence. There may be permanent damage of the harvested follicular units, leading to loss of hair density. Scarring may be hypertrophic or keloidal.

As discussed previously, hair restoration procedures have been shown to improve psychosocial health of recipients as well as others' perceptions of them.[15,17] Although alopecia is a dynamic and lifelong process, the transfer of androgen-insensitive hair to the fronto-parietal scalp can help mitigate its effects. Studies directly comparing outcomes between FUT and FUE are limited, given the relatively recent advent of the latter. However, each can be successful in the appropriate patient when proper surgical planning and technique are used.

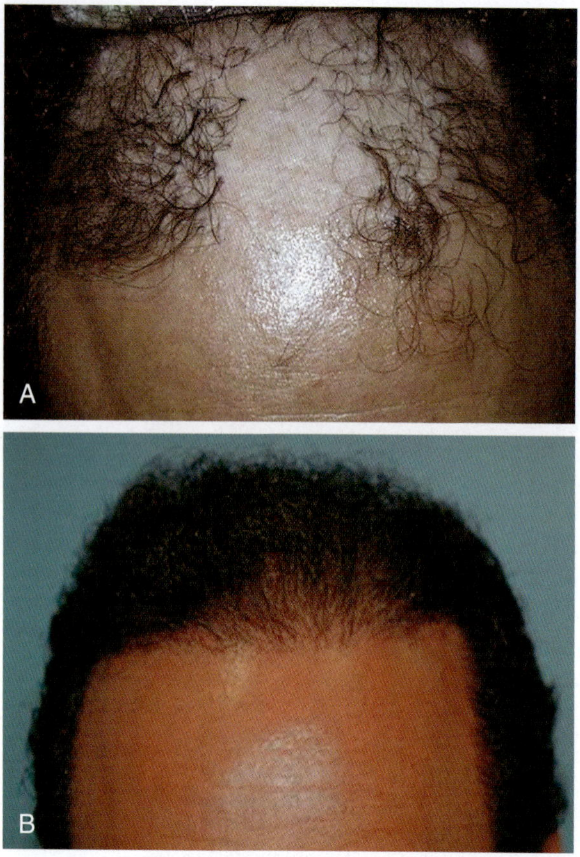

Fig. 9.6 Corrective hair transplantation (From Dermatology. Avram, Marc R.; Keene, Sharon A.; Stough, Dowling B.; Rogers, Nicole E.; Cole, John P. Published December 31, 2017. © 2018.)

REFERENCES

1. Han SH, Byun JW, Lee WS, et al. Quality of life assessment in male patients with androgenetic alopecia: result of a prospective, multicenter study. *Ann Dermatol.* 2012;24(3):311-318.
2. Davis DS, Callender VD. Review of quality of life studies in women with alopecia. *Int J Women Dermatol.* 2018; 4(1):18-22.
3. Rhodes T, Girman CJ, Savin RC, et al. Prevalence of male pattern hair loss in 18–49-year-old men. *Dermatol Surg.* 1998;24(12):1330-1332.
4. Birch MP, Lalla SC, Messenger AG. Female pattern hair loss. *Clin Exp Dermatol.* 2002;27(5):383-388.
5. Olsen EA, Messenger AG, Shapiro J, et al. Evaluation and treatment of male and female pattern hair loss. *J Am Acad Dermatol.* 2005;52(2):301-311.
6. Tai T, Kochhar A. Physiology and medical treatments for alopecia. *Facial Plast Surg Clin North Am.* 2020;28(2): 149-159.
7. Paus R, Cotsarelis G. The biology of hair follicles. Epstein FH, ed. *N Engl J Med.* 1999;341(7):491-497.
8. Lolli F, Pallotti F, Rossi A, et al. Androgenetic alopecia: a review. *Endocrine.* 2017;57(1):9-17.
9. Banka N, Bunagan MJK, Shapiro J. Pattern hair loss in men: diagnosis and medical treatment. *Dermatol Clin.* 2013;31(1):129-140.
10. Ho CH, Sood T, Zito PM. Androgenetic Alopecia. In: *StatPearls.* StatPearls Publishing; 2020. Accessed September 29, 2020. Available at: http://www.ncbi.nlm.nih.gov/books/NBK430924/.
11. Kaufman KD. Androgens and alopecia. *Mol Cell Endocrinol.* 2002;198(1-2):89-95.
12. Gupta M, Mysore V. Classifications of patterned hair loss: a review. *J Cutan Aesthet Surg.* 2016;9(1):3-12.
13. Alfonso M, Richter-Appelt H, Tosti A, Viera MS, García M. The psychosocial impact of hair loss among men: a multinational European study. *Curr Med Res Opin.* 2005;21(11):1829-1836.
14. Girman CJ, Rhodes T, Lilly FR, et al. Effects of self-perceived hair loss in a community sample of men. *Dermatology (Basel).* 1998;197(3):223-229.
15. Bater KL, Ishii M, Joseph A, Su P, Nellis J, Ishii LE. Perception of hair transplant for androgenetic alopecia. *JAMA Facial Plast Surg.* 2016;18(6):413-418.
16. van der Donk J, Passchier J, Dutree-Meulenberg RO, Stolz E, Verhage F. Psychologic characteristics of men with alopecia androgenetica and their modification. *Int J Dermatol.* 1991;30(1):22-28.
17. Abt NB, Quatela O, Heiser A, Jowett N, Tessler O, Lee LN. Association of hair loss with health utility measurements before and after hair transplant surgery in men and women. *JAMA Facial Plast Surg.* 2018;20(6):495-500.
18. Konior RJ, Simmons C. Patient selection, candidacy, and treatment planning for hair restoration surgery. *Facial Plast Surg Clin North Am.* 2013;21(3):343-350.
19. Harrison S, Sinclair R. Telogen effluvium. *Clin Exp Dermatol.* 2002;27(5):389-385.
20. Rebora A, Guarrera M, Drago F. Postpartum telogen effluvium. *J Eur Acad Dermatol Venereol.* 2016;30(3):518.
21. Sperling LC. Hair and systemic disease. *Dermatol Clin.* 2001;19(4):711-726, ix.
22. Lee JA, Levy DA, Patel KG, Brennan E, Oyer SL. Hair transplantation in frontal fibrosing alopecia and lichen planopilaris: a systematic review. *Laryngoscope.* 2021;131(1):59-66. doi:10.1002/lary.28551.
23. Dinh HV, Sinclair RD, Martinick J. Donor site dominance in action: transplanted hairs retain their original pigmentation long term. *Dermatol Surg.* 2008;34(8):1108-1111.

24. Orentreich N. Autografts in alopecias and other selected dermatological conditions. *Ann NY Acad Sci*. 1959;83:463-479.
25. Parsley WM, Perez-Meza D. Review of factors affecting the growth and survival of follicular grafts. *J Cutan Aesthet Surg*. 2010;3(2):69-75.
26. Uebel CO, da Silva JB, Cantarelli D, Martins P. The role of platelet plasma growth factors in male pattern baldness surgery. *Plastic Reconstruct Surg*. 2006;118(6):1458-1467.
27. Justicz N, Derakhshan A, Chen JX, Lee LN. Platelet-rich plasma for hair restoration. *Facial Plast Surg Clin North Am*. 2020;28(2):181-187.
28. Tekiner H, Karamanou M. The forgotten hair transplantation experiment (1897) of Dr. Menahem Hodara (1869-1926). *Indian J Dermatol, Venereol Leprol*. 2016;82(3):352-355.
29. Headington JT. Transverse microscopic anatomy of the human scalp. A basis for a morphometric approach to disorders of the hair follicle. *Arch Dermatol*. 1984; 120(4):449-456.
30. Limmer BL. Elliptical donor stereoscopically assisted micrografting as an approach to further refinement in hair transplantation. *J Dermatol Surg Oncol*. 1994; 20(12):789-793.
31. Rawnsley JD. Hair restoration. *Facial Plast Surg Clin North Am*. 2008;16(3):289-297, v.
32. Sand JP. Follicular unit transplantation. *Facial Plast Surg Clin North Am*. 2020;28(2):161-167.
33. Rassman WR, Bernstein RM, McClellan R, Jones R, Worton E, Uyttendaele H. Follicular unit extraction: minimally invasive surgery for hair transplantation. *Dermatol Surg*. 2002;28(8):720-728.
34. Epstein GK, Epstein J, Nikolic J. Follicular Unit Excision: Current practice and future developments. *Facial Plast Surg Clin North Am*. 2020;28(2):169-176.
35. Harris JA. Follicular unit extraction. *Facial Plast Surg Clin North Am*. 2013;21(3):375-384.

10

Vaginal Rejuvenation: Nonsurgical Options

Lina Triana and Esteban Liscano

INTRODUCTION

- In the aesthetic world, nonsurgical aesthetic procedures have been increasing.
- Today, 50% of aesthetic procedures are surgical and 50% nonsurgical.
- Vaginal rejuvenation: today's trend in aesthetic procedures.
- Nonsurgical genital/vaginal aesthetic options are an essential part of our armamentarium.
- Innovation is key, not only in new technologies but also by bringing something we already do elsewhere to the genital/vaginal area.

BACKGROUND

International Society of Aesthetic Plastic Surgery (ISAPS) statistics have shown that nonsurgical procedures began to increase in popularity in 2015 and have surpassed surgical aesthetic ones. The American Society of Aesthetic Plastic Surgery (ASAPS) 2017 statistics showed that since 1997, there was an unprecedented increase in nonsurgical procedures of almost 500% versus only 80% increase in aesthetic surgical procedures, showing not only that our plastic surgery practices were expanding toward nonsurgical procedures but also showing a patients trend toward seeking nonsurgical treatments.

According to ISAPS 2016 to 2018 statistics, vaginal rejuvenation procedures, labiaplasties, and surgical vaginal tightening are the aesthetic procedures that have increased the most, with 56% in 2017 compared to only 8% of the rest of aesthetic plastic surgery procedures and 23% in 2018.

Since 2017, this tendency was secondary to labiaplasties, but in the past statistics labiaplasties only increased in 1%, making it clear that today's increase in vaginal rejuvenation procedures are secondary to vaginal tightening surgical procedures.

It is clear that patients seek nonsurgical options, and that there is a trend toward vaginal rejuvenation procedures, so it is unsurprising that the sector has started producing nonsurgical devices as a complement for our practice. In addition, these have been pretty popular, especially vaginal tightening procedures, where many plastic surgeons are still likely to use surgical vaginal tightening options.

ANATOMY

It is important to understand that the vagina is like a corridor that connects the uterine cervix with the outside; it has slim walls, and the pelvic muscles give it support. These walls, although slim, have distinctive layers such as mucosa, fascia muscularis, and adventitia (Fig. 10.1).

When performing a procedure in the vaginal area, it is important to consider that the bladder and the urethra are located on its anterior aspect, and the rectum is located in the posterior aspect, and that these structures are only millimeters away from the vagina itself (Fig. 10.2).

Also, it is important to differentiate some structures from the genital area such as the labia majora, two lateral skin folds, where hairs are naturally located. During early years of life these have a puffy appearance because of subcutaneous/fatty tissue. More medially are the labia minora, one on each side and surrounding the externa introitus. The hymen is located in the vaginal entrance and can be ruptured during sexual intercourse or

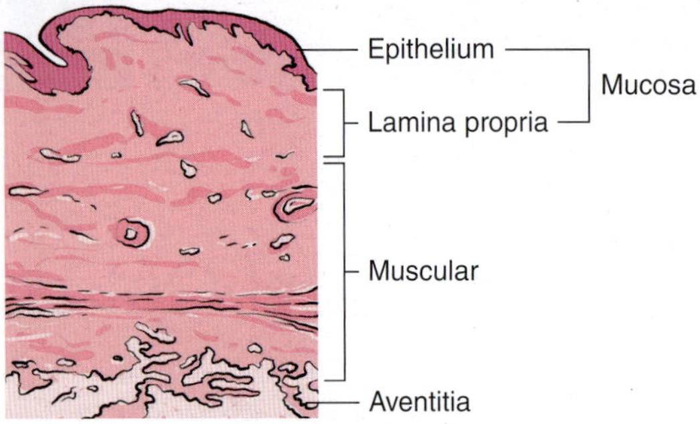

Fig. 10.1 Vaginal layers.

trauma. The mucosal extension of each labia minora join posteriorly to form the posterior fold and anteriorly to become the clitoral hood, and inside it, the clitoral body. The urethral opening is located anterior to the vaginal entrance, and the perineum skin and the anus are posterior (Fig. 10.3).

PREPROCEDURE CONSIDERATIONS

According to ISAPS statistics, today's trend in aesthetic procedures is related to vaginal rejuvenation, both genital aesthetics such as labiaplasty and vaginal tightening surgical procedures.

In the aesthetic world, nonsurgical aesthetic procedures have been increasing, to the point that today 50% of the aesthetic procedures are surgical and 50% are nonsurgical. This fact, along with the increase in vaginal rejuvenation procedures, demonstrated the need to develop vaginal nonsurgical alternatives. This is why we currently have such a large range of nonsurgical techniques for vaginal tightening, many that come from machines and technologies initially invented for skin tightening in areas such as the face that have been adapted for intravaginal use.

Similarly, many options that are currently used for rejuvenating facial skin could be used in genital area such as hydrating and depigmentation lotions, since the labia majora are covered with skin. Also, as we age, every area of our body is affected by earth's gravity and labia majora are no exception, so skin tightening methods can be used to improve and tighten skin of the labia majora. With time also, the puffy appearance of the labia majora decreases as subcutaneous tissue is lost, so fillers and fat lipoinjections can be used in this area for a rejuvenated look.

PROCEDURAL TECHNIQUE

Improving Labia Majora

Skin Texture Treatments

For this area, cleansers and hydrating creams with acidic pHs are good alternatives. Special master formulas are advisable by the author according to patient requirements:
As cleanser: Calendula, amamelis, lactic acid
For hydration: Hyaluronic acid 1% + alfa bisabolol 1%
For older skin: Vitamin E 1%, arnica 5%, alfa-bisabolol 1%
For depigmentation: Rucinol 4%, nicotinamide 1%

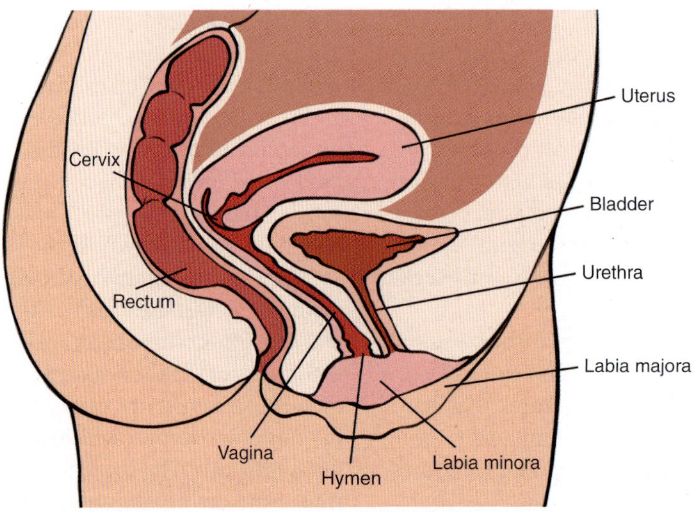

Fig. 10.2 The vagina and its relationships.

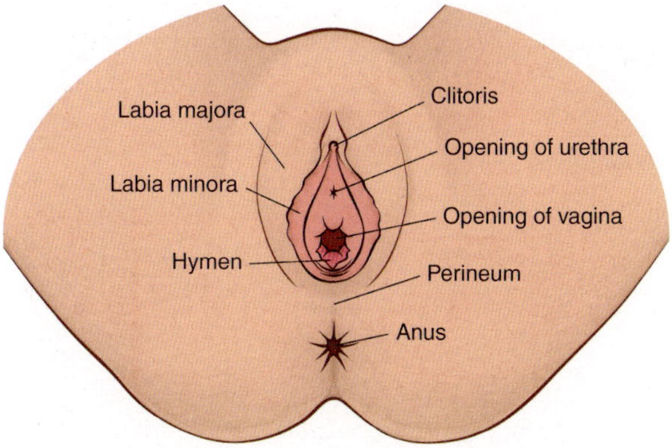

Fig. 10.3 External female genitalia.

Platelet Rich Plasma

Blood is drawn from the patient for platelet-rich plasma (PRP) preparation in laboratory (centrifugation for 5 min; nothing is added to the plasma).

Topical anesthesia is applied to the labia majora every 20 minutes for 1 hour before the procedure is performed.

The area is cleaned with an iodine solution.

The plasma is applied to the labia majora with a mesotherapy gun for a more precise injection and less pain for patient (Fig. 10.4).

> **TIP**
> For better results, three treatments with 1 month between treatments are recommend.

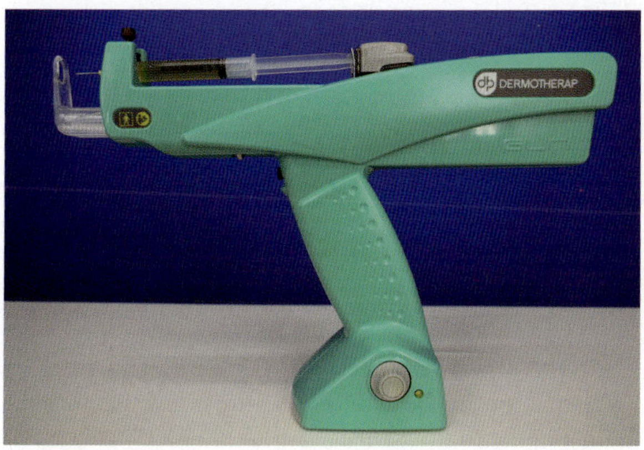

Fig. 10.4 Applcation of the plasma on the labia mayora skin

Fillers—Hyaluronic Acid

Topical anesthesia is applied to the labia majora every 20 minutes for 1 hour before the procedure is performed.

The area is cleaned with an iodine solution.

Injection is performed with a needle; no canulae is used in this area by the author.

What filler should I use?

The author only uses high-density hyaluronic acid, the same brand as the one used for the face.

Other absorbable fillers have been described, but the author has no experience with them on the face or genital area.

Only absorbable fillers are recommended by the author. In her experience, nonabsorbable substances, such as silicone and others, will bring future problems in the area.

How much should I inject?

Since hyaluronic acid is expensive, never promise that flaccid labia majora will become puffy with the injections of hyaluronic acid.

Expectations of the procedure must be regarding decreasing wrinkles but without giving the impression that there will be real restorations of volume. When volume restoration is desired, other methods must be advised.

It is important to advise the patient that the filler will eventually be reabsorbed. The amount of time it will last depends on the used product.

> **TIP**
> It is advisable to complement fillers in the labia majora with radiofrequency skin tightening in the area for better results.

Lipoinjection

Asepsis and antisepsis are done in the genital area and inner thighs and knees.

The fat graft is taken out with a 2.0-cannula and 20-cc syringe from the thighs of inner knees.

Fat is decantated only.

Fat is reinjected with disposable 18-gauge canulae with 10-cc syringes.

Injection is done in a spaghetti-like, multilayer manner, preventing fat lakes.

Massage is done in the area.

Keep the natural anatomy of the labia majora: wider anterior.

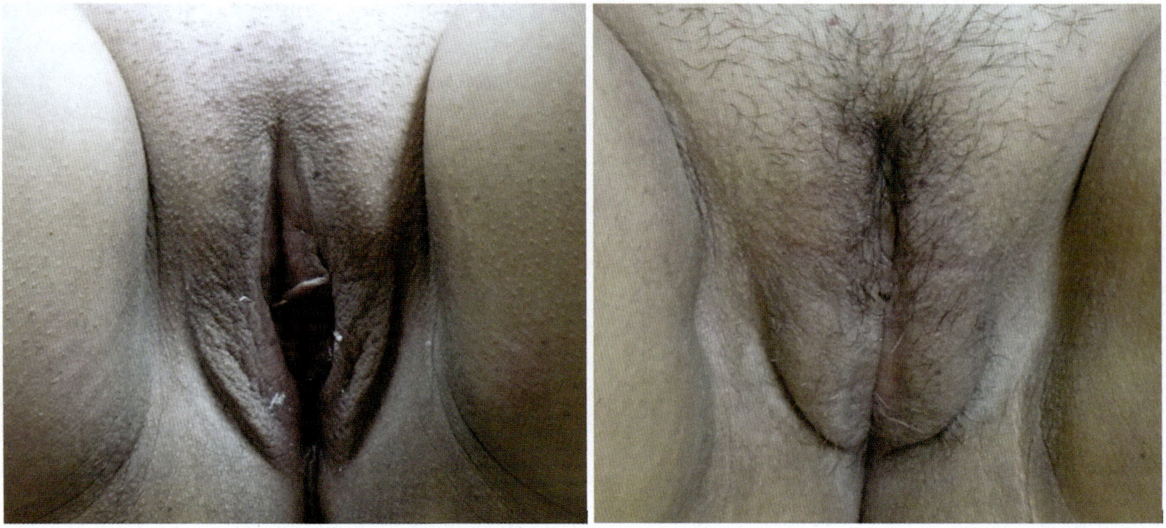

Fig. 10.5 G zone.

How much fat should I inject?

The author advises that an average of 30 cc of fat is injected in each labium majora, with no less of 15 cc in each side (Fig. 10.5).

> **IMPORTANT**
> Inform the patient that some fat will be reabsorbed. The author always tells the patients that 50% of the fat that is injected will be reabsorbed.

> **TIP**
> If there is too much lose skin, do not attempt to compensate for it by overinjecting the area. The more fat you inject, the higher the complication risk, and also the result will look unnatural.

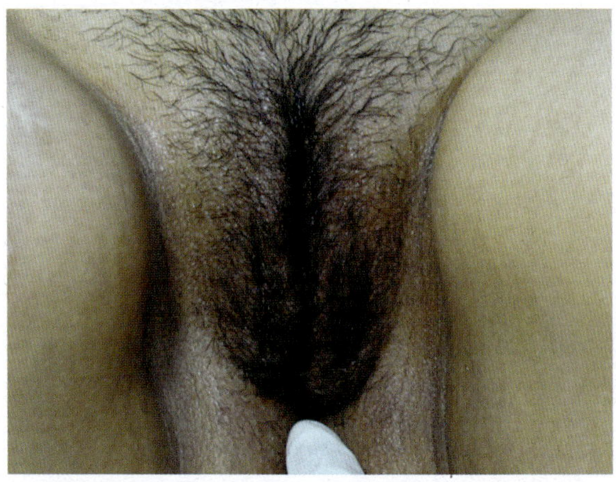

Fig. 10.6 Radiofrequency device used in left side of labia minora where a clear skin tightening is seen after 5 sessions with one week in between of each session.

Labia Majora Skin Tightening

Radiofrequency and focalized ultrasound devices can be used in the area with good results (Fig. 10.6).

The author prefers monopolar rather than bipolar radiofrequency devices and recommends applying the device to one area with constant circular movements until it feels hot, then moving to another area, before returning to the first area. According to the skin temperature (no thermometer is used), two to three passes are done in each area.

One weekly treatment, for a total of five treatments, is advised when using a monopolar radiofrequency device.

The author does not recommend the use of laser for skin contraction in the area. The laser settings for skin tightening produce more heat that will result in more inflammation in the area, and Latin skins, the author's main population, will have a higher risk of hyperpigmentation because of the inflammation.

Improving Labia Minora

The author's experience is that nonsurgical devices for labia minora retraction are not suitable. When there is excess mucosa on the labia minora or clitoris hood, a surgery must be planned for resection.

SKIN LIGHTENING

Skin lightening can be done with lasers or depigmentation creams.

Lasers for Genital Depigmentation

Carbon dioxide or erbium laser devices can be used.

Topical anesthesia is applied every 20 minutes for 1 hour on the labia majora before the procedure is done.

The area is cleaned with an iodine solution.

A fractionate skin resurfacing of the area is recommended; three passes are generally used.

Settings will vary according to the machine used.

> **IMPORTANT**
> One treatment will not be enough; usually, more than three are needed to see a result, and whitening is never promised.
> Time between treatments should not be less than 6 weeks, since the more inflammation, the higher the risk for hyperpigmentation, especially in Latin skins (the author's patient population).

> **TIP**
> Always use rucinol 4% after the procedure for at least 3 to 6 months to prevent secondary hyperpigmentation because of inflammation.

Depigmentation Creams

The author has two preferred depigmentation creams. Both are master formulas.

Cream 1: Glycolic acid 5% + arbutin 3%

- This is used only at night and sun exposure must be avoided.
- Once it is discontinued, there should be no further application of the cream, and sun exposure must be avoided for at least the next 4 months.
- Time expected to see results: more than 3 months of use.

Cream 2: Rucinol 4% + nicotinamide 1%

- Less problems with sun exposure, but still should only be applied at night.
- Rucinol acts on melanocytes, making them less prone to produce color.
- Time expected to see results: more than 6 months of use.
- Important for any depigmentation procedure.
- With lasers or depigmentation creams, the skin condition that predisposes to hyperpigmentation is not cured, so with friction and time, hyperpigmentation can recur.
- Depigmentation can be done on the labia majora, the anal area, the perineum, or other nearby areas.

> **TIP**
> Set the right expectations when using a depigmentation procedure. The dark color in the area will be less dark but it will never be white.
> Once depigmentation is achieved, treatment will be stopped; however, the patient should be informed that future treatments are often needed.

VAGINAL TIGHTENING

Laser Devices

Different lasers are available but the most common used are CO_2, erbium, and diode lasers.

Anesthesia may or not be needed according to the machine used.

Vagina must be clean, and preferably dry, for best results.

The laser settings will vary according to the machine, as well as the number of passes.

Radiofrequency Devices

Different radiofrequency devices can be used, monopolar, bipolar, tripolar, and combinations.

Usually, anesthesia is not needed but can vary from machine to machine.

Conductive gel is used during the procedure.

Machine settings and number of passes also vary according to the used machine.

> **IMPORTANT**
> It has been said that a radiofrequency device is more effective because it can go deeper, but the vaginal wall is only millimeters wide so this is not relevant.

> **TIP**
>
> **When purchasing a laser**, the machine can be used with a different hand piece for skin resurfacing in other body parts such as the face and can also be used for skin depigmentation on the genital area and other body parts.
>
> **When buying a radiofrequency device**, the machine can be used with a different hand piece for skin tightening and also, depending on the machine, to decrease fat deposits.

Fat Injections for Vaginal Tightening

The author considers the technique challenging when trying to inject on the vaginal walls.

Usually, fat injections are done on the vaginal entrance and do not benefit the woman who is the patient; rather, they only produce more friction at the vaginal entrance, which increases pleasure for the male sex partner only.

Sexual gratification during sexual intercourse for females is all about friction on the anterior vaginal wall, and for these, the woman needs to contract the whole vaginal corridor and not only the entrance.

G-SPOT ENHANCERS

Can be Done with Hyaluronic Acid or Platelet-Rich Plasma

Although many experts say the so-called "G zone" does not exist, and no good scientific data have shown it, when we as physcians utilize an energy-based device for a vaginal tightening nonsurgical procedure, the patient refers pain when the energy force device is applied on the anterior vaginal wall, pointing toward the existance of more sensitivuty recepters in this area.

It is said that the G spot is located 3.8 to 4.2 cm above and behind the pubic muscle on the anterior vaginal wall (Fig. 10.7).

First identification of area with more sensitivity receptors is done manually.

Topical anesthesia is applied.

Cleaning of the area is done.

Speculum is introduced sideways.

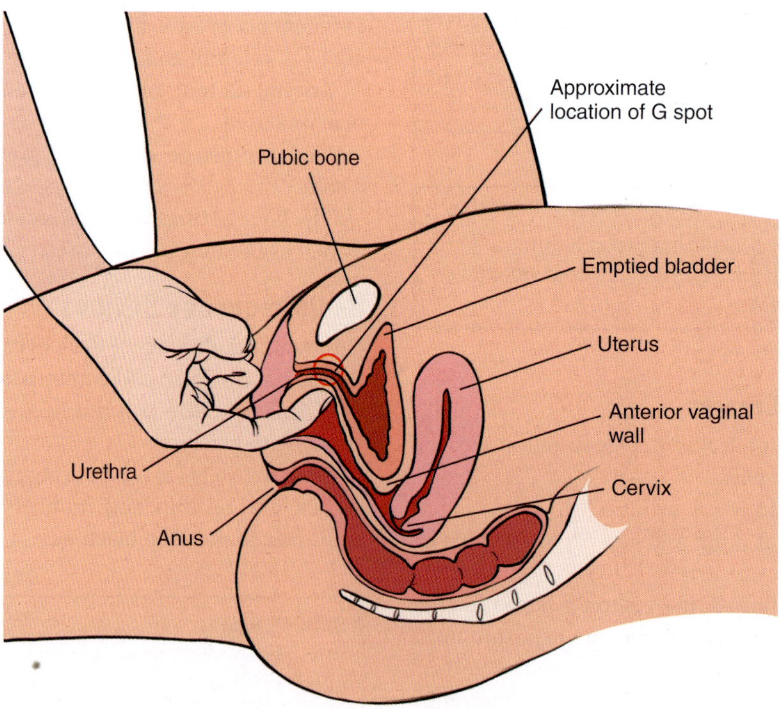

Fig. 10.7 Area where you can identify the G spot.

Spinal catheter #21 is used for injection on the previously identified area.

One cc of hyaluronic acid is injected in the previously identified area.

When PRP is being used, 2 cc are injected on the previously identified area and 1 cc around the vaginal introitus.

When PRP is used, more than one procedure is recommended, usually three and ideally 1 month apart.

> **IMPORTANT**
> It is important to set expectations with the patient.
> The procedure will not change her maximum erogenous zone; she will simply feel more during sexual intercourse when friction is applied on the previous identified area.

> **TIP**
> Always examine the patient carefully. If the vagina is not tight, she is not a good candidate for a G-spot enhancer procedure, as she will not be able to push the penis toward this G zone.

Stress Urinary Incontinence

Both lasers and radiofrequency devices can be used to temporarily improve this condition.

> **IMPORTANT**
> Inform the patient that the condition will not be cured, and she will need a follow-up treatment once her stress urine incontinence is corrected. This repeat procedure will generally be done in about 1 year or less.

> **TIP**
> Never say how many treatments will be needed to correct stress urinary incontinence, but stress that more than one will be needed.

Dry Vagina

A combination of laser treatment and PRP can be a good option for this condition.

At least three treatments are recommended, with 1 month between treatments, for better results.

When the plasma is performed with the laser treatment, no needle is needed, the plasma is applied by introducing the plasm in the vagina and massaging the area.

POSTPROCEDURE CONSIDERATIONS, COMPLICATIONS, AND OUTCOMES

Improving Labia Majora

PRP: No special consideration is needed.

Fillers: No special consideration other than it will be reabsorbed with time.
- Reabsorption varies according to the product.

Lipoinjection: More than 50% will be reabsorbed.
- The more fat that is injected, the higher the risk of fat cyst.
- How do I prevent a fat cyst? By avoiding injecting fat lakes.
- What to do with a fat cyst? Massage vigorously, as they usually are not visible.
- Has a higher risk of infection because it is used in the genital area.

Skin tightening: No sun exposure to prevent dark color on the skin afterwards.

Skin lightening with laser: No sun exposure for at least 4 to 6 months.
- Higher risk of secondary hyperpigmentation in Latin skins.
- Always use rucinol 4% between procedures and for at least 4 to 6 months once no more laser treatments will be done.
- Peeling skin will happen between days 4 and 8 according to how deep the resurfacing was done.

Depigmentation creams: The arbutin base cream will lighten quicker, but rucinol base cream is safer (has less risk of secondary hyperpigmentation).
- Can also produce secondary hyperpigmentation, especially arbutin base cream.

Vaginal Tightening

Lasers and radiofrequency: Never promise how many treatments will be needed, but usually more than one.
- No sexual intercourse for 3 days after treatment.
- Can engage in sports from the day after treatment.

G-Spot Enhancers

Hyaluronic acid: Needs to be repeated on a yearly basis.
- A tampon is used for 4 hours and no down time is required.

PRP: More than one treatment is needed for better results.

A tampon is used for 4 hours only if bleeding is present.
No down time is required.

Stress urinary incontinence: More than one treatment is needed; never promise how many.
Prepare the patient for retreatment after a year.
No sexual intercourse for 3 days after treatment.
Can engage in sports from the day after treatment.

Dry vagina: No sexual intercourse for 3 days after treatment.
Can engage in sports from the day after treatment.

CONCLUSIONS

If we want changes to happen, we cannot keep doing more of the same, and with this in mind the word innovation appears. Innovation in our day-to-day practice is key. Innovation is key not only in new technologies but also by bringing something we already do elsewhere to the genital/vaginal area.

Ten years ago, the ASAPS published a study called the 747 effect, which clearly stated that plastic surgeons were losing their patients because they did not offer them nonsurgical options, and when these patients went to non–plastic surgeons to have these nonsurgical treatments done and were happy with their doctors, they ended up having their aesthetic surgical procedures with these same doctors, although they knew they were not plastic surgeons. This forced plastic surgeons to innovate in their practices and start aquiring the knowledge, training, and experience in these nonsurgical procedures to be able to catch up with the trend.

Today, with the vaginal rejuvenation trend, and with patients seeking surgical and nonsurgical aesthetic options for their genital and vaginal areas, it is time to not only dominate the sector but to have an open mind and innovate not only with new technologies but especially with nonsurgical options used in the body areas such as our face, or if we do not, we will start losing our patients. The future of our practice is in our hands.

REFERENCES

Triana L. *Aesthetic Vaginal Plastic Surgery: A Practical Guide.* New York: Springer: 2020.

D'Amico RA, Saltz R, Rohrich RJ, et al. Risks and opportunities for plastic surgeons in a widening cosmetic medicine market: future demand, consumer preferences, and trends in practitioners' services. *Plast Reconstr Surg.* 2008;121(5): 1787-1792.

ISAPS International Survey 2016. Available at: www.isaps.org.

ISAPS international survey 2017. Available at: www.isaps.org.

ISAPS international survey 2018. Available at: www.isaps.org.

ASPAS survey 2009. Available at: www.surgery.org.

Cosmetic surgery national data bank statistics 2012. *Aesthet Surg J.* 2013;33(suppl 2):1S-21S.

Dobbeleir J MLCL, Van Landuyt K, Monstrey SJ. Aesthetic surgery of the female genitalia. *Semin Plast Surg.* 2011;25(2):130-141.

Triana L, Robledo AM. Aesthetic surgery of female external genitalia. *Aesthet Surg J.* 2015;35(2):165-177.

Braun V. In search of (better) sexual pleasure: female genital "cosmetic" surgery. *Sexualities.* 2005;8(4):407-424.

Shaw D, Lefebvre G, Bouchard C, et al. Female genital cosmetic surgery. *JOGC.* 2013;35(12):1108-1112.

Qureshi AA, Tenenbaum MM, Myckatyn TM. Nonsurgical vulvovaginal rejuvenation with radiofrequency and laser devices: a literature review and comprehensive update for aesthetic surgeons. *Aesthet Surg J.* 2018;38(3):302-311.

de Assis Florentino AV, Bicalho Bretas TL, Almeida Issa MC. *Clinical Approaches and Procedures in Cosmetic Dermatology.* New York: Springer Book Series; 2017-2019.

INDEX

R

S